STEALTH HEALTH

How to sneak age-defying, disease-fighting habits into your life without really trying

Reader's Digest Association (Canada) ULC
Montreal

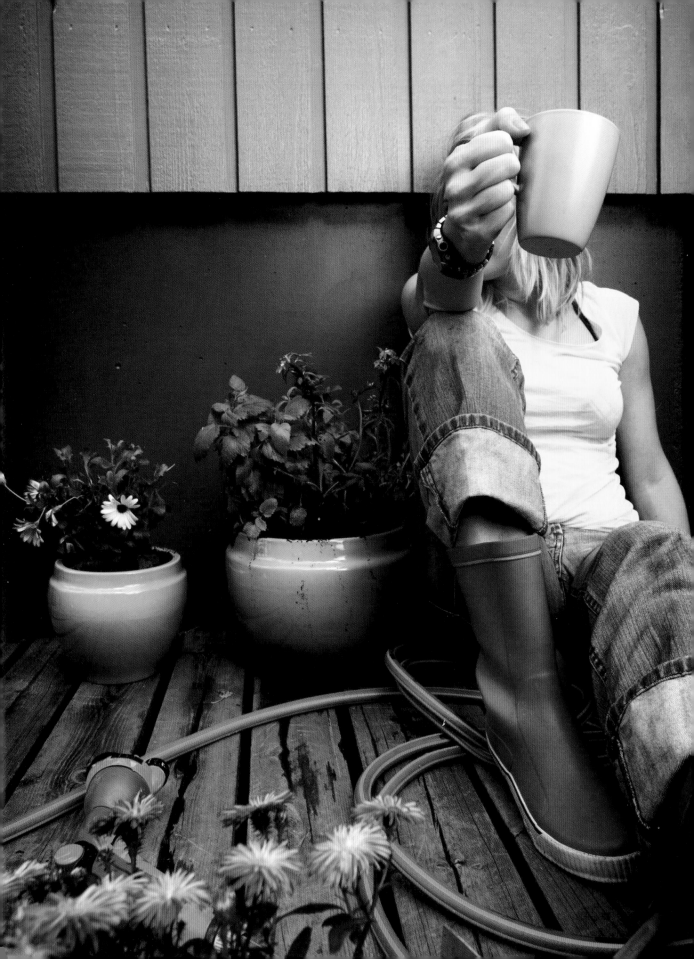

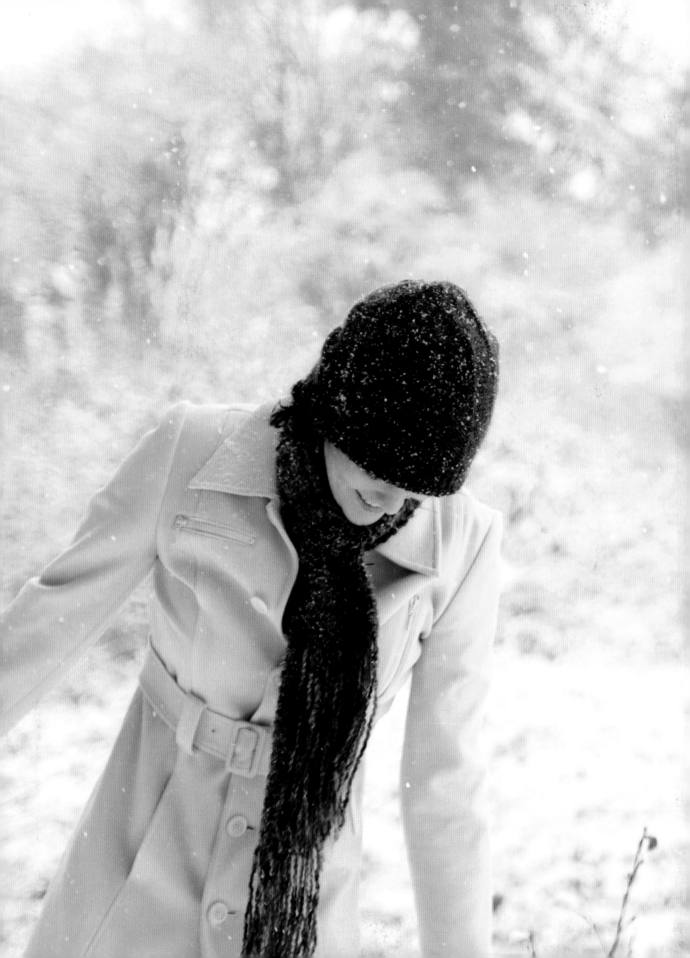

STEALTH HEALTH

Introduction

Better living, without big changes

Everyone knows the old proverb "prevention is better than cure" – but it's not always the easiest advice to put into practice. All the things you're supposed to do to prevent disease seem to require a lot of effort – and that in itself is enough to put you off trying. It's also difficult to see immediate benefits - prevention's reward is that a disease does *not* appear, so how will you know if it's effective? Combine the two problems and it's easy to see why people are often so reluctant to take active steps to ward off ill health.

The *Stealth Health* team has tackled this head-on by reviewing hundreds of valuable acts of disease prevention and health promotion. The book explains how they work and the evidence that backs them up, and offers quick and easy ways to put them into practice and reap the benefits.

The result? Health promotion in tiny acts you can fit into your life, every day. Each tip is about one thing: improving the quality of your life, and the quality of your health.

As a full-time GP advising on preventative medicine every day, I know this approach makes sense, and that even the smallest act of health promotion is worthwhile. This book is about prevention you can practise on a daily basis. It's not about making room for health with laborious add-on effort: it's about finding room for prevention in the nooks and crannies of your life as it is right now.

Healthy living is something everyone can enjoy. With every bit of advice you act on in this book, the scales of health and happiness will tip ever further in your favour as *Stealth Health* provides the elusive bridge to transport you from merely accepting the way you are living to leading a life you can love and cherish, in good health, for many years to come.

I am pleased and proud to recommend this book as an effective tool for reshaping your future health, putting control of your well-being and your own destiny firmly into your own hands.

Dr. Vince Forte

Contents

part 1   STEALTH HEALTH THROUGH THE DAY   14–75

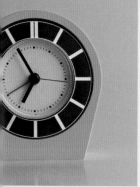

part 2   STEALTH HEALTHY COOKING   76–113

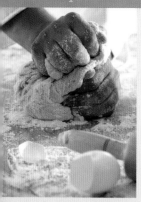

part 3   STEALTH HEALTHY DINING OUT   114–131

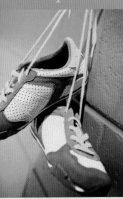
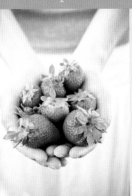
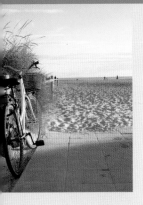

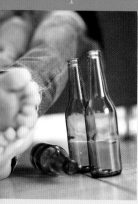
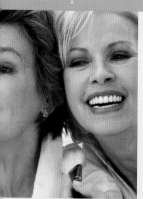
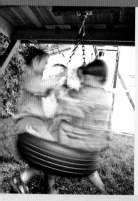

What is STEALTH HEALTH?

Small changes that quickly add up

Pick up any health or diet book these days and you come away with two impressions. First, it would appear that very few of us lead healthy lives and, secondly, there's a lot that needs to be corrected. On top of that, there's only one way to correct things – the hard way: with a complete lifestyle overhaul. Take, for example, a number of popular weight-loss programs, which start with frightening "induction phases" that involve a complete change in the way you eat, including the banning of whole categories of popular foods. The discomfort and discipline involved are on a par with military boot camp – which is exactly how some popular fitness programs bill themselves.

Desire something a little more gentle? Pilates and yoga are terrific, but to reap the maximum benefits they require lessons, teachers and practice. And if a doctor discovers something wrong with our bodies – the regimen of pills, tests, diets and scary talk about healthy living can often seem worse than the problem itself.

But what if there were another way – a way to get the benefits of a lifestyle overhaul without the top-to-bottom revamping? An easier way. A way of making tiny change after tiny change (so tiny you barely notice you're making them), yet emerging in the end with the kind of major transformation that dramatically improves your health? That wouldn't be so bad and might really deserve some serious consideration.

Welcome to *Stealth Health*, which redefines health as you know it. Living life the health-boosting way means choosing the raisin bran, not the toast and jam. It's taking a 5 minute walk when you're bored with your computer, rather than eating a chocolate bar. It's laughing when someone does something stupid, instead of shouting. It's going to sleep instead of watching the late film. It's snacking on a peach, not a cake. It's kissing your partner instead of walking out the door with only a goodbye.

After all, what is health, anyway? As defined here, health includes feeling relaxed rather than stressed; loving rather than getting irritated. It's finding time for yourself and your priorities that you didn't think you had. And, of course, it's also about healthier, glowing skin and steady, sustainable weight control. It's having more energy in the afternoon and evening, less likelihood of developing diabetes and heart disease, measurably lower cholesterol and blood pressure levels, higher self-esteem, a greater sense of personal safety and an enhanced ability to handle things without falling apart.

Health is about feeling good today and the probability of being well tomorrow. And that's not an either/or – but both. It's about taking good care of your body, mind and soul.

Easy changes

Stealth Health is the ultimate guide to the little decisions we make that add up to an enormous influence on our health. It contains more than 2,000 choices and tweaks that you can make to your day, some so small as to seem almost inconsequential, yet guaranteed to make you healthier. The ideas are fresh, unusual, simple and fast. Best of all, they work.

And they're designed for the way you live your life. For instance, you're not being told to give up all salt. Instead, you'll find two dozen ways to reduce the amount of salt in your diet incrementally, until, ever so slowly, almost without noticing, you find that your salt intake has reached healthy levels – and your blood pressure has dropped as a result.

No time to exercise because you spend too much time driving? Find out how to combine the two. Too stressed to sleep, and too sleep-deprived to handle stress? There are dozens of simple remedies for both. Unhappy about overeating,

down to context. For example, coffee is great for you if your goal is mental sharpness and alertness. But for a good night's sleep, coffee is nothing but trouble. So try not to be confused by any occasional conflicts; instead, make choices that are most sensible for your particular goals.

A lifetime journey

The biggest problem with intense, highly defined health programs is that they end – perhaps after as little as two weeks, or maybe as long as six months. And when they end, you're back to your old ways. Which is why our obesity rates

Health isn't merely the absence of disease. You're not healthy if you're perpetually stressed, frustrated or dissatisfied.

and overeating because you're unhappy? Learn some easy tactics that work during even the most frantic days to improve your mood and control your appetite.

There may be times when you'll ask yourself, "How can this advice possibly help my health?" It's a legitimate question. When you encounter tips that seem pretty far removed from the topic of health, such as how to organize your day or do chores more efficiently, the chances are they're about achieving calm or a positive attitude.

There are two reasons why they're here. First, health isn't merely the absence of disease. It involves mental and spiritual aspects as well. You're not healthy if you're perpetually stressed, frustrated or dissatisfied. Second, your mental and spiritual health have a direct link to your physical health. Research confirms it over and over. Stress, anger and other hostile emotions and attitudes are significant risk factors for everything from heart disease to obesity.

So even if some of the advice doesn't seem to have a direct health benefit, be assured that it does help. And remember that every tip in this book has come from a doctor or is doctor-approved.

Finally, you may find the occasional piece of advice that seems to contradict what's been said in a different place. In each case, it all comes

continue to rise, despite the many millions of dollars spent on weight-loss books and programs. And why heart disease, diabetes and stroke – all lifestyle-influenced diseases – are rampant.

You'll find that the pursuit of better health has a momentum all of its own – when you do it the right way. One health-promoting habit will reinforce others. The chances are, after you've hit the threshold of making subtle, little adjustments to your lifestyle, you will, in fact, have introduced the sweeping improvements in your health that once seemed so elusive and intimidating. In other words, take enough small steps, one at a time, and you've accomplished the equivalent of reaching Everest's peak or circling the globe – without even getting out of breath.

Stealth Health is the road map for your journey. It's the directions that enable you to take one small step, followed by more small steps, to introduce health promotion into the nooks and crannies of your life.

The bottom line: improving your health doesn't have to be difficult. In fact, it's mostly about common sense. Pick three tips to do a day, every day, and you'll be well on your way to a lighter, more attractive, more disease-resistant and more contented you.

The everyday
HEALTH PLAN

Just say "THREE A DAY"!

As with any program designed to overhaul your health, *Stealth Health* could seem overwhelming. After all, there are more than 2,000 tips on improving everything from the way you look to how much you weigh to your heart-health measurements to your relationships with loved ones.

Don't worry. The last thing this book does is overwhelm you – for that would be stressful and quite contrary to the book's optimistic, healthy philosophy.

So here's the proposal: every day, make three good-health choices that are outside your regular routine. That's all. Just three.

For instance, have a cup of tea instead of coffee in the morning. Substitute a bottle of water for your afternoon can of cola. Spend 5 minutes stretching in the morning while you watch the news. That's three. Call it a day. You'll do three more tomorrow.

Go ahead and make the same choices for tomorrow if that is what you wish. But here's the one and only rule in this program: once you've followed a choice for four days in a row, it no longer counts as one of your three choices. Instead, you should consider it a habit. It's time to add to it with a new and different good-health choice.

While you will recognize that habits are formed over months, not days, you also know that limiting yourself to three simple changes for weeks on end won't add up to much in the long run. Your goal is to sample new health tips, slowly and steadily. If they feel right, integrate them into your daily routine – again, slowly, steadily, over the days, weeks and months. Given time, you'll find that nearly every aspect of your life has changed in healthier ways – without you even noticing it!

That's it: the entirety of the everyday health plan. Make three healthy choices every day. With more than 2,000 to choose from in these pages, that should be easy.

The best tips for you

Just as there is only one rule to the program, there's only one bit of expert advice to get you going: focus your efforts on the areas where you need the most help. For instance, if your major health concern right now is weight, choose three from the chapters that focus on healthy eating and weight loss. Having trouble sleeping? Three tips from the sleep chapter on page 72 should guarantee you a peaceful night's slumber. Which three? You choose. In all cases, it's your choice. For the book focuses on the idea that getting and staying healthy is an option and an opportunity, not an obligation. So you decide – as long as you do something, you've taken a small step towards better health. And through an accumulation of these small steps, you will reach your goal.

As you add three more healthy choices each day, the cumulative effect will be substantial. The outcome: a sustainable, healthy lifestyle marked by fewer colds, greater energy, a leaner, more attractive body, a happier outlook and greater resistance to chronic disease.

The stealth health
PROMISE

Benefits that are proven and substantial

So just what is the stealth health promise? Well, to start with, here's what it's not. It's not a promise that you'll lose 10 lb in two weeks. Nor is it a guarantee that living the stealth health way will provide you with boundless energy until a painless death, during your sleep, at the age of 107. But here's what medical studies suggest a stealth health lifestyle *can* provide:

● **A leaner, healthier body for the rest of your life.** Of course, fad diets may kick-start your weight loss, but, as many of us have found out the hard way, in practice they're nearly always impossible to sustain over a lifetime. Instead, *Stealth Health*'s weight-loss tips are based on studies which show over and over again that the best way to lose weight and, most importantly, maintain the loss is simply through moderate daily exercise and healthy eating. Plus, there are some lesser-known research-based tips. Such as eating in front of a mirror. Cutting out soft drinks. Wearing blue while you're eating. All of these tips will help you to eat less and/or lose weight.

● **Better control of your blood sugar levels.** Just a brisk half-hour walk every day, or skipping sugary soft drinks and juices, or switching to whole grains, can decrease your risk of developing diabetes regardless of your weight.

● **A healthier heart.** It doesn't take much. One study found that a mere 30 minutes of walking three or more days a week could slash your risk of heart disease by more than a third.

● **Better control of your cholesterol levels.** Simply changing your eating habits from two large meals to six small meals a day, switching over to olive oil in your salad dressings, sipping

Special advice

There are more than 2,000 pieces of health advice in this book, all of them proven, valid, quick and effective. Of course, it's asking too much to suggest you consider each and every one. So, to help, certain tips are marked for quick spotting. These are the tips that you might wish to consider first, and they are identified as follows:

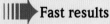 **Fast results**
These are tips that deliver benefits particularly quickly – in some cases, immediately.

 Easy gains
These are health boosters that offer the best value for the least amount of effort.

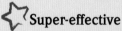 **Super-effective**
This is advice that scientific research or widespread usage by experts has shown to be especially effective.

part 1

STEALTH HEALTH THROUGH THE DAY

From the morning shower to the evening news, your days are full of regular tasks and routines. Here's how to make each a little calmer, a little healthier.

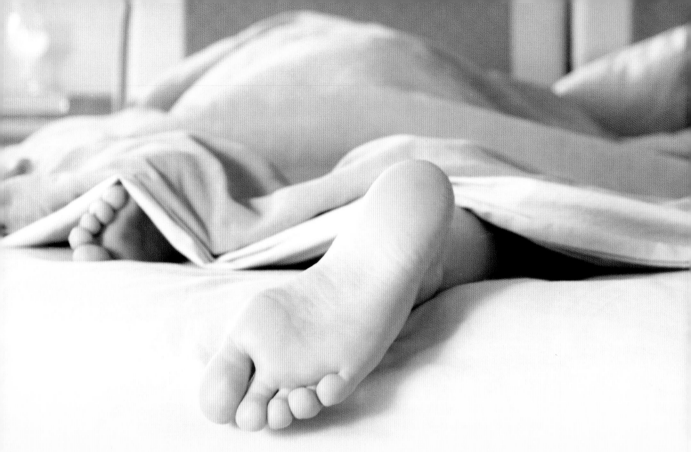

The **WAKE-UP** routine

OK, it's probably no one's favourite time, particularly if you stayed up late the night before, but there are plenty of good reasons for starting each and every day as well as you possibly can. Here are some ways to make sure you get out of the right side of bed and ease yourself into things with a positive, calm attitude. Remember: stress and anxiety wreak havoc on your immune system. If you start out happy and relaxed, you greatly increase your chance of having a healthy, productive day.

19 WAYS TO BRIGHTEN UP YOUR MORNING

In winter, sleep with your blinds or curtains halfway open. That way, the natural light of the rising sun will send a signal to your brain to slow down its production of melatonin and bump up your levels of adrenaline, an indication that it's time to wake up. When the alarm goes off, you'll already be half awake. In summer, ensure your curtains are dark enough to keep out 5 a.m. sunlight, but leave your window open so you can wake to birdsong.

Set your alarm to go off 15 minutes earlier. That way, you don't have to jump out of bed and rush through your morning. You can begin the day instead by lying in bed, slowly waking up. Have a stretch, listen to the news headlines and mentally run through what you're going to wear, what you're going to do, what you're going to have for breakfast. It's just as important to prepare yourself mentally as well as physically for your day. These few minutes in bed, before anyone else is up, are all yours.

Stretch every extremity for 15 seconds. Try this even before you open your eyes. Lift your arm and begin by stretching each finger, then your hand, then your wrist, then your arm. Next, move on to the other arm. Then your toes, feet, ankles and legs. Finally, end with a neck and back stretch that propels you out of the bed. You've just limbered up your muscles and joints, and enhanced the flow of blood through your body, providing extra oxygen to all of your tissues.

Read a motivational quote every morning. This can provide a frame for the day, a sort of self-help talk that keeps you motivated, unlike the negative impact of the morning news. Another option: use a motivational mantra that provides a

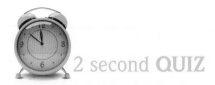

2 second QUIZ

Mouthwash or toothpaste?
ANSWER: **TOOTHPASTE.**

Mouthwash will not keep your breath fresh for more than 20 or 30 minutes (tests with garlic revealed this), and some mouthwash contains alcohol, which can dry out your mouth.

meditation-like burst, or read or recite a poem that helps you to focus. A good one to use is Rudyard Kipling's "If."

Take a vitamin. If you have a well-balanced diet and are generally healthy, taking a multivitamin may offer no additional benefits, but if you are in the habit of skipping meals or are going through a period where you're not eating healthily, a daily multivitamin will ensure you get all the essential micronutrients your body needs. Think of it as a sort of insurance policy. Keeping a supply visible on the kitchen counter will remind you to take one every morning.

Avoid any decisions. For truly relaxing mornings, reduce the number of choices and decisions you make to zero. Go about this in two ways: first, make your morning decisions the night before – what clothes to wear, what to have for breakfast, what route to take to work and so on. Second, make as much of your morning as routine as possible. Really, there's no need to vary your breakfast, timetable or bathroom ritual from one morning to the next.

Cuddle your children. Few things are more stressful in the morning than waking up an overtired seven-year-old

Healthy INVESTMENT

A sunrise alarm clock

You can find these intriguing alarm clocks in some electronic stores and department stores or buy them online. In addition to the typical radio/alarm, the clock can be set to become brighter gradually, as it gets closer to your wake-up time. The increasing light prompts your brain to begin making the stress hormone adrenaline, which helps you to wake up. You can also buy clocks that allow you to wake up to pre-recorded messages, to slowly building music coupled with an aromatherapy diffuser, or to an alarm that gradually increases in volume.

or a snoring teenager. Yet this is one of the few times when you can catch your children still vulnerable. Sit beside them and gently smooth their hair as you softly waken them, one by one. Or, if you're dealing with very young children, gently hug them awake. Such moments will send a quiet surge of joy through your entire day and will become all too rare in much too short a time.

Spend 5 to 10 minutes each morning listening to music or sitting just pondering. This allows the creative thinking that takes place during the night to gel and form into a plan of action, grounding you for the day.

Wake up to the smell of coffee. Buy the best coffee you can afford – fresh beans are best – and put twice the amount you've been using into your coffee-maker. Treat yourself to a machine with an alarm that can be set to start brewing at a specific time. The scent of strong coffee will pull you out of bed like a fish-hook in the back of your pyjamas. Morning is the best time to take caffeine – this central nervous system stimulant acts in many ways like other stimulant drugs such as amphetamines, waking you up and increasing your muscular activity. Even better: a study of 18 men found that caffeine improved their clear-headedness, happiness and calmness, as well as their ability to perform tests requiring them to pay attention, process information and solve problems.

Brush your tongue for 1 minute. There's no better way to rid yourself of morning breath and begin your day minty-fresh and clean. After all, more than 300 types of bacteria take up residence in your mouth every night. A quick brush over the teeth won't vanquish them all.

Drink a large glass of water. You've been fasting all night, so you wake up each morning dehydrated.

Fit in enough time to cuddle your children.

Check your morning calendar. First, hang a large white board in a prominent position in your kitchen. On it, write everything you need to know for that particular day, from the children's activities to whether someone is coming to fix the furnace to whether it's time to pay the bills. Check it carefully while you sip that first cup of coffee or tea; it will help you to structure the day in your mind and avoid the stressful effects of forgetting something important.

Create a checklist for your children. If you don't have children, skip this one. But if you do, to cut down on morning chaos, hang a white board or blackboard in the hallway or kitchen and list all the things that must be done before the children can leave: brush teeth, eat breakfast, get schoolbag together, make bed and so on. Have them score through or erase each item once it's completed. You can do the same thing with lists printed out from your computer. Set a consequence: if all the items aren't ticked off 5 minutes before you need to leave, there's no TV/PlayStation/dessert/computer time that night.

Keep a wicker basket for yourself and each child by the front or back door. Into it go your keys, wallet and bag, along with the child's schoolbag, papers, gloves, hats, etc. This will prevent that frantic last-minute search for lost items.

Wash in a stress-free way. We spend an average of about 12 minutes in the shower. That's fine when you're preparing for a date, but in the morning you need to get in and out quickly. If you don't like showering the night before (it can do strange things to your hair!) try using two-in-one products such as a combination shampoo and conditioner.

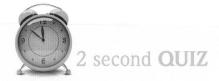

2 second QUIZ

Shower or bath?
ANSWER: SHOWER.

It's a healthier way to clean your body than soaking in the water you wash in. But baths are an excellent way to relax; for extra cleanliness use your shower attachment to rinse off afterwards.

When you wash your body, just hit the hot spots – your groin area and underarms. Everything else can just be rinsed off. The health benefit: reducing stress by saving time.

Prepare an emergency outfit in your closet. Include socks, jewellery, tights, etc., so on those mornings when you sleep through the alarm or simply need an extra 10 minutes, you can just pluck it off the hanger and go.

Dry more efficiently. Start with an oversized 100 per cent cotton bath sheet for maximum blotting. Towel-dry your hair and let it air-dry while you do your make-up or put on your underwear. Then, if you use a hair dryer, make it a high-energy one, at least 1,600 watts.

Hop on the treadmill for 30 minutes. Studies find that people who work out in the morning are more likely to stick to their exercise regimen because they get it out of the way first thing and don't have to come up with excuses later on. Plus, you'll produce endorphins whose mood-boosting effects will last most of the day.

Kiss all the people you love in your house before you leave, including pets if you like. Connecting with the ones you love soothes stress and helps you to focus on what's really important.

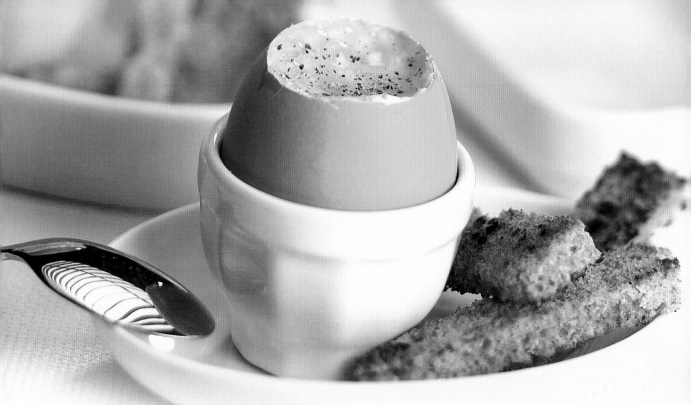

The **BREAKFAST** routine

There's a reason it's called the most important meal of the day. Not only is breakfast the first food and drink your body has had in more than 8 hours, but studies find that what you have for breakfast influences what you eat during the rest of the day. Additionally, people who eat breakfast are significantly less likely to be obese and have diabetes than those who don't. The most important tip is to have breakfast every day. Without exception. This one action alone can make a huge, positive difference to your health. But a doughnut or chocolate muffin won't do. The key is to choose energy-enhancing, health-invigorating foods. That's the focus of this part of the book.

23 WAYS TO KICK-START YOUR MORNING

Be consistent with your portions.
For most people, a perfect breakfast
has three components: one serving of a
whole-grain carbohydrate, one serving
of a dairy or high-calcium food and
one serving of fruit. Together, that
would add up to roughly 300 calories.
A high-protein serving (meat or an egg)
is unnecessary but certainly acceptable,
as long as it doesn't add too much fat
or too many calories to the mix. Here
are a few winning combinations, based
on this formula:

● A bowl of high-fibre, multigrain cereal,
with strawberries and low-fat milk on top.
● A cereal bar, an apple and a glass of
cold milk.
● Fat-free yogourt with fresh blueberries
mixed in, and a slice of whole-wheat toast
with a fruit spread.
● A mini whole-wheat bagel, spread
lightly with cream cheese and jam, and a
peach plus 150 g of yogourt.
● A scrambled egg, a whole-wheat roll,
fresh-fruit salad and a cup of low-fat milk.
● A bowl of oatmeal with chopped
banana or dried fruit.

**Have a bowl of sweetened brown
rice.** Consider this unique take on
prepared cereal. Brown rice is full of
energy-providing B vitamins, as well as
being a great source of filling fibre. Cook
the rice the night before, then, in the
morning, put it in a bowl with a spoonful
of honey, a handful of raisins, a cut-up
apple and a sprinkle of cinnamon for
a unique yet delicious treat. Don't like
rice? Try other cooked grains instead.
Some tasty ones include barley, oats,
buckwheat, quinoa or millet.

Pour a cup of fruit smoothie. Simply
whirl a cup of strawberries and a banana
in the blender, add a cup of crushed
ice, and you've got a healthy, on-the-

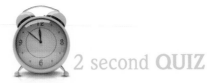

2 second QUIZ

Bacon or sausage?
ANSWER: **BACON.**

A slice of bacon, cooked thoroughly, has fewer
calories than a typical sausage. Your best bet is a
slice of lean back bacon with the rind and fat cut
off, rather than fatty streaky bacon.

Orange juice counts as one of your five-a-day
and may cut the risk of Alzheimer's.

go breakfast filled with antioxidants.
Toss in some plain yogourt, and you've
just added a bone-strengthening dose
of calcium too. Or, for a dairy-
free alternative, whirl up the
strawberries with fruit juice. In
winter, when fresh berries are not
in season, use frozen. An added
bonus: you've just crossed two of
your daily fruit servings off the list.

Use omega-3-rich eggs. They're
not much more expensive than standard
eggs but are much higher in all-important
omega-3 fatty acids, shown to benefit
everything from your mental health
(reducing the risk of depression) to your
heart health (reducing the risk of blocked
arteries and irregular heart rhythms).

**Sprinkle on a teaspoon of ground
flaxseeds.** It could be over your cereal,
yogourt, smoothie or eggs. Next to fish
and omega-3-rich eggs, flaxseeds are one
of the best sources of omega-3 fatty
acids. Lightly grind the seeds in a coffee
grinder or with a mortar and pestle before
adding them.

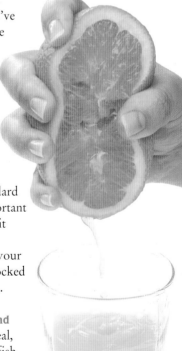

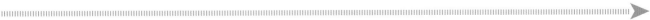

Healthy INVESTMENT

A blender

Why? Because blenders are great for making breakfast smoothies. You can toss in any kind of fruit – fresh, canned or frozen – along with cottage cheese or yogourt for your calcium portion, a handful of nuts or seeds for heart-healthy fats, and a sprinkle of cinnamon for extra flavour. Add a glass of crushed ice in the summer for a cool drink, or warm it in the microwave for 30 seconds on cold winter mornings.

☺ **Try some all-natural peanut butter instead of butter.** Whether you prefer smooth or crunchy, peanut butter is lower in saturated fat and has far more good monounsaturated fat, which your body needs.

☕ **Make your own granola.** Many store-bought brands are filled with sugar and fat. To make your own, mix two parts rolled oats to one part dried fruit and seeds with a little brown sugar. Store in an airtight container. Not interested in do-it-yourself? There are a few store-bought brands with reasonable sugar and fat levels – just read the labels carefully before you buy.

☕ **Eat half a grapefruit twice a week.** Grapefruit contains a good amount of folate and vitamin C, which are believed to help reduce the risk of heart disease and stroke. According to a review of eight studies in *The Lancet*, adding folic acid to your diet may cut your stroke risk by a fifth. But be cautious if you're taking regular medication. Grapefruit and its juice can interact with medicines that have to be processed through the liver, so check with your doctor first about any possible interactions between the grapefruit and any medication you're taking.

☺ **Sip a cup of green tea with your breakfast.** In addition to its heart-protective benefits, green tea may also have some weight-loss benefits, with one study finding that it appears to raise the rate at which you burn calories and increase the speed at which your body uses fat.

☕ **Top your cereal with soy milk.** Packed with potent phytoestrogens, soy has been credited with everything from protecting your heart to promoting stronger bones. But make sure that it's fortified with calcium for even more of the bone-building stuff.

☕ **Build your own breakfast and have great fun.** Who says breakfast has to be boring? Choose a selection of sliced fruit, yogourt, whole-grain cereals and/or whole-grain toast, and let everyone mix and match to create their own toppings. If you're in a hurry, lay everything out on paper plates to make cleaning up easier.

☕ **Add a vitamin.** If you are taking supplements, take them with breakfast, suggests nutrition expert Shari Lieberman, PhD, author of *The Real Vitamin & Mineral Book*. Taking supplements with food reduces the chance that they'll upset your stomach, as well as improving the absorption of minerals.

☕ **Spread apple slices with peanut butter.** The protein and fat in the peanut butter provide a good start to the day, while the apple and the quercetin it contains provide fibre and may protect against some cancers and heart disease.

☕ **Have a breakfast sandwich.** Top a whole-wheat roll, bread or toast with melted low-fat cheese (low-fat mozzarella is a good choice), a sliced tomato and a sliced, hard-boiled egg.

Eat when you get to work. If you really haven't got time or you simply can't face eating breakfast before you leave the house in the morning, keep a box of cereal in your desk at work, or buy a low-fat sandwich on your way to work to eat when you arrive.

Visit the vegetarian section of the supermarket. Veggie bacon, sausages and burgers are good sources of protein for breakfast without the saturated fat of their meat alternatives.

Sprinkle a handful of blueberries on your cereal. Studies find the tiny purple berries are loaded with valuable antioxidants that can slow down brain aging and protect your memory. Not into cereal? Try baking blueberries into oatmeal to create your own oatmeal and blueberry granola bar, or mix them into whole-wheat pancake batter.

Drink a glass of unsweetened orange juice every morning. A small glass (²/₃ cup/150 ml) of unsweetened fruit juice will count as one of your five-a-day. Plus, American researchers who followed almost 2,000 people for up to ten years found that the risk of developing Alzheimer's disease was 76 per cent lower in those who drank juice more than three times a week, compared to those who drank it less than once a week.

Eat a bowl of sliced strawberries three times a week. Strawberries are packed with vitamin C and have numerous health benefits, one of them being protection for your eyes. One study of 247 women found that those taking vitamin C supplements were 75 per cent less likely to get cataracts than those who didn't take it. It's better, though, to get your vitamin C from food. Like other berries they're also rich in a wide variety of antioxidants, low in calories and even have a low glycemic index (shown to keep blood sugar levels steady).

Slice two kiwis into your morning smoothie. You may have just reduced your risk of premature death by as much as 30 per cent. A British study found that every 30 g of these vitamin C-rich fruits you eat a day reduces your risk of premature death by 10 per cent. Just slice the top off and scoop out.

Get at least 5 g of fibre during breakfast each morning. If you don't get off to a good start with your daily fibre intake, you'll never reach the recommended amount (24 g per 2,000 calories). Plus, fibre is quite filling with no extra cost in calories. You can get 5 g in just a few bites with a large raw apple, a small bowl of high-fibre cereal, 80 g of blackberries or two slices of dark, whole-grain rye bread.

Choose these toppings for your (whole-wheat) toast or bagel:
- A tablespoon of low-fat soft cheese topped with a couple of tablespoons of mashed fresh raspberries or blueberries.
- One heaped teaspoon of peanut or almond butter.
- Mashed banana.
- One tablespoon of cottage cheese or low-fat cream cheese topped with a thin slice of smoked salmon.

Shave 30 g of dark chocolate over 250 g of fat-free yogourt, then mix. The calcium-rich yogourt can actually help you to lose weight, while the antioxidant-loaded dark chocolate can help to reduce the effects of "bad" LDL cholesterol, keeping your arteries more flexible.

Add two vitamin C-rich kiwis to your morning smoothie.

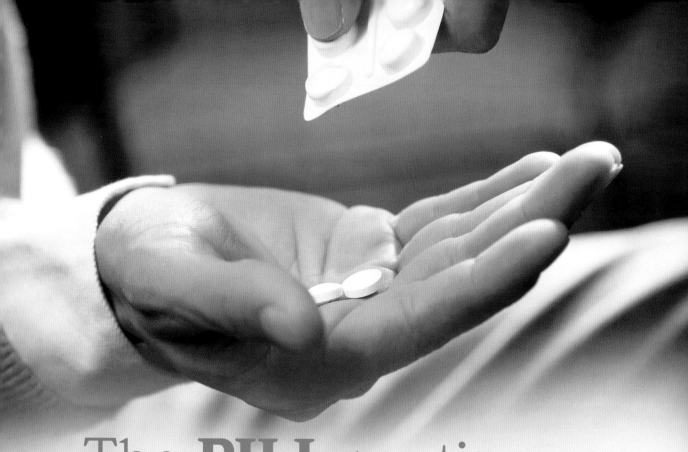

The **PILL** routine

Between us, we take a lot of pills. The numbers may surprise you.
More than $19 billion was spent on pharmaceuticals in Canada in 2007, according to IMS Health. That works out to $578 per capita spent on prescription drugs. Age plays a part. Canadians over age 65 spent twice as much as did 45- to 64-year-olds. The largest age grouping, 45–64, which includes baby boomers, was responsible for 36 per cent of retail spending on prescription drugs in 2007.

Worryingly, hospital admissions among elderly people are sometimes the result of medication reactions, which suggests that too often we're taking our medicine incorrectly. By following these tips, you can make sure you take your drugs properly, avoid interactions and learn what to look for when buying over-the-counter drugs.

9 WAYS TO MANAGE YOUR MEDICINES AND SUPPLEMENTS BETTER

Each time you visit a new doctor, or revisit your existing doctor after a period of several months, bring every pill you're currently taking with you. Simply put each prescription medicine, vitamin, herbal product, supplement and over-the-counter drug – even the Aspirin – that you take in a typical day into a bag. Then ask your doctor to look over it all to see if there are any problematic combinations or if anything is redundant.

● Ask your GP if there is a way to streamline the medication you take. Some medicines can be taken once a day in sustained release, rather than three times a day. Others can be taken once a day or in a combination product that can decrease the numbers of drugs you're taking overall. Some can even be taken once a week.

● Ask your doctor these questions about any new prescription:
● What is this medicine for?
● What side effects might I encounter?
● What side effects are dangerous and should cause me to stop taking this medicine and call you?
● If I have to stop taking this medicine because of side effects, is there another that I can take instead?
● What are the dangers for me if I don't take this medicine?
● What time of day should I take it?
● Should I take it with food or without?
● Can I take it with any kind of liquid, or only with water?
● How will I know if it's working?
● How long should this medicine take to begin working?
● For how long should I continue taking this medicine?
Remember: while only a doctor can prescribe medicine, you are the one ultimately responsible for your health.

Choosing the
RIGHT VITAMIN

Been vitamin shopping lately? If you have, you probably needed a pain-reliever for the ensuing headache triggered by all those choices. Here's what clinical nutritionist Shari Lieberman, PhD, author of *The Real Vitamin & Mineral Book*, recommends to make it easier to pick the right ones:
● Choose natural versions, rather than chemically synthesized options, when buying fat-soluble vitamins, for example, A, D, E and beta carotene.
● Avoid additives such as coal tars, artificial colouring, preservatives, sugars, starch and other ingredients that you simply don't need with your vitamin.
● Don't bother about chelated minerals. Chelation means the minerals have an added protein to enhance absorption. But they're often more expensive, and studies that examine whether they really are absorbed faster than non-chelated minerals are sparse.
● Don't buy time-release formulations. These supplements may actually take longer to be absorbed and provide you with lower blood levels of the vitamin or mineral.

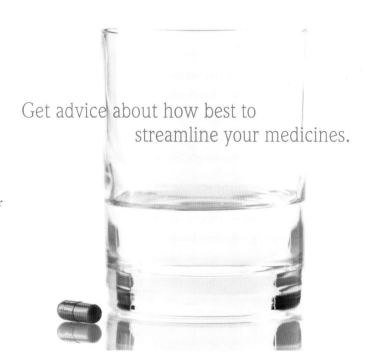

Get advice about how best to streamline your medicines.

Medicines for sale
OVER THE INTERNET

The Internet has boosted sales of many over-the-counter drugs and supplements – and, more worryingly, prescription medicines, too. Since it's hard to know exactly whom or what you're dealing with in cyberspace, you need to take some special precautions.

● Check the validity of the pharmacy website. With the exception of getting discount deals on established over-the-counter medicines from truly recognized suppliers, such as major supermarkets and pharmacy chains, buying medicines over the Internet is a risky business. The Canadian Pharmacists Association (CPhA) discourages buying medicines online. Some websites look like legitimate pharmacies when in fact both the seller and the products are illegitimate. Purchasing medicines from an illegal website puts the user at risk of receiving a contaminated or counterfeit product, the wrong product, an incorrect dose or no product at all.

● Beware of purchasing drugs that aren't normally available in Canada. If in doubt, don't do it.

● **Get all your prescriptions at one pharmacy,** and talk to the pharmacist. Pharmacists are more than just prescription fillers. They are specially trained in understanding possible medicine interactions, including interactions with herbal supplements. When you consolidate all your prescriptions, be sure to enlist your pharmacist's help to look out for these very things. In addition, pharmacists can provide advice on a great number of illnesses and diseases, including hypertension and diabetes. They are also a great source of insider information on the most effective and best value over-the-counter drugs.

● **Then keep all your medicines in one place at home.** It is generally better to have everything together in one place rather than scattered around your house, car, bag or briefcase. Choose a space that is dark, and which is perpetually at room temperature (unless instructions call for medication to be refrigerated). It should be accessible to adults, but not children. While you are doing this, check each container to see if any has passed its expiry date. Take them to any pharmacy and ask a staff member about disposal. Saving antibiotics for the next infection is the wrong thing to do.

☺ **Create a rigid pill-taking routine.** Aim to take your pills at the same time and place every day, and find a trigger to remind you to take them. Some pointers:

● Buy a pill box or other medication container and each Sunday evening re-stock it for the coming week. Place the pill box in a spot where you normally take your pills, and do not move it.

● Link your pill taking to a part of your morning ritual, such as brushing your teeth or drinking your first glass of water or juice of the day.

● Set the alarm on your watch, computer, mobile phone or personal organizer to beep when it's time to take a pill. Then, no matter where you are, or how busy you are, you'll get a reminder.

● **Watch out for shift work.** Working different shifts can create timing problems when taking your medication. Try to take it when you would normally have a shift change so the timing is similar whether you're going to bed or at work.

● **Buy measuring spoons just for your medicine,** and store them with your medicine. A kitchen teaspoon or tablespoon is rarely accurate.

☆ **Always follow the golden rules of medicine.** None of the following tips is particularly clever or surprising, but they all bear repeating – and adhering to:

- Disclose everything to your doctor and pharmacist: that you have allergies, that you are pregnant, that you have particularly high or low blood pressure, that you are prone to nausea, that you are on a diet. All are factors that can affect a drug's efficacy.
- When you collect your prescription, open the bag immediately to verify that the medication you received is the correct one, at the right dosage and for the correct duration.
- Ask your doctor or pharmacist if a medicine or supplement should be taken with or without meals.
- Take only the amount of medication prescribed or listed on the label.
- Get your prescriptions made up during slow times for the pharmacist, to avoid mix-ups.
- Whenever you purchase a supplement, ask your pharmacist if it has any potential interactions with any prescription or over-the-counter drugs you're taking.
- Don't use or share medication prescribed for someone else.
- Don't take your medicine in the dark or without glasses on or contact lenses in if you need to wear them.
- Keep your medicines in their original packaging with the full instructions; do so even for over-the-counter and herbal products.

Do **THREE** things...

Here are three useful pieces of advice on managing your medicines:

1 Find out from your pharmacist if the medication can be put into different containers such as a day-by-day pill box. Some medicines are light-sensitive or may not be compatible with plastic.

2 Try to fit in taking your medication with your daily routines. It's best to be able to associate your medication with a daily activity, such as washing your face.

3 Make a chart or have a pharmacist make a chart of each of your medicines and the times at which you take them. Put the chart on the fridge door.

Buy a pill box and keep it in a prominent place.

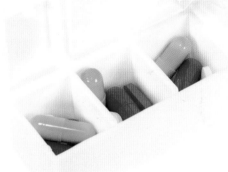

Reminder

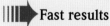 **Fast results**
These are tips that deliver benefits particularly quickly – in some cases, immediately.

 Easy gains
These are health boosters that offer the best value for the least amount of effort.

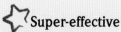 **Super-effective**
This is advice that scientific research or widespread usage by experts has shown to be especially effective.

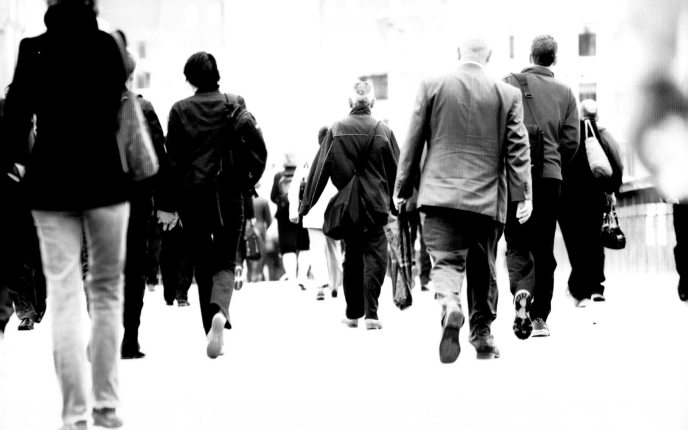

The COMMUTE

If you're like most people in Canada, it takes you about 65 minutes to get to and from work. This means that over the course of a year, you're spending about 275 hours – or a total of nearly 12 days a year – getting to work and returning home! So it should come as no surprise that in one of the few major studies ever conducted on commuters, researcher Meni Koslowsky, PhD, a psychology professor from Bar-Ilan University in Israel, found that commuters experienced significantly high levels of tension. However, Koslowsky also found that stress is not a forgone conclusion.

The tips that follow are designed to help you make your commute less of a strain, saving precious wear and tear on your heart, brain, immune system and emotions.

21 TIPS FOR A HAPPIER JOURNEY

● **If at all possible, use public transport.** Here's why. Meni Koslowsky's research found that it's not the commute per se that is so stressful. The real stress comes from the issue of control. If you drive your own car to work, part of the reason you do it is to feel that you're in control. So if you get stuck in traffic, you feel that you have lost control of your commuting experience, which is where the stress comes in. By taking public transport, be it the train or bus, you have already given up control of your commute. If you get stuck, you won't be blaming yourself for the delay. Nor will you be torturing yourself to solve the situation.

● **If it's a viable option, take the train.** Going back to that control issue again, Koslowsky found that another major cause of commuter stress is uncertainty. And there is far more uncertainty in driving a car, or even commuting via bus or car-sharing because of traffic accidents, jams, etc., than in taking a train, as arrival times are more concrete.

● **Consider carpooling.** It's not for everyone, and the research is ambiguous, but it is worth considering. On the one hand, Koslowsky's research finds that carpooling can reduce stress, both in terms of the "giving up" of control and in terms of the social interaction that occurs. But if you're an introvert who prefers a quiet commute so you can read, think or listen to music, then carpooling with people who expect conversation could just stress you more. The bottom line: if you're an outgoing people-person, try carpooling. If you're an introvert, stick to your usual mode of transport.

● **Avoid rush hour, whenever you can.** It's such an obvious way to improve your commute, yet the fact that streets

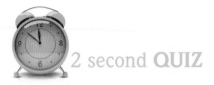

2 second QUIZ

Manual or automatic?
ANSWER: **AUTOMATIC.**

The two main arguments for driving a manual car – you'll burn more calories and less gasoline – don't hold up. Changing gears and using a clutch pedal don't add up to exercise unless you're driving an 18-wheel truck. And on new cars, automatic transmissions have become increasingly fuel-efficient. From a stress point of view, an automatic will make driving much easier.

and trains are packed every rush hour shows that few people manage to find an alternative. What are the viable options, other than moving or getting a new job?
● Ask for a 1 hour shift in the time you start and end work.
● If your company has satellite offices that are closer to home, see if you can work there sometimes.
● Drive in before the crowds, and create a constructive pre-work ritual for yourself, such as exercising, eating a leisurely breakfast, running errands.

● **If you drive, take the route with the least stop-and-go traffic.** Longer is better if the traffic flows smoothly and you avoid too many lights, turns and crosswalks. For most of us, no form of driving is as stressful as trying to move quickly on crowded main roads.

☺ **Above all, lose the "race" mentality.** All that weaving, darting and surging rarely gains you more than a few minutes, but at a huge price to your stress levels (not to mention the extra wear and tear on your car and lower gas mileage). Drive calmly, without abundant lane changes or speed surges, and your commute will become so much more pleasant.

Don't judge other drivers who play their music too loud or forget to signal. Get over it!

● **Don't be judgmental about thy fellow driver.** It's a funny thing about high-stress drivers. When someone passes them, they get angry. When someone is going slower than they are, they get angry. They get angry when others forget to signal a turn, or if their car is larger or they're playing their music too loudly. Get over it! Overreacting to other drivers is a sure road to stress, headaches and anger. Instead, be a defensive driver, and never let what other drivers do bother you.

● **Learn while you commute.** If you've always been meaning to learn to speak Spanish or read the latest best-sellers, now's your chance. You can borrow audio books on CD from the library or download them from the Internet to burn onto CDs or upload onto your MP3 player. Even coming to a standstill is bearable when you're in the thick of an exciting story.

● **Use your mobile phone for personal conversations only.** While cellphones are definitely a boon to the commuter, Meni Koslowsky's research finds that using them for work-related tasks, such as setting up meetings, only increases your stress because it increases your working day. The best thing is to turn it off.

● **Leave 10 minutes earlier than you have to.** Do this both coming and going. Studies find that the less sense of "time urgency," or worry about being late, you have, the less stressed out you'll feel during your commute.

● **Create a selection of music just for the commute:** one for going to work and one for relaxing on the way home from work. Workout experts know that music can serve many purposes and that each selection needs to be tailored to an individual's needs. Play the selection on an MP3 player if you take the train or bus or in the stereo of your car. Sing along if you're in your car. There's no need to be shy. The music has another benefit if you're driving: one study found that people who listened to music when stuck in a traffic jam were less likely to get angry and violent than those who didn't.

● **Practise good car ergonomics.** That means more than just buckling up. Before you head out, make sure your headrest is set directly behind your head, aligned with the top of your ears. Adjust your seat and steering wheel for maximum comfort. Check each mirror to make sure you don't need to lean or crane your neck to get the best vision. Now you can belt up.

● **Play a game.** Remember the old "I Spy" games you used to play as a child on interminable trips? Invent your own version. Maybe you count the number of women you see applying make-up while driving. Or the number of people you see scratching their head. Start counting them each day and see if you can beat your previous day's record.

▐▐▌➡ **Equip your car.** Make sure you have the following with you: a spill-proof coffee cup filled with your favourite brew, a bottle of water and a bag of non-perishable snacks (try granola bars and dried fruit) in case you get caught in traffic just as your blood sugar plummets. An audio book in the event of traffic coming to a complete halt and a fully charged cellphone will also come in handy.

● **Develop five alternative routes for your commute.** Again, this goes back to the control issue. If you know you can go a different way, you automatically have more control over the situation.

● **Prepare for your commute the evening before.** Check the weather and traffic reports on local websites for information on possible hold-ups and delays. Listen to local radio for warnings and updates. Again, this puts the control back into your hands.

● **Relax before you begin your journey.** Instead of gulping down a scalding cup of coffee and choking down toast en route, get up early enough to enjoy a leisurely breakfast. Once you arrive at work, take another few minutes to sip a cup of tea or coffee before diving into your work. On the way home, go to the coffee area before you set out and just sit quietly with a drink for 5 minutes before heading home.

● **Work out in your car.** Do isometrics while driving by tensing and relaxing your leg muscles, tensing your arm muscles against the resistance of the steering wheel and/or tensing your abdominal and chest muscles. When done correctly for bouts of 10 to 15 seconds, these toning exercises can make an appreciable difference to your appearance, improve your fitness and relax you without distracting you or adding an extra minute to your schedule.

● **Lift your legs up and stretch them for 30 seconds.** This is one to do if you're on public transport or, if you're driving, when you've stopped in traffic. But this movement is important because it reduces the risk of blood clots from sitting too long in one position. Also put one arm behind your neck and stretch it by holding on to the elbow with the opposite arm. Switch sides. Do one every time the traffic comes to a halt.

● **Sniffed your car lately?** If you use your car as a moving garbage can, you're putting more than your upholstery at

risk. Dirty cars can become a rolling Typhoid Mary, filled with insects, germs, mould, pollen and other irritants and pathogens destined to leave you sneezing, itching, watering and feeling sick. Even if you spend just an hour each day in your car, that's several times longer than most people spend in the bathroom!

● **Set your mood using the radio.** Tune into a music station and a news station. Use your travel time to catch up with the news, then switch to music before you arrive to relax or energize yourself.

In PERSPECTIVE

Why stress affects your health

You might think commuting has little to do with health, but the stress that comes from commuting almost certainly affects your well-being. Here's why.

Every time you're confronted with a stressor – whether it's a traffic jam, or something more serious, such as a fire – your body releases stress hormones such as adrenaline and cortisol. They, in turn, send signals to various parts of your body to ready them for action. For instance, your liver releases glucose to provide instant energy to muscle cells. Your lungs expand, your heart beats faster and your blood pressure rises to send more oxygen-rich blood throughout your body. All of this can lead to common stress-related conditions ranging from chronic hypertension, angina and gastric reflux, to constipation and irritable bowel syndrome, to depression, anxiety and fatigue.

Stress can even make you fat. Cortisol is not only a powerful appetite trigger; chronically high levels actually stimulate the fat cells in the abdomen to fill with more fat, creating a life-threatening form of fat called visceral fat, which puts you at higher risk of heart disease and diabetes.

Being tense can also inflict damage on your immune system. Like most body systems, it has a feedback loop. After the immune system has finished attacking foreign invaders, the brain sends out cortisol, to suppress the immune response. If your body is releasing cortisol all the time, as it does under chronic stress, then your immune system is constantly being suppressed, increasing your risk of illness.

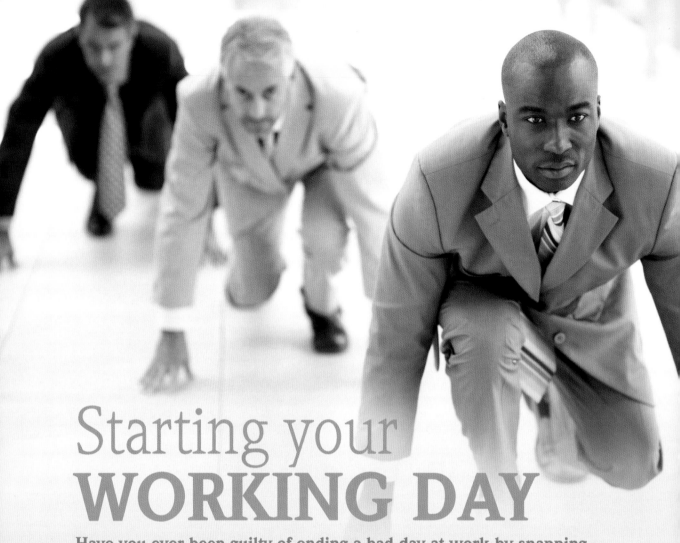

Starting your WORKING DAY

Have you ever been guilty of ending a bad day at work by snapping at the children, being rude to your partner, gorging on junk food, slumping in front of the TV or turning to alcohol? A bad work day may not seem unhealthy in itself, but it can serve as the domino that starts off a whole chain of destructive actions.

    The way you begin your working day sets the tone for the rest of the day, not only in your workplace but also at home. A few simple measures taken at the start of your day can make all the difference to how it ends. Here are some tips to help you get off to the right – and healthy – start.

19 IDEAS FOR LAUNCHING A CALMER, MORE PRODUCTIVE DAY

Limit your work-starting routine to 15 minutes. Don't spend more than a quarter of an hour getting coffee, settling in, looking at newspapers or reading e-mails. You are often at your freshest and most productive at the beginning of the day. A prolonged morning routine takes the positive edge off and makes your afternoon more stressful. Better to jump into the important work quickly, and read the non-essential e-mails after you've covered lots of ground.

● **Write two to-do lists.** The first should contain everything that you need to get done soon. It should be a comprehensive list of short, medium and long-term projects and work, and you should constantly adjust it. The second to-do list should be what you can reasonably expect to get done today, and today only. Be fair to yourself. Factor in the likely disruptions, meetings, phone calls and travel hassles. Make the tasks as specific as possible (for example, conduct online research for a particular market) and assign a time you plan to devote to it (20 minutes). Print the list out on brightly coloured paper; this keeps it from getting lost on your desk. By prioritizing your work and breaking it down into small, achievable pieces, you greatly increase the chances that you will be satisfied with your day's accomplishments.

☆ **Take a few moments to assess the day's emotional challenges.** Almost as important as your to-do list is a "be-prepared-for" list. Make an inventory of tough phone calls, boring meetings, challenging customers, frustrating red tape, infuriating rush-hour commutes, droning detail work and other mental challenges you are likely to face. Then accept that they are inevitable and prepare yourself to get through them

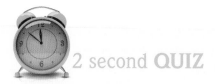

2 second QUIZ

E-mail or walk down the hall?
ANSWER: **WALK DOWN THE HALL.**

You'll get your blood circulating better, burn calories and, most likely, have a more productive, personal and satisfying conversation than you would have had via the computer.

without anger, frustration or impatience. Remember: it's usually not work that gets us down, but rather the challenges that lie along the periphery of the job.

● **Visualize your day.** Taking that last point a little further, you might wish to start each day by closing your eyes for 10 to 20 seconds and visualizing how you want it to go. See yourself making a stellar presentation at the board meeting. Experience the great feeling you're going to have when you finally make the sale or get that report off your desk. Hear yourself providing positive feedback to your employee, or even your boss. If you are religious, make this a prayer.

● **Schedule some social time for midmorning.** You probably work with people whom you like and know well. In fact, camaraderie is what makes many jobs great. So build a ritual into each morning in which you can spend a few moments of social time with colleagues. Make it short, at an appropriate time, and don't let a day go by without it. But avoid personal phone calls if you can; they can unexpectedly turn into big time-eaters.

● **Likewise, schedule some reading time.** There's not a job that doesn't require at least some reading, be it about the company, the industry, the marketplace, the economy. Create a ritual

Healthy INVESTMENT

A large freezable water bottle
Use it to keep cold water on your desk all day long. This ensures that you stay hydrated with a healthy, non-calorific liquid rather than sipping sugar-filled soft drinks or juices.

that gives you 15 minutes or so to review newspapers, electronic newsletters, industry magazines, company memos and other reading. Be disciplined – this is not the time to do online shopping! You'll find that being up to date with your business has many advantages, just one of them being a sense of control about your own situation.

Keep essentials nearby. If you have some private storage space where you work, stock up on the following:
- A box of low-fat granola bars (the perfect snack or substitute breakfast).
- A snack pack (containing an array of other nutritious snacks).
- A supply of bottled water (keeps you away from the soft drink machine).
- Bags of sugar-free mints or candy (helps to prevent needless snacking).
- A box of tissues (always handy).
- At least five family photos (which always lift the spirits).

Make sure you have the right equipment for a healthy day in the office. If you're deskbound, that means:
- Headphones for the telephone, so that you're not leaning your neck to one side when you talk on the phone.
- An antiglare filter on your computer screen. One study found filters improved the quality of the screen image and significantly reduced the percentage of people suffering from tired, dry, itchy or watery eyes, fatigue and headaches.

- A wrist-rest for your computer so that you can keep your wrists elevated, thus avoiding pressure on the nerves that go through your wrist, which can cause carpal tunnel syndrome.

If you're in sales or customer service, you're likely to be on your feet for much of the day. Comfortable, supportive shoes are just a start. Good socks and underwear, a steady supply of breath mints, and braces or some other support for your back, knees or any other problematic joints are also important. Finally, establish a safe place to keep your keys, cellphone and other bits and pieces. Full pockets can affect your posture and movement.

Set your watch or computer alarm to go off (quietly) every hour. This will be your signal throughout the day to take a break, get up and stretch, walk around the building, etc. But, in an open-plan office, for instance, keep the volume low so that it doesn't upset your colleagues.

Sit up straight. One common cause of fatigue, carpal tunnel syndrome and back pain is our tendency to slump while typing or sitting. Every time your alarm beeps or your phone rings, consider it a reminder to straighten your back, throw back your shoulders and lift up your neck.

Loosen your tie (if you're wearing one). Researchers at the New York Eye and Ear Infirmary found that tighter ties increased eye pressure, which is a risk factor for glaucoma.

Spend a few moments sparking your creativity. Here's a good way if you have a computer. Each morning, pick a random word or name and spend 5 minutes exploring the word on the Internet, or go to www.wikipedia.org and read "Today's featured article." Don't have a computer? Then pick up a dictionary, open it to a random page and look for interesting words. Simple exercises such as these blow the cobwebs from your mind and set your brain up to embrace new information – even in a job you've been doing for years.

⊕ **Record your message for the day.** If you're often interrupted by phone calls, use your voicemail to help improve your efficiency at work. Change your message frequently so that people don't miss you or disturb you when you're busy. For instance, you might leave a message saying that you're in the office, but in meetings for most of the day, so won't be returning calls until the next morning. Or leave a message saying that you're in the office, but working on a major project all day, and will be checking messages only at 4 p.m. Your phone system may even allow you to leave a voicemail for one person if you know that someone is calling for specific information.

⊕ **Keep a cellphone charger at work.** That way, you'll never be caught out if your cell's battery runs down. You could also buy yourself an emergency phone charger – a handy little gadget that fits in your pocket and gives you backup power when it is really needed.

☆ **Start your day with a cup of hot cocoa** while you tackle your most creative work. Research shows that one cup of pure cocoa a day for five days can increase blood flow in the brain, hands and legs, as well as helping to regulate blood pressure. Choose pure cocoa to get the full effect.

⊕ **Get to work an hour or half-hour before everyone else.** That precious calm time – before the e-mails start pouring in,

the phone starts ringing and the problems start piling up – is more valuable than diamonds in terms of your overall work performance and accomplishments. An added bonus: you may get to leave early.

⊕ **Find a compliment you've received from a colleague** or boss via e-mail, print it and tape it inside your top drawer. If you're feeling overwhelmed, take a peek to remind you of what others think of your abilities.

⊕ **Keep fresh flowers or plants at work.** One U.S. study found that live plants increased creative thinking. Keep them within sight, near your computer. Other studies find that plants significantly lower workplace stress and enhance productivity – possibly because they release extra oxygen and remove carbon dioxide from the air during photosynthesis.

☺ **Block off 30 minutes on your calendar at the end of the day.** It may seem strange to do this at the start of your day, but this will be your time to begin the transition from work to home. During this last half hour of your working day, you can finish answering any e-mails, update your to-do list for the next day and tidy up your desk.

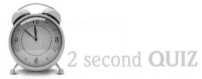

2 second QUIZ

A packed lunch or a purchased lunch?

ANSWER: A PACKED LUNCH.
It'll be healthier, it'll probably have fewer calories, it'll be cheaper and it'll save you lots of time that you can use for walking, reading or socializing instead.

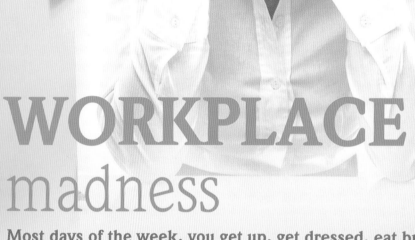

WORKPLACE
madness

Most days of the week, you get up, get dressed, eat breakfast and head out into one of the unhealthiest places in the world. Problems at work are more strongly associated with health complaints than any other cause of stress – even more than financial or family problems. In fact, U.S. researchers have found the first-ever link between stress and back pain. It turns out that people who get upset when they're criticized in the workplace use their muscles in ways that might lead to injury over time. Here is a wide spectrum of health-boosting tips to help you to cope with stress at work.

31 WAYS TO CALM THE CHAOS

☎ **Work on one thing at a time.** Today's office worker changes tasks an average of every 3 minutes. Such a lightning-speed day of interruptions is helped along by the multi-tasking made possible by computers. Working on eight things at once might seem impressive, but it isn't. Rather, it is exhausting, inefficient and highly stressful. So, instead of constantly checking e-mails, having two or three documents open on your screen, or returning e-mails as they come in, structure your day to focus on one thing at a time. In particular, start your day by blocking out 2 hours for uninterrupted hands-on work. During this time, do not answer your phone or check e-mails. Then check e-mails and respond all at once. Go to lunch. Structure your afternoon in the same way. Designate a time immediately after lunch and an hour before you leave for returning calls.

▮▮▮▶ **Work in short bursts.** The flip side to multi-tasking is that it is hard to sustain creativity or intensity on one task for long stretches. Rather, our brains work in cycles of creativity, then take a rest. So try this: after an hour or so of concentrated work, get up for 5 minutes, walk around, do some stretches. Not only will this help the quality of your work – by the time you finish your day, you'll have fitted in 30 minutes of stress-reducing exercise.

☎ **Deal directly, but constructively, with difficult workplace relationships.** "Toxic people" are those whose negativity or demeanour seems to drain or annoy you. This might be your boss, your assistant, your colleague – in other words, they are people with whom you frequently interact. After a negative encounter with a toxic person, the temptation is to be angry and accusatory. But that leads nowhere. Instead, try this direct, honest

and disarming approach: "I am finding our interactions stressful because of —— and am feeling bad about ——. I would like our working relationship to improve. What suggestions do you have for me?" Even if you feel that the other person is the one who should change, by asking for his or her suggestions, you avoid putting that person on the defensive. If your colleague is even a little bit reasonable, this might make him or her admit, "Well, I suppose there are some changes I could make too."

☆ **Praise yourself at least once a day.** Most of us don't take enough time to praise ourselves for doing things well. So when you've completed an interim or long-term goal, tell yourself – out loud – what a good job you've done. You'll get a burst of confidence that will go a long way towards helping you to maintain your cool amid the workplace madness.

☎ **Be creative in motivating yourself.** Here's a good one: write a cheque to an organization you loathe, put it in a stamped, addressed envelope and tell a trusted friend to post it if you fail to meet an important deadline or complete a vital task. Or take the positive route: give the friend something you really cherish or desire and let your friend give it back to you only if you achieve your goal.

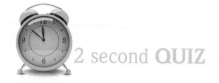

Shout or walk away?
ANSWER: **WALK AWAY.**

Shouting means the disagreement has become overly personal and emotional. Little good will come of it. Cut off the conversation firmly by saying this is an unacceptable way to resolve an issue and that you'll reconvene the discussion when your colleagues have regained their composure, thoughtfulness and perspective.

☎ **Forego the coffee during team meetings or group work.** A study sponsored by the British Economic and Social Research Council found that when men drank coffee while working together in a group, it tended to make the group less effective. The study also found that just the perception that the drink contained caffeine – whether or not it actually did – also increased the men's feelings of stress and their heart rates.

☎ **Stand against the wall and slide down it as if you were sitting** in a chair. Stay there for a few minutes without looking down, just feeling your spine against the wall. Breathe deeply (in through your nose, out through your mouth) and focus on one peaceful thought (waves crashing on the shore, a glass of wine by a roaring fire). Press your feet into the ground as you hold this position and picture the stress oozing out of your body. When you stand up, shake out your arms and legs and return to work refreshed.

☎ **Keep a vacation file on your desk.** Fill it with brochures of places you'd like to visit. When you're feeling stressed, daydream your way through it. It will remind you of one reason you're working, and provide a little virtual vacation.

☎ **Read a poem out loud twice a day.** The cadence, words and images will soothe your soul. Not into poetry? If you're religious, try reading a psalm or other sacred writings. If you love music, listen to a few of your favourite songs.

☎ **Make an altar or display in your office to remind you of your life** outside the office. Include pictures of your spouse, children and/or pet, a photograph of yourself doing something fun, plus a memento that reminds you of a special occasion. When you feel yourself getting overwhelmed and stressed out, take 5 minutes and simply stare at the display. Recall the day each picture was taken. Hold the memento and return in your mind to the place where you got it. Now you're ready to return to work.

☎ **Keep a work journal.** This is a journal you keep in your desk drawer (preferably locked). Write in it whenever you feel your temper rising, your frustration growing or your despair increasing. In it, you can write all the things you'd like to say to the boss/client/colleague so you get it out of your system without losing your job. It will also help you to understand what it is about your job and your day that really drives you crazy – and what you actually enjoy. Do not, however, keep said journal on your computer, and always, always keep it out of sight.

☎ **Take an impromptu vacation.** If you're experiencing an unusual number of headaches, a sore neck, sore back or other aches and pains; find you have trouble falling or staying asleep; or are snapping at your colleagues for no reason, it's time for a day off. Check your calendar for the coming week and find the first available day you can take. If you really are feeling unwell, take it as a sick day rather than a vacation day - there's no shame in admitting that you are unwell. Whether you do something special or simply rest, make sure you take days off when you need them – if you don't you can bet you'll be really sick before long.

☺ **Schedule 10 minutes of "worry time."** Close your office door or go to an empty conference room and focus on what stresses you. You can bring your journal or just a sheet of paper. Divide the paper into three columns: My Worry; Why It Worries Me; Worst Thing That Could Happen. Once you confront the worst thing that could possibly happen – and realize that it's highly unlikely it ever will happen – you can get back to work with your worry load lightened.

☆ **Manage your e-mail.** With the increasingly massive number of e-mails sent each year, this electronic form of communication has become a major source of stress. A study by the University of Western Ontario found that managers spend more than an hour a day on e-mail, extending their working week by an average of 5 hours. The study also found that only 17 per cent of e-mail users can answer their e-mails in the same day. To cope:
● Read e-mails once, answer immediately, delete if possible or move them to folders. Overflowing inboxes are depressing and take too long to read and sort.
● Insert e-mail responses in the subject line whenever possible rather than composing a new message each time; reply only when you have something to say.
● Use the automatic signature function in your e-mail so that people can phone you or send you information via snail mail.
● Don't waste time acknowledging receipt of e-mail. Also, don't e-mail and phone with the same message.

Are you a **WORKAHOLIC?**

Sharon Lobel, PhD, professor of management at the Alber School of Business and Economics at Seattle University, has an interesting perspective on workaholism. Rather than saying that all workaholics have a problem, she divides them into two types: Happy Workaholics, who don't wish for a different lifestyle, and Unhappy Workaholics, who complain regularly.

"Happy Workaholics value work more than other aspects of life and arrange their lives accordingly," she says. "If people love to work and spend most of their waking hours at work, that's not a problem. On the other hand, if other people wish they had more time to devote to family, fitness or hobbies but are prevented from doing so because they work too many hours, those people are Unhappy Workaholics." So how can you tell which category you fit into?

"People who say they're working to 'advance in my job' or 'to buy a house' are probably not Unhappy Workaholics," says Lobel. "Unhappy Workaholics are likely to say their employer makes them work long hours and they're likely to express resentment towards the employer." So what do you do if you find you're in this latter category?

"I think everyone needs to ask themselves what really matters in their lives," says Lobel. "Which values are most important? Achievement, wealth, social justice, health, relationships? Then you need to look at how you're living your life. Do you devote time and energy towards what you most value? If the answer is yes, there isn't much of a problem. If the answer is no, it's time to implement some change."

● Don't insert the recipient's address first before composing the e-mail message. You might mistakenly send a message before it's finished or when it's saying something you didn't want it to say.
● Use the "rule of three": if you've gone back and forth three times on a topic and you're still confused or have questions, pick up the phone.
● Never send an e-mail if you're angry. You can write it (either as a draft, or preferably in your word-processing program) then save it and look over it when you feel calmer.

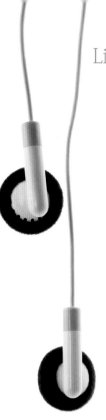

Listening to music in the office makes you more positive.

☎ **When things feel as if they're falling apart all around you, take 5 minutes and draw.** Seriously. Grab a pencil and some blank paper and sketch the chaos around you, or something funny, something peaceful or a caricature of the office villain. Using another part of your brain and focusing on something outside the chaos will provide a much-needed break.

☎ **Listen to music in your office.** A study by Sheffield University found that listening to music in an office-based working environment led to workers having a more positive mood, which they believe improved their overall work performance. One thing: it was important that the workers were able to choose the music themselves.

☎ **Talk to your best friend at work.** Studies find that social support at work is associated with lower blood pressure during the working day and smaller blood pressure surges even during work-related stressful moments.

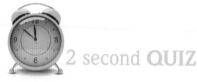

2 second QUIZ

Complain or keep quiet?
ANSWER: **COMPLAIN.**
Complain effectively, by being specific and positive, focusing on how correcting the problem will help the company and by providing at least one viable solution to the problem. Any sensible business wants to do things better. If your boss or company is so insecure or political that you can't speak honestly about things that need to be fixed, it's time to move on.

☎ **Rub a drop of lavender oil on your inner wrist.** The aroma of lavender (or cucumber oil) is a known relaxant. Close your eyes, hold your wrist up to your nose and sniff deeply, picturing as you do a field of lavender in Provence, the purple stalks waving in the breeze.

☎ **Leave the office for lunch every day.** Getting out of the office, away from the stress and into a totally different environment, clears your mind and helps you to put some perspective on whatever hassles are dogging your day.

☎ **Build rewards into your working week.** Having something to look forward to makes every difficult task more bearable. It might be a special dinner, a film, a game of tennis or a massage. Put it in your schedule wherever it will help the most and think of working hard in advance to get to that reward.

☎ **Eat three Brazil nuts.** They're an excellent source of selenium, a mineral that may help to prevent depression.

☎ **Munch on a handful of pumpkin seeds.** A useful source of iron and micronutrients, these taste delicious and are a healthy way of providing a distraction from stressful moments in the working day.

▐▐▐▶ **Eat peppermint chocolates.** Treat yourself now and again to some peppermint chocolate – particularly good if it's dark chocolate. The chocolate itself is stress relieving, the peppermint provides a burst of minty energy and the tiny sugar rush might be just enough to get you over the hump. At the very least, it's better than slamming your office door or reacting in otherwise self-defeating ways to a madness-filled workplace.

☎ **Pour a cup of boiling water over a handful of camomile leaves** or a camomile tea bag. The herbal mix, long known for its gentle, soothing properties, will help to de-stress and centre you.

☎ **Hold one nostril closed with a finger and blow strongly out** through the other (blow your nose first!). This is a yoga movement believed to reduce stress.

☎ **Walk and talk slower.** This tricks your body into thinking that things are calmer than they actually are.

☎ **Examine your real feelings.** If you love what you do, the stress related to your job will be far less damaging than if you don't. But if you hate your job, it's time to explore other options. Spending a few minutes each evening rewriting your CV and researching other job options or employers can help you to handle the stress at your current job.

☎ **Offer feedback.** As they say, it's better to give than to receive. Provide praise and recognition to others at work whenever it is appropriate. You will feel good by making others feel good, and the good feeling will tend to spread.

☎ **Have a "perspective reminder" handy.** Work may seem overwhelmingly stressful at times, but your troubles are likely to be smaller than they seem. Keep a picture in your office – the earth taken from space, a starry night or the ocean – and look at it whenever you feel overwhelmed. Amid countless stars and the timeless crashing of waves against the shore, how important is that deadline, really?

☎ **Plan ahead.** When work is challenging, devote some of your down time –

In PERSPECTIVE

Why is work so stressful?

There are lots of reasons. The experience is so widespread and affects so many workers in all sectors of the economy. Here is a list:

● **How tasks are designed.** Overloaded or too little work, too few or infrequent breaks, long working hours, shift work and hectic and routine tasks with little inherent meaning, can all cause stress.

● **Management style.** If your workplace (or manager) discourages worker participation in decision making, micro-manages, has poor communications skills, this is a potentially harmful environment.

● **Interpersonal relationships.** Do you get support and help from colleagues and supervisors? Do you feel that there is a threat of violence? Is there harassment?

● **Work roles.** If you have conflicting or uncertain job expectations, if too much is expected of you, if you feel that your skills are being wasted, you're working in a toxic waste dump when it comes to stress.

● **Career concerns.** Job insecurity, lack of opportunity for growth, advancement or promotion; rapid, unexpected changes; and continued rumours of layoffs and belt tightening can all land you with stress-related illness.

● **Environmental conditions.** Unpleasant or dangerous physical conditions such as crowding, noise or air pollution can turn any work environment into a stress pool.

weekends and evenings – to delineating a sequence of tasks. Make a list, place boxes next to each item and tick off the boxes as you move through the list (which is in itself very satisfying). You'll avoid forgetting anything, you'll stay focused on the job, you'll be more efficient and it's very satisfying to tick off those boxes.

☎ **Socialize your work.** Suggest a once-a-week lunch with colleagues where you can talk about a particular work issue. Use the collective brain to figure out how to do something better, improve your work facilities, perhaps, enhance productivity or improve relationships.

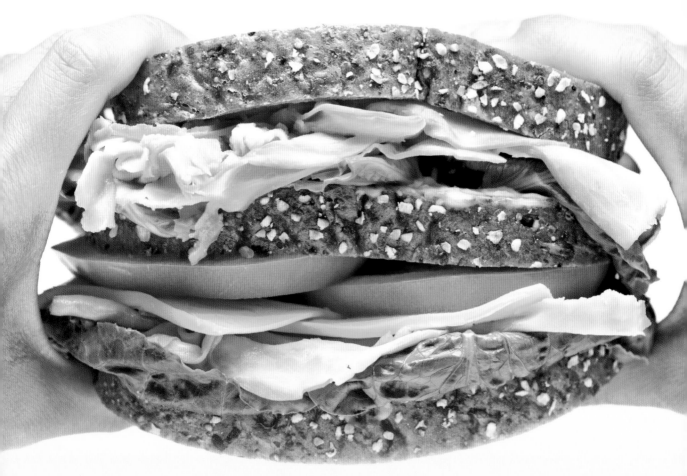

The **LUNCH** hour

For too many of us, the lunch break has become just another extension of our already overburdened day. Although the lunch hour was originally designed for just that – lunch – today we spend our time at midday running errands, pecking away at a computer keyboard or returning personal phone calls. When we do actually sit down to eat, it's often to consume whatever comfort food we can scrape together from the company vending machine or cafeteria. Yet your lunch hour offers the perfect time to break this hectic cycle. Rather than spending the time stressing over what you still need to accomplish or wolfing down fatty, salty, high-calorie foods, consider the following advice.

15 WAYS TO MAXIMIZE YOUR MIDDAY BREAK

☺ **Go outside.** If you work in an office or a retail establishment, you're likely to be stuck in the same building all day long. Now's your chance to escape. Soak up the sun, watch the rain or feel the wind. Breathe some real air and disconnect for a moment from the job. At least once every day you should make the time to step outside, even if just for 2 minutes. It will recharge your body and mind.

● **Daydream for 15 minutes – then eat, run errands or return to work.** Creative daydreaming is not only a way to get out of the daily lunch-hour grind, but it's also a way to put your creative juices to work. If you're feeling particularly stressed about a project, spend your quarter of an hour exploring ways you can tackle it. If you feel mentally stale and burned out, spend the 15 minutes in la-la land, on a mini vacation. Imagine yourself strolling along the beach, climbing a mountain or generally spending time in a location that makes you happy.

● **Nap for 10 to 15 minutes.** Studies increasingly show the value of short naps during the day, and progressive employers are becoming more lenient about them. So if you can, curl up under your desk, nod off in your car (unless you're driving!) or otherwise arrange yourself in your office chair so you can snooze without anyone noticing. Your nap will refresh your mind and put a whole new perspective on the afternoon, because it breaks the tension of the day.

● **Pack a frozen dinner.** They're not just for dinner. You can pop your meal into your break room microwave for a quick-and-easy lunch that allows plenty of time to run errands or power walk during the rest of your lunch hour. Today's frozen food aisles include organic, vegetarian,

low-fat, low-carbohydrate and numerous other healthy food options. Look for a frozen dinner that supplies fewer than 400 calories and less than 15 g total fat, 5 g saturated fat and 750 mg salt.

☆ **Practise the art of preparing a quick and healthy packed lunch.** Making your own lunch need not take a lot of time or creative energy. Include a source of lean protein, fruit or vegetables (raw carrots, celery, broccoli or cauliflower florets with a bit of low-fat salad dressing work well) and whole rather than processed grains. Leftovers from last night's dinner work wonders, as do the following quick-and-easy sandwich options:
● Peanut butter and banana sandwich: two slices of whole-wheat bread topped with 2 tablespoons of peanut butter and half a sliced banana.
● Chicken or tuna salad sandwich: 170 g of water-packed tuna or cooked chicken breast pieces mixed with 1 tablespoon of light mayonnaise and relish or grated carrots, served between two slices of whole-wheat bread.

Peanut butter and banana sandwiches – quick, easy and healthy.

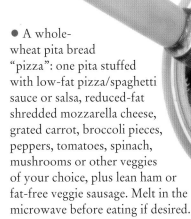

● A whole-wheat pita bread "pizza": one pita stuffed with low-fat pizza/spaghetti sauce or salsa, reduced-fat shredded mozzarella cheese, grated carrot, broccoli pieces, peppers, tomatoes, spinach, mushrooms or other veggies of your choice, plus lean ham or fat-free veggie sausage. Melt in the microwave before eating if desired.

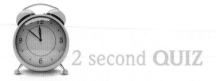

2 second QUIZ

Lunch or graze?
ANSWER: GRAZE.

Nibble food throughout the day, rather than having a large, formal lunch. Spreading out your calories stabilizes blood sugar and insulin levels, provides more frequent relief from stress, tension and boredom, and avoids the post-meal fatigue, because you don't have a big meal. Plus, you never get really hungry, and so are less likely to make the regrettable food choices that you might when you're starving. Best reason: all-day grazing frees up lunchtime for other things, such as a walk or catching up on work so you can get home a bit earlier and go for a walk then.

● Tortilla roll-up: 1 whole-wheat tortilla spread with 1 tablespoon of low-fat soft cheese, topped with 2 slices of lean ham or wafer-thin sliced turkey and various veggies such as chilis, lettuce or spinach, tomatoes, onion, cucumber, sprouts or grated carrots.

● Cheese and salad sandwich: 2 slices of whole-wheat bread spread with 1 tablespoon of light mayonnaise or mustard and filled with 1 slice of low or reduced-fat cheese, along with lettuce, sprouts and sliced avocado, tomatoes and peppers.

● **Pack ready-to-eat soup.** Your supermarket stocks numerous healthy soups sold in microwaveable cartons. One study suggests that broth-based soups help you to feel full, although they have few calories. Pack a bean and vegetable soup along with a piece of rye bread spread with low-fat soft cheese and a carton of juice. With this easy lunch you'll have put together all the protein and fibre you need to power your body and brain through the afternoon.

● **Get away from your desk – even if it's just for 15 minutes.** No matter how pressing that big project is, physically remove yourself from your office for at least 15 minutes. Walk the corridors, chat with a friend or, as mentioned before, go outside. The time away from the desk will refresh your mind, allowing you to return to work more invigorated.

▌▌▶ **Make better menu choices.** If you have arranged a business lunch or lunch in a restaurant with friends or colleagues, try to be the first to order. Studies show that we're often swayed by other people's choices, so be sure you forge ahead by picking healthy options (see page 116).

● **Don't be tempted by meal deals.** When buying lunch, especially from fast-food restaurants, don't be tempted by any "meal deal" unless it offers healthy options as part of the deal. Otherwise you may end up eating more than you actually want.

● **Create a sandwich chart and stick it on your fridge.** This prevents the early-morning haze from overcoming your better judgment and allowing you to leave the house without a packed lunch. In one category on your chart, list your bread options (whole-wheat bread, pita, tortilla wrap and so on). In the next column, list your protein options, such as turkey breast, low-fat cheese, lean roast beef, hummus or tuna/chicken salad. In another column, list vegetable toppings such as broccoli, bean sprouts, spinach, lettuce, cucumber slices, tomato slices, roasted red peppers and grated carrots. Finally, in the last column, list your condiments, ranging from mustard to low-fat mayonnaise to Italian dressing. You can also include a list of accompaniments such as cheese sticks, apples, oranges, yogourt, baby carrots, low-fat milk and ready-made soup. Then, every morning (or, even better, the night before) pick one item from each column to pack. Voilà! A quick, healthy lunch.

● **For a healthier lunch, eat a healthier breakfast.** Breakfasts composed of simple starches such as pastries, white breads or many popular breakfast cereals are quickly converted into sugar that floods your bloodstream then goes away quickly. This leaves you craving fatty, high-calorie foods at lunchtime. Far better is to eat healthier breakfast foods that are digested slowly and thus leave you feeling fuller for longer. These include whole grains and lean proteins.

● **Walk to the sandwich bar.** If you must eat out, walk to your destination. You'll burn some extra calories and refresh your mind at the same time. The short walk may also give you the will-power you need to order more healthily.

● **Improve your work performance with healthy food.** Studies have shown that serving healthy food options and replacing soft drink-filled vending machines with machines filled with juice and water leads to students behaving better and achieving more in the classroom. The students were found to pay more attention and to be better

able to focus on a task. And a report that linked temper tantrums and bad behaviour in younger children to artificial food additives, has advised parents to avoid foods containing these additives. So why not follow the lead and switch to healthy, natural lunches to find out what it can do for your mental outlook and motivation.

● **Exercise as you run errands.** If you need to run errands during your lunch break, get in some exercise at the same time. If possible, power walk to the bank, shops, post office, etc. The exercise will help to refresh your mind and reduce the stress of the day.

● **Start a lunch bunch group.** Eat with other colleagues who are interested in weight control, health and nutrition. Share foods for taste-testing, exchange tips and recipes and once a week ask each member to bring in one healthy contribution to the meal.

Reminder

 Fast results
These are tips that deliver benefits particularly quickly – in some cases, immediately.

 Easy gains
These are health boosters that offer the best value for the least amount of effort.

 Super-effective
This is advice that scientific research or widespread usage by experts has shown to be especially effective.

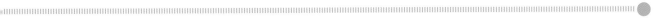

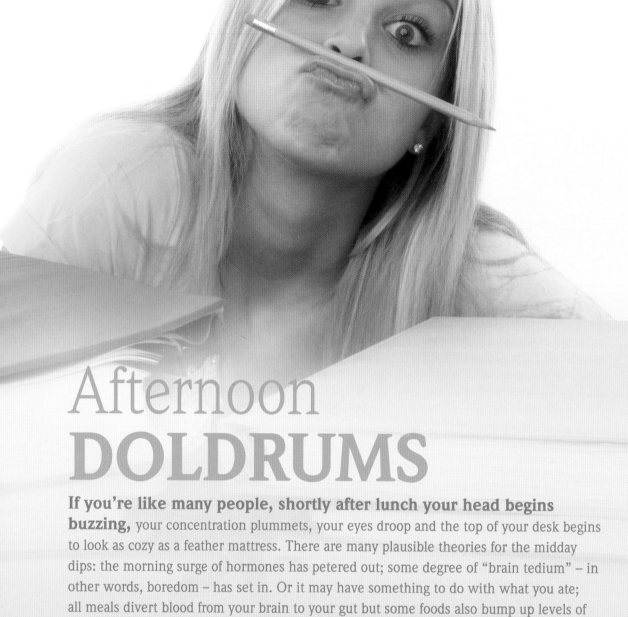

Afternoon
DOLDRUMS

If you're like many people, shortly after lunch your head begins buzzing, your concentration plummets, your eyes droop and the top of your desk begins to look as cozy as a feather mattress. There are many plausible theories for the midday dips: the morning surge of hormones has petered out; some degree of "brain tedium" – in other words, boredom – has set in. Or it may have something to do with what you ate; all meals divert blood from your brain to your gut but some foods also bump up levels of the soporific hormone serotonin. While the midday doldrums are common, they're not inevitable, especially not if you follow these tips.

20 IDEAS TO BOOST YOUR SPIRITS AND YOUR ENERGY

Before and during lunch...

● **Head outside and sit in the daylight for 10 minutes.** Better still, have your lunch outside and divide your break between eating and a walk. Here's why: your office probably has about 500 luxes of light, which is equal to about 500 candles. That compares with 10,000 luxes at sunrise and 100,000 at noon on a July day. So when the afternoon doldrums hit, go outside and sit in the sunlight. It will help reset your chronological clock, keep down the amount of melatonin (the sleep hormone) your body produces during this circadian dip and give you a valuable boost of beneficial vitamin D, reducing your risk of osteoporosis as well as various cancers.

● **Take a brief midmorning break for tea, coffee and/or a snack.** Use this time to relax and refocus, but, more importantly, to consume a few calories you might otherwise eat at lunchtime. Shrink the size of your lunch accordingly and the result will be less stupefying later.

☺ **Snack all day long.** Simply snack on nutritious foods whenever you get hungry, rather than eating lunch per se – but watch portion sizes. Then use your lunch break for some kind of exercise, whether it's in the company gym or walking around a park.

☆ **Choose activating protein not energy-sapping carbs.** So a tuna salad without the bread is a better choice than a tuna sandwich. A green salad sprinkled with low-fat cheese, a hard-boiled egg and some sliced turkey wins over a pasta salad. The change can really make a difference. When researchers compared men who ate a 1,000 calorie lunch with those who ate a 300 calorie lunch or skipped the meal altogether, they found that when given a chance to nap after lunch, nearly all of the participants did so. But while the lunch-eaters slept for an average of 90 minutes, those who skipped lunch slept for only 30 minutes. These were also high-carbohydrate lunches (carbs stimulate serotonin release, which increases sleepiness), which may have contributed to the napping. You shouldn't skip lunch altogether, but the combination of eating less and eating fewer carbohydrates should lead to less sleepiness.

After lunch...

● **Enjoy teatime.** Get into the routine of a midafternoon cup. It's a good step towards beating the afternoon doldrums thanks to that little bit of a caffeine burst and the few quiet minutes it entails. The aim is not to munch down scones and clotted cream, but you can do better than a tea bag dunked in your unwashed coffee mug. Keep a selection of exotic flavoured teas (preferably caffeinated) in your office and an aesthetically pleasing cup just for tea. When the doldrums hit, brew yourself a cup and sit somewhere quiet (not your office) to sip and reflect. The meditative time will soothe your frenzied brain, while the caffeine will give you just enough of a kick-start to get you through the rest of your day.

● **Clean your desk and clear out your e-mail inbox.** Both are relatively mindless tasks that don't require great amounts of concentration or clear thinking, and both will leave you feeling more energized because you'll have accomplished something visible as well as having reduced energy-sapping clutter.

A cup of afternoon tea hits the spot.

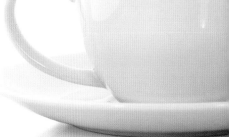

● **Make an "I was thinking of you" phone call.** To your wife, child, siblings, parents, a friend or a retired colleague. A 5 minute keep-in-touch call will lift your spirits for hours and reinvigorate you to get your work done.

● **Have an afternoon snack designed to get the blood flowing.** That doesn't mean a chocolate bar. The high glycemic index in the chocolate bar (a measure of how high it pushes up your blood sugar) might give you a temporary boost, but once that jolt of sugar is gone, you'll sink faster than the stock market after an interest-rate hike. Instead, you want a snack that combines protein, fibre and complex carbohydrates (such as whole-grain crackers or raw vegetables) to raise your blood sugar levels steadily and keep them up. So opt for snacks such as:

● Low-fat milk and high-fibre cereal. Milk provides the protein as well as valuable fluid (tiredness is an early sign of dehydration), while the high-fibre cereal will curtail any sudden blood sugar rushes.

● Peanut butter spread on whole-wheat crackers. Again, there's a good source of protein in peanut butter, a bit of healthy fat for staying power, coupled with the fibre and complex carbohydrates in the whole-wheat crackers.

● Cut-up vegetables dipped into hummus. These days, you can buy both these ingredients at just about any food shop. Eaten together, you get the high fibre, antioxidants and valuable vitamins of the vegetables, coupled with the fibre and protein of the hummus.

● Tomato or vegetable juice with a handful of unsalted nuts. The nuts provide a healthy dose of protein and monounsaturated fat, while the tomato juice provides not only the lycopene and other phytonutrients found in tomatoes, but energy-sustaining liquid as well.

● A piece of Edam or low-fat cheese and an apple. Portable, easy and a great pair. The cheese, with its fat and protein, cushions the fruit sugars from the apple, while the apple provides you with one all-important fruit serving for the day, along with a healthy dollop of antioxidants and fibre (be sure to eat the skin).

☆ **Go for a 10 minute walk and resist that chocolate bar.** When American researchers compared study participants who ate a chocolate bar or who walked briskly for 10 minutes, they found the chocolate bar subjects felt more tense in the hour afterwards, while those who walked not only had higher energy levels for 1 to 2 hours afterwards, but also reduced their tension.

● **Defer the work you most want to do to the time of day when you least feel like working.** Get through the routine work in the early morning so it's done, then stave off the midday doldrums with a task you really enjoy.

● **Drink a cup of caffeinated coffee or tea.** The caffeine will perk you up; studies also find it will enhance your memory and make you more productive on tasks requiring concentration.

● **Put a drop of peppermint oil in your hand and briskly rub** your hands together, then rub them over your face (avoid your eyes). Peppermint is a known energy-enhancing scent.

● **Roll your shoulders forwards, then backwards,** timing each roll with a deep breath in and out. Repeat for 2 minutes.

● **Consider a morsel of dark chocolate.** This is not a licence to overindulge, but dark chocolate does have some unique

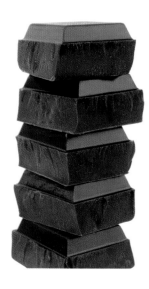

A small piece of dark chocolate is a healthy treat.

advantages. Unlike milk chocolate, it is truly a healthy food, closer to the category of nuts than candy, given the high levels of healthy fat and antioxidants it contains. Plus, it has abundant fibre and magnesium. Additionally, it provides a little caffeine, as well as a satisfyingly decadent feeling. But don't eat more than one square.

Chew some "spicy" gum. Chewing gums with strong minty flavours are stimulating, and the mere act of chewing is something of a tonic to a brain succumbing to lethargy. Plus, chewing stimulates saliva, which helps to clear out bacteria responsible for cavities and gum disease from lunch. Just be sure to choose sugar-free gum.

● **Plan group activities for midday.** If you often work on your own, try to organize work involving others at the time of day when your concentration might otherwise be waning. We are social animals, and interactions always rev us up. But make sure it's an interesting, interactive activity. Sitting in a room listening to someone else drone on and on will just send you snoozing.

● **Do your filing.** It's a physical activity that gets you up from your desk, bending and pulling and stretching. Plus, you can lose yourself in it, and any activity that enables you to get into a "flow" will help to pull you through the doldrums.

● **Take 10 minutes for isometric exercises.** Isometric exercises involve nothing more than tensing a muscle and holding it. For instance, with your arm held out, tense your biceps and triceps at the same time and hold for 5 to 10 seconds. You can do this with your calf muscles, thigh muscles (front and back), chest,

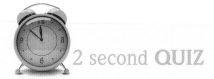

abdomen, buttocks, shoulders and back. If you wanted to, you could work a rotation, or cycle, of isometric exercises involving almost your entire body into your desk job every day. The total workout would be quite significant, despite never interrupting your work or causing you to break into a sweat. Plus, you're not only toning your body, you're toning your mind.

All day long...

● **Weave variety into your working day.** Tedium taxes the mind and induces somnolence. Most studies suggest that concentration on anything wanes after an hour, and is pretty near to pitiful at 90 minutes. So divide your tasks to maximize a balance between variety and productivity. For instance, if you have a large report you need to get out, work on it for 30 minutes, switch to something else for 30 minutes, then return to it.

● **Keep a rosemary plant in your office.** Not only will sharing your space with a live, growing thing provide its own mood boost, but studies find the scent of rosemary to be energizing. Whenever you need a boost, just rub a sprig between your fingers to release the fragrance into the air. Or, if you're really wiped out, rub a sprig on your hands, face and neck.

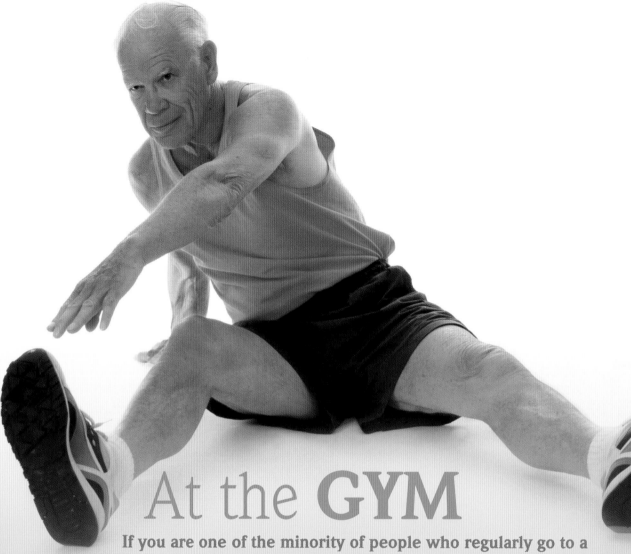

At the GYM

If you are one of the minority of people who regularly go to a gym for exercise, then congratulations! It means you have the right priorities and terrific discipline. But it's fair to say that at times, even for committed exercisers, motivation often flags, and there are days when it requires a Herculean effort just to put on your workout clothes and walk through the gym doors.

If you're lucky, the sights and sounds of exercise are all you need to motivate you to get moving. At other times, you still may not have the slightest urge to get started. For those days, this chapter is for you. Here are the easy ways to get the most out of your workout.

16 IDEAS FOR HEALTHIER, EASIER WORKOUTS

☆ **Avoid the mirrors.** Many fitness centres line exercise rooms with mirrors to allow you to watch your form as you work out. Yet a study of 58 women found that those who exercised in front of a mirror felt less calm and more fatigued after 30 minutes of working out than those who exercised without staring at their reflections. One exercise chain, Curves, deliberately designs its small gyms without mirrors so that women can concentrate on each other and the workout rather than on how they look. Other gyms are beginning to offer "reflection-free" zones. If yours doesn't, mention the idea – and the study – to the gym manager.

👟 **Try using aromatherapy oils known to enhance energy,** such as rosemary. Mix them with water and store them in a squirt bottle in your gym bag. Give your gym clothing a few squirts before leaving the dressing room so you can smell the oil as you work out. If you're in the middle of a more meditative, slower-paced workout, such as Pilates or yoga, try lavender oil instead of rosemary.

👟 **Create your own personal gym-mix tapes,** CDs or digital recordings, and listen to them as you work out. Researchers have found that people who listen to up-tempo music get significantly more out of their stationary bike workouts. They pedalled faster, produced more power and their hearts beat faster than when they listened to slow-tempo music or sounds with no tempo. Overall, they worked between 5 and 15 per cent harder while listening to the energizing beat. Although the type of music you choose is up to you, pick something with a fast beat that makes you want to start dancing. You can custom-design your own exercise music to burn to a CD or download to an MP3 player.

Pick your
VIDEO OR DVD wisely

In a study completed at McMaster University, exercise videos that featured super-skinny models with amazing muscles and revealing outfits made participants feel less confident about their fitness and less inclined to exercise in the future. Videos featuring an ultra-slender host surrounded by plumper, more normal-looking women reduced motivation even more. The researchers' hypothesis: seeing a thin instructor surrounded by fleshier participants intensified the participants' awareness of the thinness of the instructor.

To choose a motivating exercise DVD or class, look for a teacher you can trust, who has a fitness background and who must exercise to look great. In other words, DVDs created by personal trainers and exercise physiologists, or classes taught by them, will be more likely to motivate you than those hosted by supermodels and actresses.

👟 **Think of someone who irritates you.** Then step on the treadmill, exercise bike or elliptical machine and sweat out your aggression as you work out. You might even imagine that you are running an imaginary race against this person. You'll get a better workout – and blast away anger and stress at the same time.

☺ **Drink a bottle of water or juice on your way to the gym.** If you're already dehydrated, you'll feel overly fatigued during your session. When you're dehydrated, you can't work as hard, you don't feel as good and your mental function is compromised. So you won't get as much out of your workout.

👟 **Think you can and you will.** So simple, yet so often ignored, positive thinking can help you to power your way through a workout. In one study, exercisers who thought positively were more likely to stay active than those

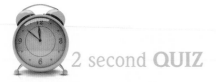

Free weights vs. machines
ANSWER: FREE WEIGHTS.

With free weights, you can always work both sides of your body separately, eliminating muscle imbalances. Only some machines allow that. Not only that, you don't need a degree in astrophysics to figure out how to operate them or adjust them to your size and strength. Also, gym machines are generally designed for a male body. If you are short and slight, your body may be too small for the machine, no matter how much you adjust it. Finally, dumbbells are inexpensive, small and nicely portable.

TV than when they were. Although TV may take your mind off your workout, it also causes you to lose touch with your effort level. You unconsciously slow down or use poor form as you get caught up in what's on screen.

Work out with a friend. If you're feeling stale and are thinking of skipping your gym workouts, ask a friend to meet you for a gym date. As you walk or run on the treadmill, you can share stories of your day and encourage each other to work a bit harder. Your friend can also help you to find the courage to approach unfamiliar gym equipment, as it's easier to laugh off your foibles when you have a trusted companion nearby.

whose minds often uttered those two evil words, "I can't." Whenever you find yourself making excuses, replace any negative thoughts with positive messages such as, "I feel great" or "Bring it on."

Turn off the TV when exercising. It's tempting to try to lose yourself in a TV program as you slog away. But one study found that women worked out about 5 per cent harder when they weren't watching

Wear the right shoes for the right class. Resist the urge to wear the old trainers you dug up from the back of the closet. Various fitness disciplines require specific types of footwear. The wrong shoes will not only make your workout feel harder, it could cause an injury. For example, wear running shoes for running, walking shoes for walking, and hard-bottomed cycling shoes for spinning (exercise on stationary bikes).

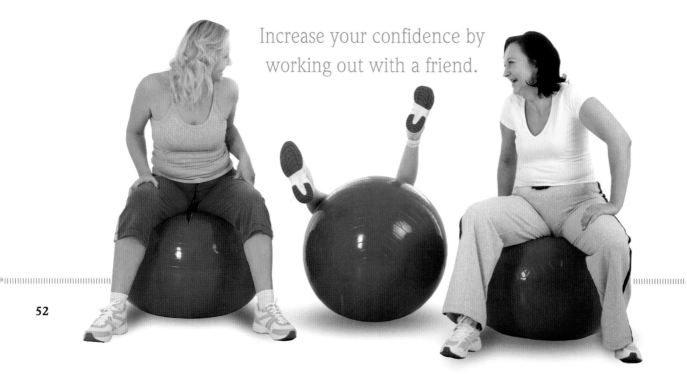

Increase your confidence by working out with a friend.

▐▶ **Set a short-term workout goal.** Of course, goals motivate you to work harder, and the best exercise programs include measurable goals to achieve weeks or months down the road. Sometimes, though, when your motivation is drooping, a goal focusing on what you can complete over the next 30 minutes is what you need. So pick something achievable: maintain a sweat for 20 minutes, give your arms a good workout or cover 4 kilometres on the treadmill. A target gives you focus to get through.

👟 **Whenever you feel as if you're out of steam,** hire a trainer. In just one session a trainer can open your eyes to a whole new world of workouts. (See "What to look for in a trainer," opposite.)

👟 **Work out during the least crowded hours.** You'll squeeze in a more effective workout in less time if you hit the gym during the slowest period of the day, often midafternoon. You won't have to wait in a line for equipment or feel hassled in the changing room.

☆ **Change your routine every three to four weeks.** This will keep your body guessing – improving your results – and fuel your motivation. In the weight room, alternate exercises and modify the way you lift weights. If you usually do two sets of 15 reps, complete one set of 15, then increase the weight for another set of 8 reps. On cardio equipment, switch from the treadmill to the stair stepper, etc. Mix up your exercise classes as well, switching around from Pilates to aerobic dance to yoga to kickboxing.

☺ **Slow down.** In one American study, participants who lifted slowly – taking at least 14 seconds to complete one repetition – gained more strength than participants

What to look for **IN A TRAINER**

Hiring a personal trainer keeps you accountable and helps you see results faster, even if you already know your way around a weight room. But be sure you know who you're hiring. To find the best trainer for you, follow these pointers:

● Check qualifications. Most personal trainers in Canada are certified by one or more accredited associations, such as Can-Fit-Pro or the American Council on Exercise (ACE). Ask prospective trainers for proof of certification – where it's from, and if it's up to date.

● What has the trainer done in the past 12 months to stay educated? Quality trainers hold professional memberships, read industry news and attend conferences or workshops.

● Do you need a specialist? Specialty areas include: weight loss for women, increased strength, sports performance, exercise rehabilitation, pre/post natal fitness and posture training.

who lifted at a rate of 7 seconds per rep. Slower lifting may help increase strength because it prevents you from using momentum or improper techniques.

👟 **Put your mind behind every move.** Rather than daydreaming through your workouts, put as much mental emphasis on what you do at the gym as you do at work – or at least should do! For example, when doing a strength exercise, feel the muscle contract as you lift. This will help you to tune into your technique.

👟 **Invent a competition with the person on the next treadmill.** If you're on the treadmill and you're bored, glance at the display on someone else's nearby treadmill. If you're walking at 5.5 kilometres per hour and he or she is chugging away at 6 km/h, see if you can increase your speed and catch up, as if it were a race. The other person won't even know you're racing.

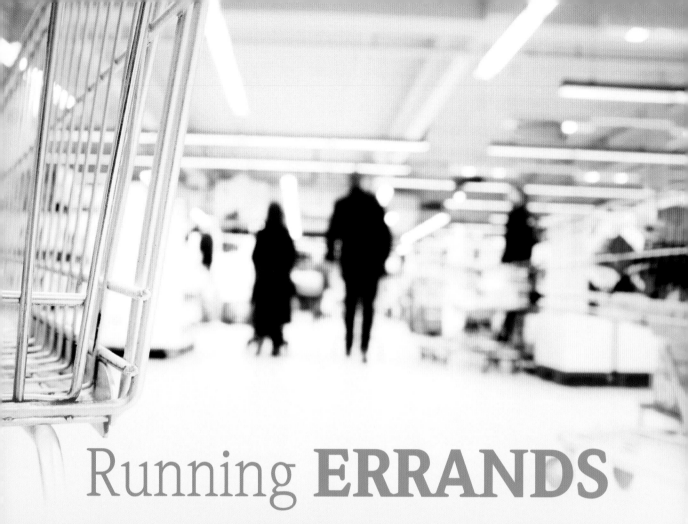

Running **ERRANDS**

Like death and taxes, there's no escaping having to run errands.
Supermarket, pharmacy, dry-cleaner, library, post office. Pick up, drop off, wait for children – or parents. If you're not careful, you can spend more than half of your leisure time in your car seat running errands.

So what does any of that have to do with health? Plenty. All of those errands stress you out and suck you dry of energy. They also eat up hours that would be better spent exercising, relaxing, cooking, having fun – the healthy stuff of life. So the goal here is to get you through your errands faster, easier and with less stress. Just be sure to use the time you gain wisely.

19 WAYS TO GET THINGS DONE QUICKER WHILE HAVING MORE FUN

▶ **Group your errands.** This is a golden rule: never run a single errand at a time. You'll save time, gasoline, energy and stress hormones by grouping your errands into batches. If you have to drop a child at a piano lesson, you can also go via the bank and deposit a cheque, pop into the supermarket for milk and bread or pick up the dry-cleaning.

☺ **Run your errands at quiet times.** In other words, not on the weekend (when the vast majority of people run their errands). Instead, make sure your dry-cleaner, bank, doctor, supermarket, etc., are near work so you can take care of these mundane tasks on your way into or out of work, or during your lunch hour. You'll avoid the packed stores and heavy traffic on the weekends, and have those two days just for you and your family. One of the best times to grocery shop? After dinner, when the children are in bed. One parent stays at home and one goes to the supermarket. You'll be in and out in half the time it takes with children in tow.

● **Create an errand centre in your house.** This is where library books that need to be returned, the dry-cleaning that needs to be dropped off, or the letters that need to be mailed, all live. Everything in one place (ideally near the door you use most often) will make it easier to run "bulk" errands. Another option: keep these things in your car, in the passenger seat. They'll be a visual reminder of all you need to do.

● **Keep an errand list with you at all times.** This includes both the ordinary errands that must be done (dry-cleaning, library, post office), but also those little things you keep forgetting (pick up socks for the six year old, make vet appointment for the dog, buy underwear for partner, find organic potting soil). Use a sturdy notebook that you carry with you at all times, and make sure the rest of your family knows where it is so they can add things to the list.

● **Buy in bulk.** The less often you have to go shopping for mundane items such as toilet paper, paper towels, dog food, cat litter, toothpaste, deodorant, tampons, etc., the less time you'll spend running errands. Storage space tight? Most of these items will fit under the bed quite nicely.

● **Always include a little fun.** List all the things you find joyful. Maybe it's reading a novel, writing in your diary or hitting a few golf balls on a spring afternoon. Now, plan to include one of these items in any extended errand run. Take a novel with you as you head to the post office; you can read it while in line. Carry your diary in your glove compartment – jot down a few lines as you're waiting for the car to be washed. Or ride your bike to the stores, then take a spin around a local park or nearby countryside.

● **Turn waiting time into you time.** Any time you're stuck in a line, shift the negative, glass-half-empty thinking ("I don't have time for this") into positive, glass-half-full thinking ("Ahhh! A few minutes of peace"). Close your eyes (yes, while you're standing there in line) and picture yourself in the most peaceful place you can imagine. It could be a desert at sunrise, the vast ocean (and you in a lone canoe) or the middle of a massage in a luxurious spa. Let your mind go and take several long, deep breaths. Now how do you feel?

Buy in bulk and you'll save precious time.

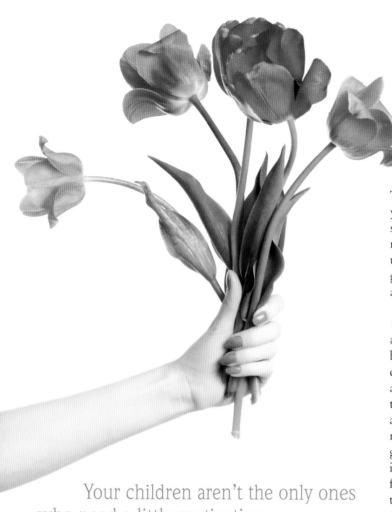

Your children aren't the only ones who need a little motivation ... buy yourself some flowers.

IIII➤ Use the Internet for as many errands as possible. These days, you can bank online, order office supplies, buy garden perennials, shop for shoes and do your grocery shopping online. The Internet, used sensibly, can save you hours of time and immeasurable stress. Worried about giving a credit card number over the Internet? If the website uses a secured server, then it is safer than giving your credit card over the phone and, in some cases, using it at a store.

● **Keep an "errand bag" in the car at all times.** This includes such things as bills that need to be paid, stationery and envelopes for writing letters (yes, letters!), a variety of greeting cards (birthdays, thank you, "just thinking of you"), pens, an envelope of coupons, your calendar, magazines that you haven't read and a good book. Then whenever you're sitting in a waiting room, stuck in traffic, waiting for a child's over-long hockey practice to end, you can also be completing other tasks on your list and/or catching up on your reading.

● **Keep a cooler and a basket in your trunk.** The cooler is to keep frozen and cold foods cold while you run errands; the basket is so you can carry parcels into the house without making umpteen trips.

● **Offer to run errands for an elderly neighbour or a mother with young children.** Studies find that helping others actually reduces our own stress hormones and makes us feel better.

☆ **Keep your grocery list on the computer.** Most weeks, you're buying the same things anyway; having a master list on your computer makes it easy to add and subtract items. Organize the list in the same order as the store you usually use. So, for instance, if the produce section is the first area you see, fruit and vegetables should be first on your list. Hit the print button and off you go!

● **Learn to run errands with your kids and not go crazy.** There are few things more stressful than being stuck in traffic with ice cream melting in the trunk and a two year old melting down in the back seat. But today you're more likely than ever to be running your errands with children in tow. To cope:
● Run your errands at the right time of day for the child. If you've got a toddler, that's morning, before naptime.

- Stock the car with snacks, juices and toys. Keep a cooler in the front with cold drinks and cut-up fruit that you can hand back to your toddler when he or she gets grumpy. Have stocks of toys that come out only when you're running errands.
- Keep an extra diaper bag in the car. Make sure the bag is stocked with diapers, wipes, a change of clothes and diaper cream.
- Combine errands for you with a treat for your child. It could be lunch out, an ice cream or a trip to the park.
- Play games while you're shopping. Give a school-age child a calculator and ask him or her to add up the cost of the groceries as you go along. Let pre-school children put non-breakable items into the shopping cart. Toddlers can pick the colour of the tissues you buy, and will enjoy a game of peekaboo as you go around the aisles.
- Bring the right carrying equipment for babies and infants: a backpack type of carrier, or a front sling, both of which leave your hands free.
- Play a thinking game with older children to keep them disciplined and you relaxed. A good game is "jotto." You each pick a word with five letters, no two the same, and have to guess the other's word by stating five-letter words and being told how many letters match. Keeping track in your head is challenging, but fun.

● **Pay attention as you run your errands.** That is, rein in your racing mind and focus solely on the task at hand. Start by walking slowly and deliberately to and from your car to the stores. As you shop, focus on the colours and shapes of the produce and the rich scents from the bakery. Notice each step, each movement you make. By living mindfully in the moment – even while picking out Brussels sprouts – you are performing what relaxation experts call walking meditation. Do errands this way and you'll find yourself far more calm and engaged and, at the end, less exhausted and frustrated.

☺ **Buy yourself a treat.** Your children aren't the only ones who need a little motivation during errand running. So make sure you add one more item to your list – something nice for you. It could be flowers, a scented bath soap, an imported brand of beer or a fancy cheese.

● **Keep several bottles of water in the freezer.** When it's time to run errands in the summer, grab one of them to take with you. You'll have plenty of icy-cold water to drink as you go along.

● **Listen to inspirational tapes or books on CD** in the car while running errands. It's a lot more relaxing than the commercials, the DJs and the overall intensity of everyday radio.

● **Alternate tasks with your neighbours or children's friends.** For instance, one week you do the grocery shopping for your neighbour; the next week, she does it for you. Or she watches your children while you do the errands for both families (or vice versa). Another option: do errands with a friend. Not only will you benefit from the social support, but your children might just be better behaved if there's another adult there.

● **If you're a dad, run errands with your child.** A University of California study has found that children who clean, cook and do household errands with their fathers are better behaved and have more friends. An added bonus: the wives of these men find them more sexually attractive.

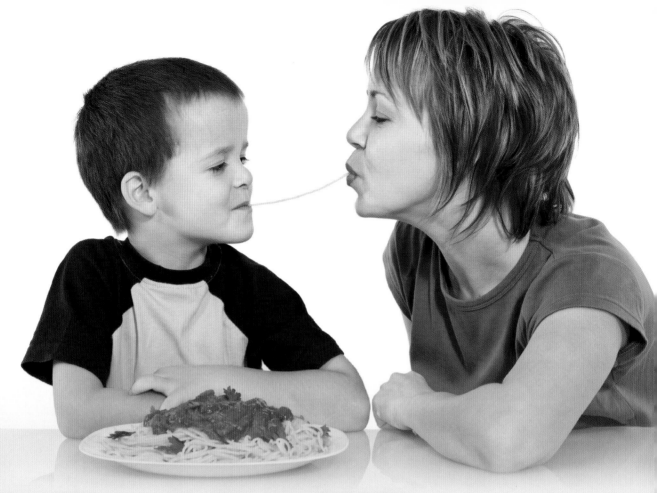

The **DINNER** routine

We're all busy. Whether it's working, caring for children, running errands, studying, volunteering or some combination of the above, we are all rushed off our feet. Too tired or unprepared to cook after 10 or 12 hours of perpetual busyness, we often take the easy path: a pizza or other takeout food, a frozen meal. Yet such pre-prepared dishes are filled with salt, sugar and fat. Then there's the shortage of vegetables, fibre and vitamins, not to mention the portion sizes – often huge. There is a better way. Here are simple, realistic, easy tips to get you eating healthily at dinner again.

24 WAYS TO MAKE SUPPER SUPREMELY HEALTHY

☺ **Keep your kitchen clean.** Families tend to congregate in the kitchen, bringing with them newspapers, mail, schoolbags, schoolwork, toys and a thousand other little things. Don't allow it. Set a new policy: the kitchen is for cooking and, if you have room, eating only. Why? It's hard to get motivated about cooking if you have to clean up a mess first, not to mention what it does to your mood. The opposite also holds true: a clean, bright, inviting kitchen can be a wonderful oasis after a day of craziness.

☞ **Speaking of which, make your kitchen a place you like to be.** Is there music playing? Do you have a glass of wine? Is the evening sun shining through the window? Are the knives sharp, the vegetables fresh, the pots good quality, the counters clutter-free? All of these contribute to your desire to make good food. If you don't enjoy being in your kitchen, do what you need to change that.

☆ **Plan a week's worth of dinners.** Many of us don't know what we're having for dinner as late as 4 p.m. in the afternoon. Yet planning ahead takes just a few minutes. Here's how to do it. Every Friday night or Saturday morning, sit down with a pad of paper and your favourite cookbooks or some cooking magazines. Think about what's in your freezer and fridge, what your family likes to eat, what your upcoming week entails. Then plan out a week's worth of menus (you can always leave one night for takeout pizzas). At the same time, write out your shopping list. Now stick the list of menus on the fridge or bulletin board so it's the first thing you see when you get home. Voilà! No more thinking ahead. If you need help or inspiration, consider an online meal planner, such as www.allrecipes.com.

Healthy INVESTMENT

A panini machine
Panini are sandwiches grilled in a machine that looks like an oversized sandwich toaster and that presses all the ingredients together. Panini machines are widely available and turn an ordinary sandwich into a real treat. Keep whole-grain bread on hand at all times (bread freezes well). When you can't think of what to have for dinner, serving panini with various grilled veggies works beautifully.

☞ **Enjoy the cooking process.** Of course, not everyone loves cooking. But there's no reason to not like doing it. If the thought of cooking fills you full of dread, you need an attitude adjustment. Cooking is a pleasure, far easier than many non-cooks realize. For the sake of your health, your pleasure and your wallet, you should learn – or relearn – the pleasures of cooking. Make it a project. Spend time with your friends and family while they cook so that you can absorb the methods and routines. Consider taking a class, or buy an introductory cookbook. Most of all, lose your fear. It is harder to be a bad cook than a good cook, particularly if you use good ingredients.

☞ **Delegate, delegate, delegate.** If you have children aged ten-plus or another adult who gets home before you do, get them started on dinner. For example, you might ask your partner to pick up ingredients on the way home, your teen to start chopping vegetables for the salad and fill the pasta pot with water, and your pre-teen to gather necessary ingredients for a given recipe and put them on the counter for you, preheat the oven and set the table. Yes, they may think of it as a chore, but if you build in a little opportunity for them to "create" (for example, with place cards for dinner,

Healthy INVESTMENT

The George Foreman grill

Although many kitchen appliances probably sit in a cupboard gathering dust, the George Foreman grill may become the one appliance that occupies a permanent spot on your kitchen counter. This device allows you to barbecue inside your house. The health bonus: a drip pan catches the grease, reducing the fat content of cooked meat, which also makes it easier to clean. One of these grills gives you the convenience of low-fat barbecuing during the winter months, when it's too cold to barbecue outdoors.

fancy napkin folding, their own recipes) it will make your children more interested in nutritious food and will encourage them to try new things.

Stock your freezer with homemade meals. Stews, soups and chili all freeze wonderfully. Work out how much of a one-pot meal you need to feed your family for one dinner, then buy plastic containers of that size. Make a pot of your family favourites on the weekend and you'll have four or five meals waiting in the freezer. A smart freezer is filled with plastic containers of several different homemade meals, each labelled with the contents and the date it was made.

Go the extra mile with freezer food. Side dishes also freeze well, particularly rices, pastas and breads. For space, put the right portion amount in freezer bags and squeeze out the air before sealing.

Base a meal on good-quality soup stock. Soup makes a great dinner. It's healthy, filling, delicious and easy to make. If you keep homemade chicken stock in the freezer, or cans of low-salt soup stock in the cupboard, it often takes just a few minutes to whip together an

impromptu vegetable soup. Use 4 cups (1 litre) of stock or low-salt chicken broth as the base. Then just toss in a variety of chopped veggies such as spinach, carrots, corn, peas, green beans and zucchini. Be sure to include lentils, chickpeas and other legumes. They provide excellent protein, lots of fibre, an array of micronutrients, and are filling and satisfying at a relatively low cost in calories. To round out the meal, have some whole-grain bread (dip it in olive oil rather than spreading it with butter) and a salad.

Or, make a pot of broth-based soup on Sundays, then start each meal during the week with a cup. Studies show watery foods such as soup tend to fill up the stomach, making you feel full quicker, despite being relatively low in calories. This also makes cooking the rest of the meal a little less demanding.

Invest in a slow cooker and/or a breadmaker. Imagine popping a few ingredients – chicken, a few vegetables, barley and stock – into a slow cooker before you leave the house in the morning and coming home to a satisfyingly healthy home-cooked meal. Or waking up to the delicious aroma of bread in the timed breadmaker. These gadgets can make life simpler and tastier.

Include three old standbys on your weekly menu. No one expects you to come up with a new meal every night. Pick three low-fuss, nutritious recipes that you and the family enjoy and, most importantly, that you can almost cook in your sleep. You might designate Monday as pasta or casserole night, Tuesday as grilled fish night and Wednesday as roasted chicken night. Include similar vegetable and grain side dishes as well. This eases

Soup is healthy, filling, delicious, cheap and easy to make.

the headache of grocery shopping – you'll need many of the same groceries from one week to the next.

⭐ **Plan which night you'll eat out – and stick to it.** Rather than eating out whenever you lack the inspiration – or groceries – to cook at home, eat out on a designated night. This makes eating out what it should be – a treat. You'll enjoy the restaurant more and eat more healthily throughout the week.

☞ **Try new recipes on weekends, when you have more time to cook.** You'll get more enjoyment from cooking if your mind feels rested and unfettered. Once you get the hang of a new recipe, you can incorporate it into your weeknight repertoire.

⭐ **Eat together as a family at least three times a week.** Children who eat dinner at the table with other family members are more likely to enjoy a healthy diet according to research by the National Family and Parenting Institute in the U.K. Shared family time, including mealtimes, may also hold the key to building successful relationships. Families that eat together are also likely to consume more fruit and vegetables and drink fewer soft drinks. Hold a family meeting and pick nights and times that work for everyone. Make eating together at the table non-negotiable.

☞ **Keep your shopping and recipe lists on the computer.** That way, you can just rotate your weekly menus (along with the shopping list) every month or every two months. Thus, once you have, say, eight weeks of menus, you're set for the rest of the year.

⭐ **Relax for 20 minutes before you eat.** If you skip breakfast, gorge through dinner, then snack until bedtime, you may have a condition known as night eating syndrome. People who eat more than 50 per cent of their calories after 6 p.m. tend to suffer from insomnia, gain weight more easily and feel more stressed than people who spread their food intake throughout the day. Try relaxation. In a study of 20 people with the syndrome, a once-daily progressive muscle relaxation session reduced stress, anxiety, fatigue, anger and depression within eight days. Participants also felt hungrier in the morning and less ravenous at night. Just sit in a chair or lie on your back. Then progressively tense and relax various muscles in your body, starting at the top of your head and moving down your body and ending at your feet. Tense as you inhale. Slowly release as you exhale. When you reach your toes, it's time to eat.

☞ **To eat less at dinner, keep your afternoon snack to a small portion.** When U.S. researchers offered study participants different-sized bags of potato chips as a midafternoon snack, participants ate the entire bag, regardless of size or calorie content. Those given smaller bags felt just as satisfied after their snack as those who ate twice as many chips from a larger bag. Even more compelling, participants who ate twice as many chips from the larger bags consumed an average of 150 calories more during dinner. If you need a midafternoon snack to get you through the day, serve up a small portion and make it high in protein and fibre (such as a piece of rye bread with low-fat cheese spread and an apple). Your body digests protein more slowly than carbohydrates, keeping your appetite under control for a longer period of time.

☞ **Turn off the television during dinner.** A study has found that the more television and videos students watched, the fewer fruits and vegetables they ate. Researchers theorize that television programs and commercials depict unhealthy foods, causing people to reach more often for soft drinks and chips rather than fruit and vegetables. A separate study found that watching television during dinner reduced fruit and vegetable consumption during the meal.

▐▐▐▶ **If your children won't eat what you put on their plate,** bite your tongue. Hassling children over their eating habits during dinner actually causes children – and their parents – to eat less well, according to one study. Both the children and their parents consumed more fat during meals when they argued over eating behaviour. The stress from the argument may have led to cravings for fatty comfort foods rather than an appetite for Brussels sprouts and spinach.

☞ **Instead of forcing kids to clean their plates, enforce a one-bite rule.** Encourage your children to take one bite out of all the foods on their plate. If, after one bite, they still don't want to eat their spinach or broccoli, let them push it aside. This technique encourages children to try new foods, but doesn't create a stressful eating experience. Also, involve young children in preparing foods you want them to try. A sense of ownership makes them bolder.

☞ **Avoid alcohol before your dinner.** In a study conducted at the University of Liverpool, men who drank a glass of beer 30 minutes before a meal ate more during the meal than men who had a nonalcoholic beverage. They also ate more fatty, salty foods and felt hungrier after the meal than men who didn't drink. Alcohol stimulates the appetite, so if you don't want to eat too much, avoid alcohol or enjoy one glass with your meal.

☞ **No ideas and need to lose a few pounds? Serve cereal.** This handy standby provides plenty of vitamins and minerals, together with some protein from the milk, and fibre, if you choose a high-fibre cereal. More importantly, it could help the entire family to lose weight. In one study, people who ate a bowl of cereal instead of lunch or dinner consumed on average 640 calories less a day and lost an average of 4 lb (just under 2 kg) of fat in two weeks. Or make up a great big bowl of granola for the whole family, mixing cut-up fruit with low-fat granola cereal with or without nuts, fat-free plain yogourt and honey.

☞ **Have breakfast for dinner.** A great "breakfast" option for dinner is an omelette. It's quick and easy to make, a good protein source and relatively low in calories. Fill it with veggies instead of cheese, and you have a complete meal in a frying pan.

☞ **Use parts of last night's dinner for tonight's meal.** This allows you to cook once and eat twice. For example, if you have roasted chicken one night, use the leftovers to serve up chicken fajitas or chicken salad the next. Prepare all key protein foods – chicken, turkey, fish, etc. – in larger-than-needed amounts so they will last two nights instead of one. Do the same with rice and other grain-based side dishes. Serve as a side dish one night and use the leftovers to make a casserole, stir-fry or soup the next.

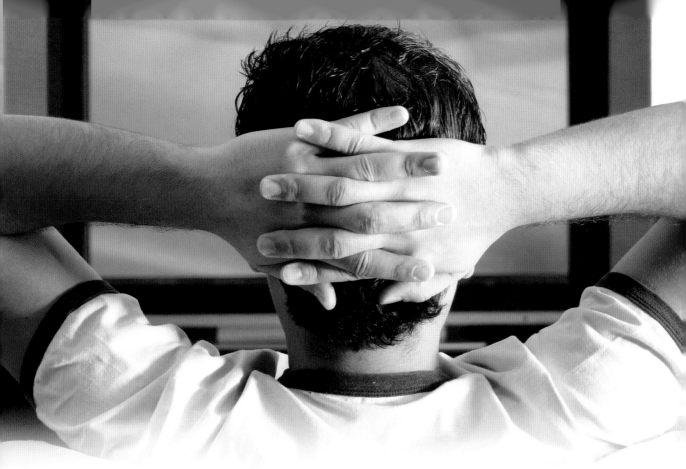

The **AFTER-DINNER** routine

Dinner is finished, the dishes are done and you're looking at a lovely 3 hours ahead of you before your body begins sending go-to-sleep signals. You could sit in front of the TV, as so many people do these days. Or you could choose to do one of the following and sneak a little health into your evening. This section starts off with pleasure-based ideas, then shifts into more practical ways to spend your evening time.

24 IDEAS FOR HEALTHIER, MORE PLEASURABLE EVENINGS

☺ **Go for an after-dinner walk.** What better time for a hand-in-hand stroll through the neighbourhood? To make it interesting, play a game of learning two new things about your neighbours on each walk, either through observation or conversation. It could be that the Smiths have painted their living room red (something you spot through the window), or that Mrs. Walker has a new car. Playing this kind of game on your walk will make it go quicker and keep it more interesting. The best bonus: the health-promoting effects of the walk.

● **Play a game with your partner or children.** Try a board game, work on a puzzle or opt for a rousing game of cards. Not only will it keep the television off, but it will make those brain cells work a lot harder. And the social bonding with your loved ones contributes mightily to emotional and physical health. Stumped for choices? Go back in time to when you were a teenager – try games such as backgammon, dominoes, checkers or chess. Crossword puzzles are great fun, as

are visual, number and logic puzzles. Do you have a dartboard, pool table or table-tennis table? Wear them out.

● **Go up to your partner, put your arms around his/her waist,** and begin kissing the back of his/her neck. Hopefully, this will lead to something more. In addition to the obvious benefits of sex, you'll also be raising your heart rate, sending immune-boosting endorphins to your brain and extending your life. One study found that sexually active men lived longer than those who made love less often. The study covered men, but it is likely to apply to women too.

● **Do something totally mindless for 30 minutes.** It could be watching the most mind-numbing program you can find on TV, holding a computer solitaire tournament with yourself, soaking in a steamy, scented bath or just lying on the couch listening to a favourite piece of music and staring at the ceiling. The idea

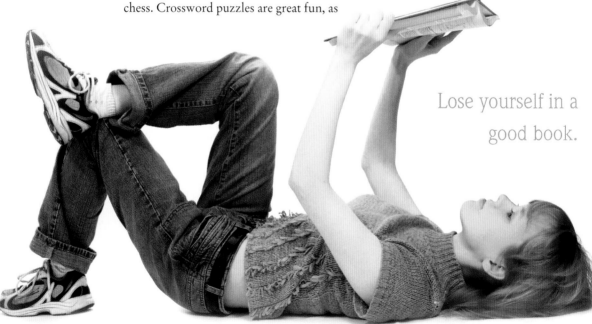

Lose yourself in a good book.

here is that your mind is disengaged; it is not focused on anything, but is allowed to run free in a kind of "active meditation."

⭐ **Slowly sip a glass of really good wine once in a while.** The definition of "really good wine" depends on your tastes. If you're used to boxed wine, then a $20 bottle of merlot is just the ticket. If you're a moderate oenophile, you might reach for a $40 bottle of Bordeaux. The idea is that you savour this one glass. While you're identifying the flavours and the elements in the bouquet, the wine, if it's red, will be providing significant heart-healthy antioxidants, shown to reduce your risk of heart disease.

● **Get lost in a book.** Or a magazine or a newspaper. Rekindle your love of reading. It's so much more rewarding for you than watching television. And it's much healthier, because it keeps your brain highly active and engaged.

⭐ **Savour a piece of dark gourmet chocolate.** Gram for gram, chocolate contains more healthy antioxidants, which repair damage to cells and prevent cholesterol from oxidizing (making it stickier), than any of the other antioxidant champions, including tea, blueberries and grape juice. Plus, it's well known for its ability to soothe a troubled mind. It takes only one piece to provide the perfect post-dinner sweetness we often crave. Keep the chocolate dark – it has the most antioxidants – and plain. You don't need the extra sugar and calories from caramel and other goodies.

● **On a dark, clear night, go outside and lie down in your backyard** and stare at the stars. Feel the immensity of the world as you view the heavens. Think about any problems you've been wrestling with and put them into context with the trillions of stars that are up there. If you find you enjoy this, consider learning about the stars with a star atlas. Or take a walk when the moon is full. The magic and mysticism of a moonlit night will energize you and provide an unexpected burst of positive thinking.

● **Go to sleep at 8 p.m.** Many of us are sleep-deprived. So every now and again, pretend you're six years old, put on flannel pyjamas, get into bed at 8 p.m. and turn off the light.

● **Give yourself a pedicure.** Fill a basin with warm water and a few drops of peppermint oil. Soak your feet in it until the water cools, then pumice away the rough skin on your soles. Massage a scented lotion all over your feet, inhaling the lovely scent and feeling your skin soften with every stroke. Trim your toenails, push back your cuticles and, if you desire, polish your toenails in a colour you'd never dare wear on your fingernails. If you can, convince your partner to give you a foot massage.

● **Ask your partner, or even an older child or a friend, to wash your hair.** Having your hair washed and your scalp massaged is an unexpected luxury that will help wash away the stress of the day.

● **Put a CD (whatever music you like dancing to)** on the stereo and dance for 20 minutes. Jazz and cheek-to-cheek dancing not your thing? Fine, slip some high-energy rock music into the CD and pretend you're in a mosh pit. Either way, you'll get 20 minutes of physical activity and, if you're doing the mosh pit thing, you'll burn as many calories as if you were jogging. An added bonus: improved coordination and, if you do a lot of dips, some good stretches. Plus, this is a great way for younger parents to engage their kids in physical activity – the whole family can let themselves go, dancing energetically until just one is left standing.

☺ **Make a yogourt smoothie for dessert.** Toss a frozen banana, 175 g of plain or vanilla yogourt, a handful of blueberries and a teaspoon of honey into the blender along with some crushed ice. Blend the mixture until it is thick and smooth. The combination of the antioxidants in the blueberries, the potassium in the banana and the live bacteria in the yogourt will give you a health boost that no vitamin can match. Specific conditions you have just helped to protect yourself against: urinary tract infection (blueberries), high blood pressure (banana) and yeast infection or irritable bowel syndrome (yogourt).

● **Sip a cup of camomile or mint tea.** The camomile will help you to sleep and the mint will aid your digestion.

● **Set a timer and write your journal for 10 minutes.** Many people don't want to keep a journal because they can't stand the sense of responsibility it brings to write in it every night. But if you know

you have only 10 minutes, suddenly what seemed like a chore takes less time than washing the dishes. Not sure what to write? Just try listing what you did that day. Write down five things that made you smile. List five things that made you angry – and why. Numerous studies attest to the stress-busting power of regular journal writing. Plus, it's fun to leaf back through your journal and see what you were doing a year before.

● **Express yourself.** Go one better than a journal: compose a letter to a friend, write some e-mails or a missive to your MP or write a short story. Writing is wonderful brain activity, and who doesn't benefit from learning how to express themselves better?

● **Write down your entire to-do list for the next day.** It takes 5 minutes, yet the peace of mind it brings is priceless. Instead of running a to-do list over and over in your mind – making your responsibilities morph into gargantuan proportions – you can enjoy the rest of your evening and have a better shot at sleeping.

● **Play with your dog or cat for 15 minutes.** Studies show significant stress-reduction benefits from pets, particularly those that, like dogs and cats, can interact with you. Looking for ideas? Find an old sock and get your dog to try to pull it out of your hand. Teach your cat to "fetch" by tossing a crumpled piece of paper. Hide treats around the house and watch your dog or cat go on a treasure hunt. Don't have a pet? Get one!

▐▐▐▶ **Pack your (or your children's) lunch for tomorrow,** and also lay out your clothes, check your briefcase and make sure the children's school stuff is by the front door. The health benefits

Interact with your pet and your stress will melt away.

are clear: this will avoid the surge in stress hormones the following morning that comes from rushing around like a stockbroker on Black Monday while screaming at the children, ripping your tights and spilling juice on your silk shirt.

 Once a week, hold a "chore-free" night. Order pizza and eat on paper plates, leave dishes unwashed, forget the laundry, don't even wipe the counter. Arrange lifts for the children to hockey practice or piano. This is your night to be as lazy (or productive in other ways) as you like. Maybe you have a hobby that you never seem to have the time to get to. This is your night for you. Don't let anything – especially your guilt – get in the way. If your life is too hectic to pull it off once a week, make it every other week or once a month. But make it some time.

● **Have a cooking fest.** Tonight, cook meals for the next two weeks to stock up your freezer. Try easy-to-double recipes such as lasagne or meatballs (use turkey to reduce the heart-clogging saturated fat) or lentil or eggplant casserole.

● **Change into pyjamas and slippers early in the evening.** Even before dinner. It will help separate the "daytime you" from the "evening you," and be a reminder throughout the evening to relax.

Healthy INVESTMENT

A journal
Don't think of journals as a private place for teenage girls to write about their newest crushes. Every single adult – be it man or woman – can benefit from having a good-quality notebook to record observations, thoughts, opinions and reminders. At the front or the back of the journal, set aside pages for lists of books to read, music to buy, restaurants to try, even friends to call. While shopping for a journal, buy a nice pen to go with it. Keep them by your bedside so they're always ready for you at bedtime (and in the morning, when dreams and ideas are fresh). Don't feel compelled to write every night, but remember: the more you write, the more you'll want to write in the future. You'll probably find that a private journal is an outstanding way to defuse stress, clear your mind and organize your thoughts.

 Clean out one closet in your house. This chore takes no more than 30 minutes, and leaves you with a sense of accomplishment, yet without any added stress because the task is simple and unchallenging, yet satisfying.

● **Do your weekend shopping and chores.** Why buy your groceries or go clothes shopping when everyone else is doing it? Make Saturday a fun day, not an errand and shopping day. The stores are much emptier and shopping is less stressful on weekday evenings.

Reminder

➤ Fast results
These are tips that deliver benefits particularly quickly – in some cases, immediately.

☺ Easy gains
These are health boosters that offer the best value for the least amount of effort.

☆ Super-effective
This is advice that scientific research or widespread usage by experts has shown to be especially effective.

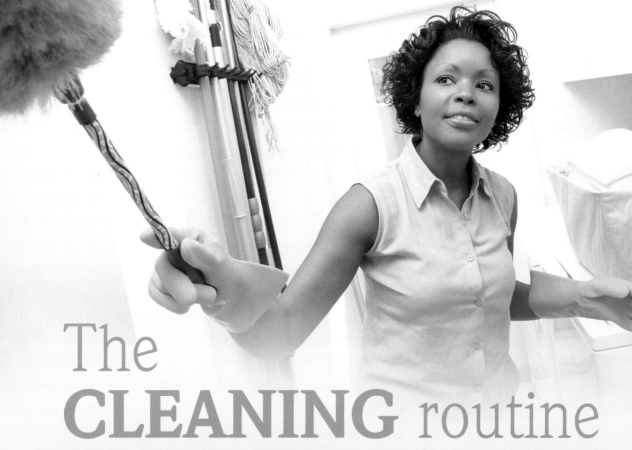

The
CLEANING routine

You may not realize it, but your house is hazardous to your health. Insect droppings, dust mites, bacteria-laden sponges, spoiled food – all can contribute to a plethora of health problems ranging from allergies and asthma to gastrointestinal upsets. In fact, an American germ guru, Charles P. Gerba, professor of microbiology at the University of Arizona, says you're more likely to get sick at home than nearly anywhere else in your life (except maybe hospitals). What's scarier is that the cure for a dirty home can be worse than the problem as we attack germs with more and more toxic chemicals. Many cleaning products contain volatile organic compounds (VOCs), which can cause eye, nose and lung irritation, as well as rashes, headaches, nausea, asthma and, in some cases, cancer. There is a solution. Here's what the leading "green" cleaners recommend.

12 TIPS FOR HEALTH-FRIENDLY CLEANING

● **Clean in an organized manner.**
There's no point in mopping the floor
only to dust the ceiling fan next and
deposit a grey film over everything again.
To clean well – and that means to clean
healthily – you need to clean efficiently,
avoiding going back and forth around a
room. Instead, work using a systematic
approach. Think in terms of left to right,
top to bottom. Begin with ceilings and
walls, and work your way down to
windows and furniture, finishing with
the floors.

✩ **Clean the things you'd never think
to clean.** For instance, your mattress is
a magnet for allergy-causing dust mites.
Washing the mattress cover in very hot
water (60°C or more) every month, and
wiping down the top of the mattress with
hot water, can go a long way towards
reducing morning stuffiness. Other areas
often ignored:
● Indoor garbage cans. Particularly those
in the kitchen and bathroom. Emptying
them isn't the same as cleaning them.
Scrub them regularly to make sure germs
aren't germinating.
● Shower curtains. They get wet most
days, and they often stay wet, making
them a perfect home for mould.
● Automatic dishwashers. Take a close
look at the edges of the door on your
dishwasher. Many are breeding grounds
for mould and mildew. The same is true
of the rubber cushioning that surrounds
some fridge doors.
● The fireplace. A clogged chimney is not
only unhealthy, it can kill you if it ignites
or, in the case of a gas fireplace, becomes
blocked, sending dangerous carbon
monoxide fumes into the house.
● HVAC filters. These filters are
designed to filter out allergy-causing
dust from the air, but if they're clogged,
they're more harmful than helpful.

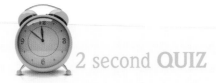

2 second QUIZ

Vinegar or bleach?
ANSWER: VINEGAR.
Health-conscious cleaners consider vinegar their
number one ally. Studies find a straight 5 per cent
solution of vinegar kills 99 per cent of bacteria,
82 per cent of mould and 80 per cent of viruses.
Chlorine bleach does a great job too, but it is
irritating to the lungs and eyes and contains
trace amounts of organochlorines – extremely
persistent and toxic chemical compounds known
to cause cancer in animals, among other serious
health problems.

● **Dust with worn-out wool socks or a
corner of an old wool blanket** or sweater.
Wool creates static when rubbed on a
surface. One wipe can keep your furniture
dust-free without polish or spray.

● **Polish silver with toothpaste.**
Some silver polishes contain petroleum
distillates, ammonia or other hazardous
ingredients. Instead, dab on toothpaste
with your finger or rub it on with a cloth.
Rinse with warm water and polish with a
soft cloth. For larger trays and bowls, use
a paste made of baking soda mixed with
water on a wet sponge.

✩ **Clean your drains the non-toxic
way.** Chemical drain cleaners (also called
drain openers) are extremely corrosive
and dangerous, containing such toxic
ingredients as lye or sulphuric acid. Even
the vapours are harmful. Instead, pour a
pot of boiling water or toss a handful of
baking soda followed by $^1/_2$ cup
(125 ml) of vinegar down the drain
weekly. Also effective, particularly in
preventing blockages, are many brands of
enzymatic cleaners found in pet stores.

Shopping list for
HEALTHY CLEANING

You can get just about everything you need for healthy cleaning at the supermarket, mostly avoiding the commercial cleaning aisle. Here's a shopping list:

- 4 litres of white vinegar
- 1 bottle of rubbing alcohol
- 1 large box of baking soda
- 4 litres of distilled water
- An oxygen-based cleaner, such as OxiClean
- Dishwashing detergent
- An enzymatic cleaner (found at most pet stores or in the pet products aisle)
- Foaming shaving cream
- Hydrogen peroxide (available from pharmacies)

Also pick up three or four spray bottles. Use each bottle for the make-your-own cleaning products listed throughout.

● **Clean windows the easy way.** Try this homemade solution: add 5 Tbsp (80 ml) of distilled white vinegar and a spoonful of dishwasher detergent to 1 litre of distilled water. And try these tips:
  - Use a sponge wand to soak the window in suds, rather than a spray bottle. Wet the windows thoroughly and let the solution do its work for about 5 minutes.
  - Avoid cleaning your windows in bright sunlight. The sun dries the solution too quickly, which can cause streaks.
  - Use a black rubber squeegee to dry the window. Make sure every iota of water comes off, or you're leaving dirt on the window.
  - For serious dirt, try an oversized razor blade and wet it with soapy water.

● **Sanitize your toilet bowl safely.** Pity germ guru Charles Gerba. He spends his days swiping cotton swabs over every conceivable household surface, then peering at the results under a microscope, identifying germs and other unpleasant things he finds there. You can only imagine what he finds in the bathroom.
  - To clean the toilet safely, turn to vinegar. Fill a spray bottle with straight white vinegar. Pour a capful into the toilet, then spray the sides of the bowl. Also, sprinkle baking soda in the toilet, wait 15 minutes, and scrub with a bit of baking soda sprinkled on the brush. Once a month pour 1 cup (250 ml) of vinegar into the toilet and leave it overnight. The vinegar dissolves any alkali build-up and prevents hard-water rings in the toilet. Whenever you go on vacation, pour 1 cup (250 ml) of vinegar into the toilet to prevent build-up while you're gone.
  - To disinfect the toilet completely, wipe all surfaces with a cloth soaked in rubbing alcohol or with some of the alcohol-based hand cleaner available in stores.

● **Clean your kitchen floor the easy way.** Don't try to disinfect it. Unless you disinfect your feet, there's no point. Instead, use these homemade cleaners:
  - Hardwood and laminated floors: add 4 Tbsp (60 ml) of white vinegar per litre of water. Use only 100 per cent cotton terry towels on hardwood floors and don't use self-wringing or microfibre mops. Microfibre is made from 80 to 85 per cent polyester, which is plastic. Plastic will eventually scratch the sealant off the floor.
  - Marble, tile and granite: just use very hot water. Cleaners of any kind will pit these.
  - Linoleum floors: use hot water with just a bit of liquid soap if needed.

You'd think your washing machine would be clean. It's not the case.

☺ **Clean out your washing machine and dryer.** You'd think they would be clean, right? Wrong. In a study of 50 homes, Gerba found high levels of coliform bacteria, an indicator of unsanitary conditions, and diarrhea-causing *Escherichia coli* in home washing machines. When researchers washed sterile cloths in non-bleach laundry detergent, they found that 40 per cent emerged contaminated with *E. coli* bacteria – with enough extra to contaminate the next load. The greatest risk from the germs comes when transferring wet laundry with your bare hands to the dryer. Try using rubber gloves when doing your wash, and add 1 cup (250 ml) of hydrogen peroxide to your loads instead of bleach.

▐▐▐▶ **Disinfect your chopping board.** In his research, Gerba found 200 times more fecal bacteria on the average chopping board in the home than on the toilet seat. To get it clean, run it through the dishwasher or spray it with straight 5 per cent vinegar and let it set overnight. Alternatively, microwave on high for 30 seconds or swab it with alcohol.

● **Microwave your kitchen sponges for 30 seconds every day.** Gerba found that the common household sponge may contain 320 million opportunistic bacterial pathogens, enough of which could be transferred from the sponge to your eyes or mouth to make you sick.

● **Make your own.** Keeping a box of borax around for extra-tough cleaning jobs is a good start. Borax is a natural product made of sodium, boron, oxygen and water and it's unbeatable for tough cleaning jobs, as a bleach substitute, or mixed with water for a disinfectant. Gerba suggests rubbing alcohol as

Spot the **BAD STUFF**

Just as important as seeking out healthy cleaning products is avoiding unhealthy ones, those that are highly toxic to the environment, human health or both. The American non-profit organization Green Seal and other experts say to watch out for the following:

● **Corrosives.** Avoid products labelled: "Danger. Corrosive." Corrosives include some of the most dangerous chemicals in the home, such as lye, hydrochloric acid, phosphoric acid and sulphuric acid – the active agents in many drain cleaners, oven cleaners and toilet cleaners. These can burn the skin, cause internal burns if ingested and explode if used incorrectly.

● **Ammonia.** Many home recipes and commercial products contain ammonia, but it is a strong eye and lung irritant and should be avoided by anyone with asthma or other lung sensitivities.

● **Bleach.** For the reasons noted elsewhere, but primarily for its toxic fumes.

● **Phosphates.** Phosphates are naturally occurring minerals used in automatic dishwashing detergents as a water softener. When released back into the environment, phosphates can cause algae blooms in lakes and ponds that kill aquatic life. Try a homemade recipe of half borax and half washing soda.

● **Petroleum.** Many cleaning agents are refined petroleum products linked with health problems. A few to avoid: diethylene glycol, nonylphenol ethoxylate, butyl cellosolve.

another good natural disinfectant. Just don't light any matches. Here are some more homemade, environmentally and health-friendly products.

● Furniture polish. Mix olive oil and vinegar together for an excellent cleaner and polish.

● Mildew remover. Mix equal parts of water and hydrogen peroxide (20 per cent strength).

● Laundry whitener. Use hydrogen peroxide rather than bleach. Soak your dingy white clothes for 30 minutes in the washer with $1/2$ cup (125 ml) of 20 per cent peroxide, then launder as usual. This removes the greying that is caused by chlorine bleach.

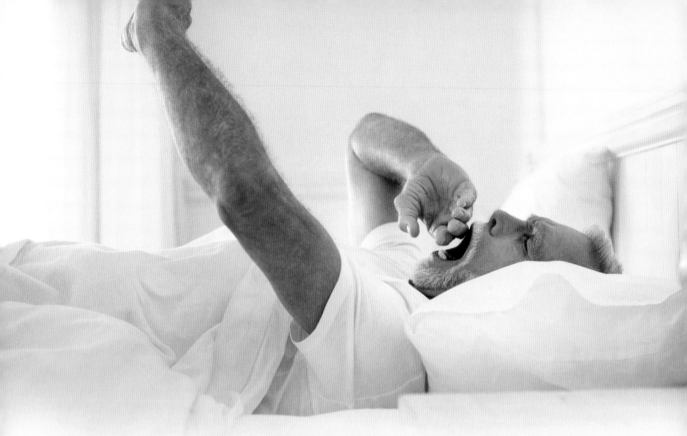

The **SLEEP** routine

Blessed sleep – the holy grail of health. Did you know that some researchers believe a chronic lack of sleep may lead to insulin resistance, a risk factor for diabetes? That's just for starters. Sleep deprivation can also alter your levels of thyroid and stress hormones, potentially affecting everything from your memory to your immune system, heart and metabolism. Of course, lack of sleep can kill you instantly. Studies from around the world show that a significant number of all road and highway accidents are sleep-related, costing billions of dollars in damage and lost workdays – and lives. A good night's sleep is one of the best things for your health, so pick three of these tips to follow each night until you get all that you need.

20 WAYS TO ACHIEVE A DEEP, UNINTERRUPTED SLEEP

☺ **Create a transition routine.** This is something you do every night before bed. It could be as simple as letting the cat out, turning off the lights, turning down the heat, washing your face and brushing your teeth. Or it could be a series of yoga or meditation exercises. Regardless, it should be consistent. As you begin to move into your "nightly routine," your mind will get the signal that it's time to chill out, physiologically preparing you for sleep.

ᶻZ **Figure out your body cycle.** Do you ever find that you get really sleepy at 10 p.m., that the sleepiness passes, and that by the time the late news comes on, you're wide awake? Some experts believe sleepiness comes in cycles. Push past a period of tiredness and you probably won't be able to fall asleep very easily for a while. If you've noticed these kinds of rhythms in your own body clock, use them to your advantage. When sleepiness comes, get to bed. Otherwise, it might be a long time until you're ready for sleep again.

ᶻZ **Sprinkle just-washed sheets and pillowcases with lavender water** and iron them before making up your bed. The scent is scientifically proven to promote relaxation, and the repetition and mindlessness of ironing will soothe you. Or put lavender water in a perfume atomizer and spray above your bed just before climbing in.

ᶻZ **Hide your clock under your bed** or on the bottom shelf of your bedside nightstand, where its glow won't disturb you. That way, if you do wake up in the middle of the night or have problems sleeping, you won't fret over how late it is and how much sleep you're missing.

ᶻZ **Change your pillow.** If you're constantly pounding it, turning it over and upside down, the poor pillow deserves a break. Find a fresh new pillow from the linen closet, put a sweet-smelling case on it and try again.

ᶻZ **Pyjamas or naked?** The answer is pyjamas. Warm skin helps to slow down your blood's circulation, cooling your internal temperature and generally contributing to a deeper sleep. Just don't overdo it. Your body goes through a few cool–warm cycles as the night passes, so you want pyjamas, sheets and covers that keep you comfortable through these changes.

ᶻZ **Clean your bedroom and paint it a soothing sage green.** Or some other soothing colour. First, remove the clutter from your bedroom – it provides a distraction and stands in the way of a good night's sleep. A soothing colour provides a visual reminder of sleep, relaxing you as you lie in bed reading or preparing for sleep.

ᶻZ **Choose the right pillow.** One Swedish study found that neck pillows, which resemble a rectangle with a depression in the middle, can actually enhance the quality of your sleep as well as reduce neck pain. The ideal neck pillow should be soft and not too high, provide neck support and be allergy tested and washable, researchers found. A pillow with two supporting cores received the best rating from the 55 people who participated in the study. Another study found that water-filled pillows

Sage green walls make a soothing bedroom.

provided the best night's sleep when compared to participants' usual pillows or a roll pillow, and yet another study rated "cool" pillows best, so choose one made of natural fibres, which release heat better and keep your head cooler than polyester. If you're subject to allergies or find you're often stuffed up when you awake in the morning, try a hypoallergenic pillow.

ᶻᶻ **Switch to heavier curtains over the windows** if you find it difficult to drop off. Even the light from streetlights, a full moon or your neighbour's house can interfere with the circadian rhythm changes you need to fall asleep.

Healthy INVESTMENT

A good mattress
A survey of 400 people found that 8 in 10 thought a bad mattress could cause sleep problems. Ironically, nearly half said they had a "bad" or "very bad" mattress. First off, you need a new mattress if yours is ten years old or even older. Also consider how lumpy it is – ditch your mattress if its topography resembles a mountain range, with its peaks, valleys and slopes. Another warning sign is waking up feeling sore or stiff, despite not being physically active the day before. Although no one mattress works best for everybody, there are some guidelines to follow:
● **Size.** Make sure you buy one that's larger than you think you will need, especially if you sleep with someone else.
● **Firmness.** This is strictly an individual decision. But make sure you try out any mattress in the store. Lie on it. Roll over. Get into your typical sleeping position.
● **Frame.** Make sure you get a sturdy, good-quality frame, one with at least ten slats and a fifth leg as a centre support.
● **Maintenance.** Turn your mattress over and upside down at least every three months.

ᶻᶻ **Move your bed away from any outside walls.** This will help to cut down on noise, which a Spanish study found could be a significant factor in insomnia. If the noise is still bothering you, try a white-noise machine, or just turn on a fan.

ᶻᶻ **Tuck a hot-water bottle between your feet** or wear a pair of ski socks to bed in winter. The science is a little complicated, but warm feet help your body's internal temperature get to the optimal level for sleep. Essentially, you sleep best when your core temperature drops. By warming your feet, you make sure blood flows well through your legs, allowing your trunk to cool.

ᶻᶻ **Kick your dog or cat out of your bedroom.** A 2002 research study found that one in five pet owners sleep with their pets. The study also found that dogs and cats created one of the biggest impediments to a good night's sleep since the discovery of caffeine. One reason? The study found that 21 per cent of the dogs and 7 per cent of the cats snored!

ᶻᶻ **Sleep alone.** One of the greatest disruptors of sleep is your loved one dreaming away next to you. He might snore, she might kick or cry out. In fact, one study found that 86 per cent of women surveyed said their husbands snored, and half had their sleep interrupted by it. Men have it a bit easier: 57 per cent said their wives snored, while just 15 per cent found their sleep bothered by it. If you won't kick your partner out (or head to the guest room yourself), consider these anti-snoring tips:
● Get him (or her) to stop smoking. Cigarette smoking contributes to snoring.
● Feed him (or her) a light meal for dinner and avoid any alcohol, which can add to the snoring.

- Buy some earplugs and use them.
- Play soft music to drown out the noise.
- Present your lover with a gift-wrapped box of Breathe Right strips, which work by pulling the nostrils open wider. A Swedish study found they significantly reduced snoring.
- Make an appointment for your partner at a sleep centre. If nothing you do improves his or her snoring, your bedmate might be a candidate for a sleep test called polysomnography to see if sleep apnea is the cause.

ᶻZ **Eat a banana before bed.** It's a great natural source of melatonin, the sleep hormone, as well as tryptophan. The time-honoured tradition, of course, is warm milk, also a good source of tryptophan.

ᶻZ **Take antacids straight after dinner, not before bed.** If you take antacids, take them after dinner – they contain aluminum, which appears to interfere with sleep.

ᶻZ **Listen to a book on tape while you fall asleep.** Just as a bedtime story soothes and relaxes children, a calming book on tape (try poetry or a biography, but stay away from horror novels) can have the same effect with us grown-ups.

ᶻZ **Simmer three to four large lettuce leaves in a cup of water** for 15 minutes. Remove from the heat, add two sprigs of mint, and sip just before you go to bed. Lettuce contains a sleep-inducing sub-stance called lactucarium, which affects the brain in a similar way to opium (but without the risk of addiction)!

ᶻZ **Use eucalyptus for a muscle rub.** The strongly scented herb provides a soothing feeling and relaxing scent.

Do **THREE** things...

If you can do only three things, try these to get a good night's sleep:

1 Allow one hour before bedtime for a relaxing activity. Watching the news or answering e-mails does not count. Better choices are reading or listening to soft music. As for sex ... some people say it just wakes them up. So factor this into the timing of your routine.

2 If your mind is relaxed but your body is tense, do some low-intensity stretches and exercises to relax your muscles, especially those in your upper body, neck and shoulders. Before you go to bed, use light weights (1-2 kg/3-5 lb for women; 2-4 kg/5-10 lb for men) to exercise these muscles calmly. Do one set of eight to ten repetitions of a basic exercise for each upper body muscle.

3 Allow at least 3 hours between dinner and bedtime. The brain does not sleep well on a full stomach. If you know that you'll be busy the following day, have your big meal at lunchtime and a lighter meal as early as possible in the evening.

☆ **Take a hot bath 90 to 120 minutes before bedtime.** A study published in the journal *Sleep* found that women with insomnia who took a hot bath at this point (with the water temperature at approximately 40°C), slept much better that night. The bath increased their core body temperature, which abruptly dropped once they got out of the bath, readying them for sleep.

ᶻZ **Give yourself a massage.** Slowly move the tips of your fingers around your eyes in a slow, circular motion. After a minute, move down to your mouth, then to your neck and the back of your head. Continue down your body until you're ready to drop off to sleep. Another option: ask your partner for a massage and massage each other on alternate nights.

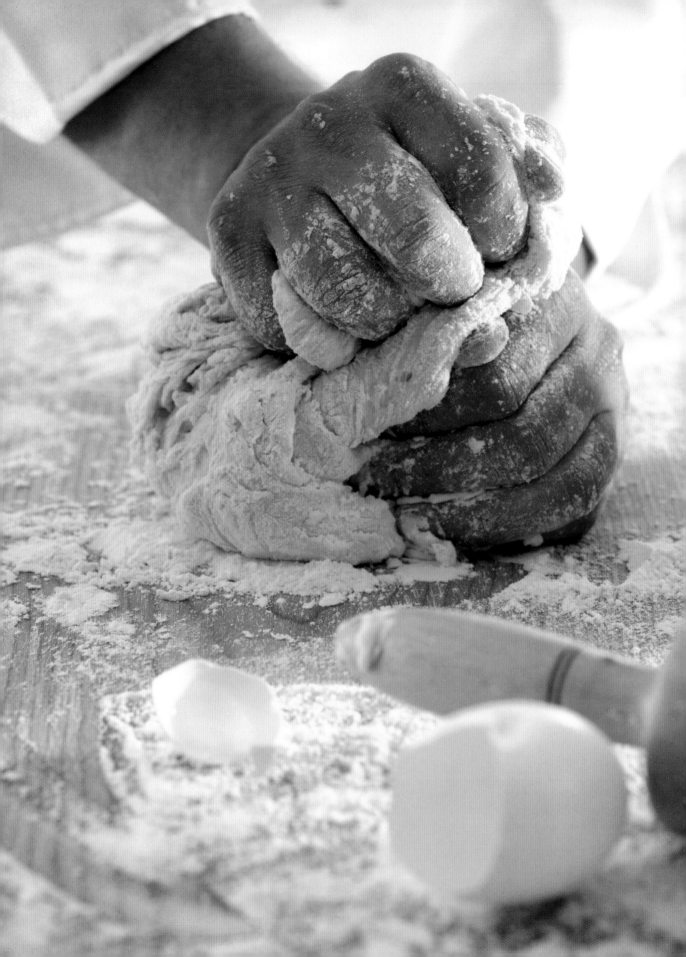

part 2

STEALTH HEALTHY COOKING

Probably the easiest and most effective way to improve your health is by adjusting your diet. Learn the best tricks for eating the right foods — and avoiding the bad.

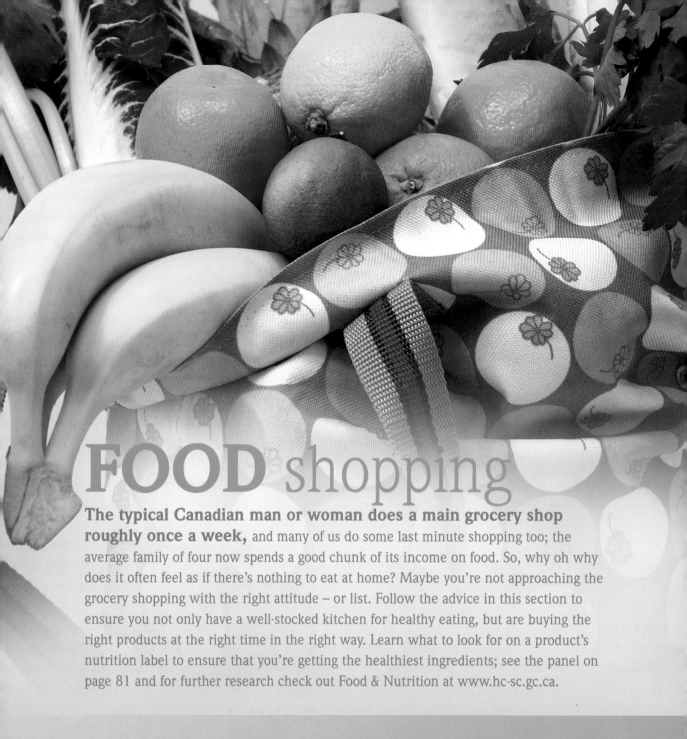

FOOD shopping

The typical Canadian man or woman does a main grocery shop roughly once a week, and many of us do some last minute shopping too; the average family of four now spends a good chunk of its income on food. So, why oh why does it often feel as if there's nothing to eat at home? Maybe you're not approaching the grocery shopping with the right attitude – or list. Follow the advice in this section to ensure you not only have a well-stocked kitchen for healthy eating, but are buying the right products at the right time in the right way. Learn what to look for on a product's nutrition label to ensure that you're getting the healthiest ingredients; see the panel on page 81 and for further research check out Food & Nutrition at www.hc-sc.gc.ca.

25 TIPS FOR YOUR GROCERY LIST

Rule number one: buy fresh food! There is no simpler, no easier, nor plainer measure of the healthiness of your food than whether it comes to you in boxes and cans or is fresh from the farm or fields. If more than half of your shopping comprises prepared foods, then you need to take your eating habits back to the healthy side by opting for more fresh vegetables, fruit, seafood, juices and dairy products.

Shop around the perimeter of the supermarket. That's where you'll find the fresh foods in many stores. If that's the case in your supermarket, avoid the central aisles and your shopping trip will be the healthier for it. Just dip into the aisles for the staples you know you need.

Think of the different sections (dairy, fresh produce, meat and so on) as separate stores within the supermarket. You wouldn't shop at every store in the shopping centre, would you? Target only those that are safe to browse through – the fresh food sections, primarily – and steer clear of the danger areas (candy, ice cream, chips …).

Shop with a list. Organize your shopping list based on the tip above – that is, order it by the individual sections of the store. This will get you out of the supermarket at the speed of light. If you're a woman, consider asking your husband or son to do the food shopping. U.S. research shows that, compared to women, men are more likely to buy only what's on the list. But shopping with a list has benefits beyond speed and spending. By sticking rigidly to a well-planned shopping list, you can resist the seductive call of aisle upon aisle of junk food, thereby saving your family and yourself from an overload of empty calories.

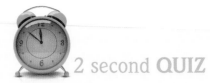

2 second QUIZ

Paper or plastic?
ANSWER: **PAPER.**

The debate over which bag is better for the environment is long and complicated. Yes, plastic can be recycled, but it's not as easy as recycling paper. And plastic production and processing require the use of toxic chemicals. Plus, plastic decomposes only when air and sunlight are present, whereas landfilled garbage is buried. On the plus side, the newer bioplastics are made from renewable sources such as cornstarch and vegetable oils, which are compostable. Meanwhile, although paper bags are made using manufacturing techniques that require water and air pollution, they are increasingly made from reprocessed materials and are more easily recycled and broken down. An even better bet: choose reusable cloth or string bags.

Food-shop on a full stomach. You've no doubt heard it before, but it's worth repeating. Walking through a supermarket with your tummy rumbling can make you vulnerable to buying anything that isn't moving. If you can't arrange to shop shortly after a meal, be sure to eat an apple and drink a large glass of water before heading into the store.

Purchase a few days before food is fully ripe. There's no point in trying to buy fresh vegetables and fruit for your family if the bananas turn brown and the peaches go mushy two days after you get them home. Buy fruit that's still a day or two behind ripeness. It will still be hard to the touch; bananas will be green. Feel carefully for bruises on apples, check best before dates on bagged produce and stay away from potatoes or onions that have started to sprout. If the fresh produce on the shelves looks a bit beyond its peak,

Healthy INVESTMENT

A cheese knife

A good cheese knife will enable you to cut paper-thin slices of your favourite hard cheeses. You'll use less cheese (meaning you take in less saturated fat and fewer calories) without losing any of the delicious flavour.

don't walk away; ask to speak to the manager. Chances are, there's a fresh shipment in the back just waiting to be put out on the shelves. For a really tasty treat, if you're going to eat them within the next couple of days, buy a bunch of vine-ripened tomatoes. There's just no comparison.

Buy in season. Of course, it's tempting to buy strawberries in December, and once in a while that's fine. But fresh fruit and vegetables are definitely best when purchased in season, meaning they've come from relatively close to home. They often cost less and are tastier. Ask around at the farmers' market to find out what's best when.

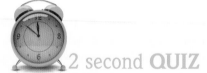

2 second QUIZ

Cash or credit?
ANSWER: **CASH.**

You'll almost certainly spend less on your groceries if you pay with cash. In one study, researchers asked several hundred families to do all of their grocery shopping with cash for three months, then, for the next three months, to use only a credit card. When the families used credit cards, they spent between 20 and 30 per cent more on their shopping.

Consider buying organic. Some studies suggest that organic produce contains higher levels of cancer-fighting nutrients. While others find no difference, organic is undoubtedly better for the environment and doesn't contain the pesticide residues sometimes present in non-organic produce. But it is generally more expensive so, when choosing what to buy, consider which non-organic foods have the worst residues. That being stated, do not let the price factor dissuade you from eating ample portions of fruits and vegetables, all of which are good for the body and mind.

Buy frozen. Frozen fruit and vegetables are often flash frozen at source, locking in more nutrients than some fresh or canned foods contain. So stock your freezer with bags of frozen vegetables and fruits. You can add the veggies to soups and stews, microwave them for a side dish with dinners or thaw them at room temperature and dip them into low-fat salad dressing for snacks. Use the fruits for desserts and smoothies, and as ice cream and yogourt toppings.

Stock up on canned tomato products. Here's one major exception to the "fresher is better" rule. Studies find that tomato sauces and crushed and stewed tomatoes have higher amounts of the antioxidant lycopene than fresh, because they're concentrated. Canned tomatoes are a godsend when it comes to rustling up a quick dinner. Warm up a can with some crushed garlic for a chunky pasta sauce; pour a can over chicken breasts and simmer; add to stews and sauces to provide flavour and extra nutrients.

Don't forget canned beans. They may have a bit more salt than you'd choose, but it's easy enough to rinse it off. Beans can be mixed with brown rice, added to soups and stews, puréed with onions and garlic to make a dip, or served over pasta for a traditional pasta e fagioli (*fagioli* means "beans" in Italian). You may have heard that pasta raises blood sugar. But the soluble fibre in the beans lowers the overall glycemic index of the meal (see page 100), reducing both the steepness of the rise in blood sugar during digestion and the surge in insulin secretion that follows. So a dish of pasta and beans is as healthy as it is delicious.

☑ **Spend some time in the condiment aisle.** With the following basic ingredients you have the foundations for tasty sauces, low-fat marinades and low-salt flavourings. Plus, you can stay away from the less-healthy ingredients such as mayonnaise, butter, margarine, creamy salad dressings and so on. Choose: flavoured ketchups, relishes, chutneys and barbecue sauces (look for sugar-free varieties), horseradish, mustards, flavoured vinegars, extra-virgin olive oil and pesto sauces (delicious spooned on top of salmon and baked), capers, jars of olives, sun-dried tomatoes, spaghetti sauce, anchovies, roasted red peppers, Worcestershire sauce, chili sauce, hot pepper sauce, soy sauce, sesame oil, walnut oil, teriyaki sauce and jars of salsa.

☑ **Choose prepared foods with short ingredient lists.** It's unrealistic to expect yourself to cut out prepared foods entirely. Just remember: the shorter the ingredient list, the healthier the food usually is. Of course, if the ingredients are sugar and butter, put the item back on the shelf.

☑ **Try new whole-grain alternatives.** Today's stores offer delicious whole-grain pastas and couscous, instant brown rice that cooks in a mere 10 minutes instead

Food-labelling **DIRECTORY**

If you learn what the information on food packaging means you'll be better equipped to make healthy choices. Many products lure us with labels of "low fat" and "cholesterol-free." But what do they really mean?

● **Fat.** "Low fat" indicates that the food specified on the nutrition facts label contains no more than 3 g of fat. Health Canada recommends that the range for fat intake is about one third of the calorie total.

● **Calories.** "Reduced in calories" indicates that the food contains at least 25 per cent fewer calories than the regular food.

● **Light.** "Light" is allowed only on foods that are either "reduced in fat" or "reduced in calories."

● **Fibre.** "Source of fibre" indicates that the food specified on the nutrition facts label contains at least 2 g of dietary fibre.

● **Sodium.** "Sodium-free" indicates that the food specified on the nutrition facts label contains less than 5 mg of sodium.

● **Cholesterol.** "Cholesterol-free" indicates that the food specified on the nutrition facts label contains less than 2 mg of cholesterol. It must also be low in saturated and trans fat.

QUICK GUIDE TO food labels

LOW FAT	less than 3 g
REDUCED IN CALORIES	25% fewer
SOURCE OF FIBRE	2 g or more
SODIUM-FREE	less than 5 mg
CHOLESTEROL-FREE	less than 2 mg

of the long 50 minutes it once took, even tasty whole-grain cookies. While you're at it, pick up a bag of whole-wheat flour to replace the white flour in your cupboard.

☆ **Reject food and drinks made with corn syrup.** Corn syrup is a calorie-dense, nutritionally empty sweetener perhaps even worse for us than refined sugar (see page 103 for more on corn syrup). A number of foods and drinks contain it, including apparently healthy foods such as fruit juices, pre-made spaghetti sauces and even bread. If corn syrup is listed as one of the four main ingredients (usually near the top), for your good health's sake, avoid it.

☑ **Look for fibre.** You want at least 1 to 2 g of fibre for every 100 calories you consume.

☑ **If partially hydrogenated oil,** or trans fats, are listed on the label, step away from the box and protect your health.

☑ **Pick up a jar of dried shiitake mushrooms.** They may look a little strange, but toss them in some hot water for half an hour and you have a meaty, healthy addition to soups, stews and sauces, not to mention a unique filling for tarts and omelettes. Plus, they keep for ages.

▶ **Whenever you find yourself reaching for a package of ground meat,** go to the poultry section instead and choose ground turkey or chicken, or try ground soy. These work just as well as ground beef in, for example, meatballs and chili. This substitution alone can cut nearly a third of the calories and at least half of the fat and saturated fat in an 85 g serving. When it's covered in a zesty tomato sauce or flavoured with seasonings, you won't be able to tell the difference.

☑ **Choose low-fat cheeses.** Instead of high-fat Gorgonzola, Cheddar, Double Gloucester or Parmesan, choose ricotta, low-fat cottage cheese or low-fat cream cheese. You can also enjoy medium-fat cheeses such as Brie, Edam, Camembert, Danish blue and feta in moderation.

☑ **Buy canola oil instead of vegetable oil.** It's rich in healthy monounsaturated fatty acids and contains the essential fatty acids (EFAs) alpha-linolenic acid (ALNA) and linoleic acid (LA). It also costs less than olive oil.

▶ **Choose whole-wheat bread.** Studies show that people who eat three or more servings of whole grains a day are less likely to suffer from diabetes. If your family will eat only white bread, choose a fibre-enriched variety.

☑ **Buy plain yogourt and flavour it at home.** Pre-flavoured yogourts contain sugars that destroy any healthy benefits. If you add fruit at home, it will still taste yummy, plus you'll consume far fewer useless calories *and* save money.

☺ **Choose healthy toppings for plain cereals.** These include raisins, fresh berries, dried berries, pumpkin seeds and bananas. Buy unsweetened cereals, then add your favourite flavours. That helps you to bypass all the empty sugary calories – and lets you enjoy the cereal more. For ease, keep a wide-brimmed, well-sealed jar of ingredients on your kitchen counter for quick mixing. Have a scoop and some sealable bags handy, and you've got a handy, nutritious meal or snack to eat at home or when you're on the go.

☑ **Read juice labels carefully.** Orange juice, though healthy, often has 20 g of sugar in the average 1 cup (250 ml) glass. Instead, try guava juice. It has three times more vitamin C and is full of potassium and beta carotene. NB If you have kidney disease or are on a blood pressure-lowering medication, avoid potassium-rich foods as extra potassium may be harmful.

Shiitake mushrooms are a versatile addition to any kitchen.

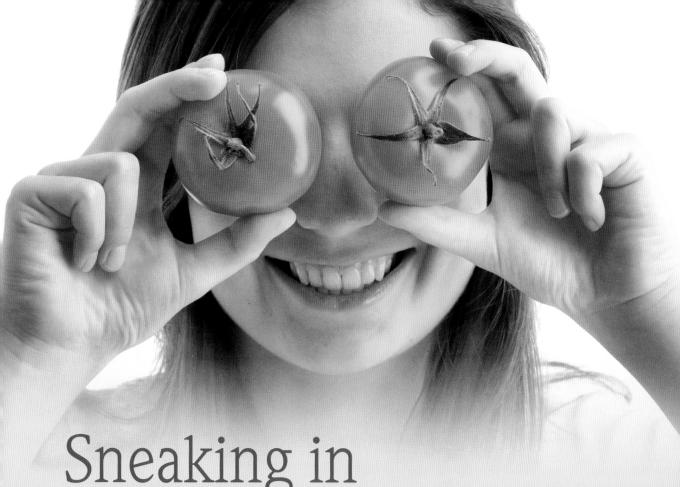

Sneaking in
VEGETABLES

The average Canadian does not eat enough vegetables, yet nutrition experts would advise us to eat four to five helpings every day. This is pretty much our health problems in a nutshell. If we ate more vegetables and fewer processed foods, we'd lose weight, clean out our arteries, balance our blood sugar and shut down a large number of hospitals. But getting four to five servings doesn't come without planning or effort. Here's the health-boosting and *painless* way to sneak more veggies into your daily diet.

23 WAYS TO GET YOUR FILL

Do your health and digestion a favour and ask for extra veggies on your pizza.

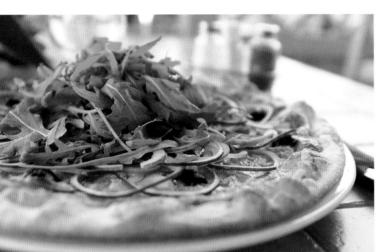

Serve raw vegetables at every meal. Nearly everyone likes carrot and celery sticks, cucumber slices, string beans, cherry tomatoes and/or green pepper strips. They're healthy, they have virtually no calories, they have a satisfying crunch and they can substantially cut your consumption of the more calorie-dense main course. So make this a routine: place a plate of raw vegetables in the centre of the table, no matter what the meal is.

● **Sneak vegetables into breakfast and lunch.** One reason we don't get enough vegetables is that many of us consider

Healthy INVESTMENT

A vegetable grater
Grating vegetables such as carrots, cabbage, celery, cucumber and so on adds volume to your meals, meaning you take in fewer calories while eating more food. Plus, grating helps you to "hide" your veggies in casseroles, sauces and other dishes.

them merely as a side dish to dinner. If you really want to increase your vegetable consumption, you have no choice but to eat them at other meals. But how? Easy:
● Choose salad as part of your everyday lunch.
● Make scrambled egg a regular breakfast, using the egg to hold together sautéed vegetables such as peppers, mushrooms, zucchini, asparagus or onions.
● Eat leftover veggies from last night's dinner with breakfast or lunch.
● Snack on cherry tomatoes, cucumbers, carrots and celery – all the time.
● Make vegetable sandwiches using almost any vegetable that won't roll out of the bread.

☺ **Start each dinner with a mixed green salad** before you serve the main course. Not only will it help you to eat more veggies, but by filling your stomach first with a nutrient-rich, low-calorie salad, there'll be just a bit less room for the higher-calorie items that follow.

● **Purée veggies into soup.** Potatoes, carrots, cauliflower and broccoli – just about any cooked (or leftover) vegetable can be made into a creamy, comforting soup. Here's a simple recipe: in a medium saucepan, sauté 160 g of finely chopped onion in 1 tablespoon of vegetable oil until tender. Combine the onion in a blender or food processor with cooked vegetables and purée the mix until smooth. Return the purée to the saucepan and thin it with broth or low-fat milk. Simmer and season to taste.

● **Order your weekly pizza with extra veggies.** Instead of the same old pepperoni and onions, do your health and digestion a favour and ask for the artichoke hearts, broccoli, hot peppers and other exotic vegetables that many takeout pizza places offer these days.

● **Once a week, eat a main-course salad.** A salade niçoise is a good example: mixed greens, steamed green beans, boiled potatoes, sliced hard-boiled egg and tuna drizzled with vinaigrette. Serve with crusty whole-grain bread. Bon appétit!

☺ **Pack your spaghetti sauce with vegetables.** Take a jar of low-salt prepared sauce and add in green beans, peas, corn, peppers, mushrooms, tomatoes and more. Like it chunky? Cut them into big pieces. Don't want to know they're there? Grate or purée them with a bit of sauce in the blender, then add.

☆ **Follow the golden rule:** half of your dinner plate should be filled with vegetables. That leaves a quarter of the plate for a healthy starch and a quarter for lean meat or fish. This is the perfectly balanced dinner, say experts.

● **Make a sandwich that has more lettuce and tomato than meat.** Stack the meat component in the sandwich to no higher than half the thickness of a standard slice of bread. Then pile on low-calorie slices of lettuce and tomatoes to the combined height of both slices of bread.

● **Eat a veggie burger for lunch** once a week, and top it with a sliced tomato and lettuce. Veggie burgers taste better than you might imagine.

☺ **Open a can of low-salt soup** and add a bag of pre-cut broccoli and carrots, either fresh or frozen. Voilà! You have a superfast and easy lunch or starter course that's bursting with good nutrition and fibre. Flavour it with your preferred

The **COOKING** corner

Vegetables are easier to cook than chicken, burgers or pork chops. But they do require a little more creativity. Here are four mini-recipes to give you some initial ideas:

● Add grated carrots and steamed spinach to 450 g of ground beef or turkey, then shape into patties and grill for your own version of a veggie burger.

● Serve celeriac instead of mashed potatoes or white rice as a side dish. Peel it and slice it into chunks, drizzle with olive oil, then roast in a hot oven until soft. Or boil it and mash with seasoning and a little olive oil.

● Substitute sweet potatoes for potatoes – peel them, slice into bite-size chunks, then boil until soft and mash with seasoning and olive oil. Alternatively, roast them (as for celeriac above), or make sweet potato wedges as a healthy change from fries (peel and slice the sweet potatoes into wedges, parboil them, then drain and coat with a little olive oil and fajita or spicy seasoning before baking in a hot oven for 15 to 20 minutes).

● Cut an eggplant in two down the middle and stuff each half with tomatoes. Top with slices of Parmesan, drizzle with olive oil, wrap in foil, then bake or grill until softened.

spices, herbs or spicy sauce and, as the soup simmers, it will simultaneously cook the veggies.

● **Move your veggies to the top shelf of the fridge.** As long as they're bagged properly, they'll last as well as they would in a vegetable crisper. More important, now they'll be visible and enticing. In particular, keep quick-to-eat vegetables such as baby carrots, red and green pepper strips, broccoli florets, tomatoes and cucumbers as accessible as possible.

● **Eat vegetables like fruit.** Half a cucumber, a whole tomato, a stalk of celery or a long, fresh carrot are as pleasant to munch on as an apple. It may seem unusual, but who cares? A whole vegetable makes a terrific snack.

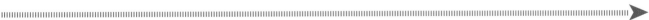

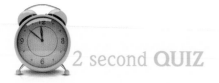

2 second QUIZ

Fresh or powdered garlic?
ANSWER: **FRESH.**

Technically, the jury is still out. A large American study on fresh garlic by Christopher Gardner, PhD, of Stanford University Medical Center, found that fresh garlic failed to reduce cholesterol levels, although further research is needed on its other possible medicinal benefits. But, Gardner notes, the active ingredient in garlic is allicin, which can easily be destroyed if you mess with it too much, which suggests that fresh is best. Other tests indicate that you'd usually need more powdered garlic than fresh to get the same benefits.

● **Add chopped kale or other hearty greens** to your next soup or stew. Just a couple of minutes is all that's needed to steam the greens down to tenderness and add quantities of potassium, fibre and calcium to your soup.

● **Use low-sodium vegetable juice** as the base for soups instead of chicken or beef broth.

● **Incorporate grated carrots and shredded cabbage in your soups,** salads or casseroles. These coleslaw ingredients add flavour, colour and lots of vitamins and minerals.

☆ **Go vegetarian one day a week.** You can do this by merely replacing the meat serving with a vegetable serving (a suggestion: make it a crunchy, strong-flavoured vegetable such as broccoli). Or you can dabble in the world of vegetarian cooking, in which recipes are developed specifically to make a filling, robust meal out of vegetables and whole grains. For those times, you should get yourself a good vegetarian cookbook. Try Reader's Digest's *The Vegetarian Cookbook* or an old vegetarian cookbook standard to get you started.

☺ **Use salsa liberally.** First, make sure you have a large batch of tomato salsa filled with vegetables. One good approach: add chopped yellow peppers and zucchini to store-bought salsa. Then put salsa on everything: baked potatoes, rice, chicken breasts, sandwiches, eggs, steak, even bread. Don't save it just for tortilla chips. It's too tasty and healthy not to be used all the time.

● **Roast your vegetables.** Here's a great side dish that's easy to make, delicious to eat and amazingly healthy. Plus, it tastes surprisingly sweet, and lasts well as a leftover, meaning you can make large batches to serve throughout the week. Cut hearty root vegetables such as parsnips, turnips, carrots and onions into 3 cm (1 in.) chunks and arrange in a single layer on a baking sheet. Drizzle with olive oil and sprinkle with sea salt, freshly ground pepper and fresh or dried herbs. Roast in the oven at 450°F (230°C) until soft, for about 45 minutes, turning once.

● **Use vegetables as sauces.** How about puréed roasted red peppers seasoned with herbs and a bit of lemon juice, then drizzled over fish? Why not purée butternut squash with carrots, grated ginger and a bit of brown sugar for a yummy topping for chicken or turkey? Cooked vegetables are easily converted into sauces. It just takes a little ingenuity and a blender.

● **Lose the bitterness of healthy veggies with a sprinkle of salt.** There's more about how to reduce the salt in your diet later, but the chemical reality is that salt helps to neutralize bitterness. For an added kick, try capers, olives or mashed anchovies instead of salt.

 Grill your vegetables. If you use your grill only for meats, you're missing out! Peppers, zucchini, asparagus, onions, eggplant, tomatoes – they all taste great when grilled. Generally, all you need to do is coat them with olive oil and throw them on. Turn every few minutes and remove when they start to soften. Or put chunks on a skewer and turn frequently.

● **Go exotic.** Every week, try to buy a slightly exotic vegetable, perhaps something that you've never eaten before. Here are some ideas, and some preparation and cooking suggestions:
● **Endive.** This type of lettuce has a mild, slightly bitter flavour, and is packed with fibre, iron and potassium. Use it in salads and with vegetable dips.
● **Bok choy.** An Asian cabbage, bok choy is excellent chopped and stir-fried in a bit of peanut oil and soy sauce. Or add it to the soup just before serving.
● **Kohlrabi.** A member of the turnip family, this is also called a cabbage turnip. It's sweeter, juicier, crisper and more delicate in flavour than a turnip, and the cooked leaves have a kale/collard flavour. Trim and pare the bulb to remove all traces of the fibrous underlayer just

Counting **TO TEN**

Learning that you need to get eight to ten servings of fruit and vegetables a day can be daunting. But consider the definition of a serving below (from Health Canada's *Canada's Food Guide* website), and you'll see that it's perfectly do-able:
● One medium-sized fruit (such as an apple, orange, banana or pear), half a grapefruit, 1 large slice of pineapple or half a mango.
● $^1/_4$ cup (50 ml) of dried fruit, such as raisins or apricots or mixed fruit.
● $^1/_2$ cup (125 ml) broccoli, cauliflower or green beans.
● $^1/_2$ cup (125 ml) of cooked vegetables such as carrots, peas or corn.
● Salad vegetables such as 1 stalk of celery, 1 medium tomato, 7 cherry tomatoes or $^1/_2$ cup (125 ml) of cucumber.
● $^1/_2$ cup (125 ml) of 100 per cent pure fruit or vegetable juice or smoothie.
● One large kiwi, one guava or ten lychees.
● $^1/_2$ cup (125 ml) of frozen or canned vegetables.
● $^1/_2$ cup (125 ml) of cooked leafy vegetables, such as kale or bok choy.
● One cup (250 ml) of raw leafy vegetables.

beneath the skin, then eat the vegetable raw, boiled, steamed, microwaved or sautéed, or add to potato casseroles.
● **Fennel.** Also known as sweet anise, fennel has a mild licorice flavour. The feathery fronds can flavour soups and stews, while the broad, bulbous base can be eaten raw, or sliced/diced for adding to stews, soups and stuffing.

Reminder

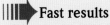 **Fast results**
These are tips that deliver benefits particularly quickly – in some cases, immediately.

 Easy gains
These are health boosters that offer the best value for the least amount of effort.

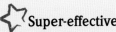 **Super-effective**
This is advice that scientific research or widespread usage by experts has shown to be especially effective.

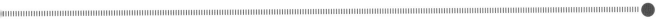

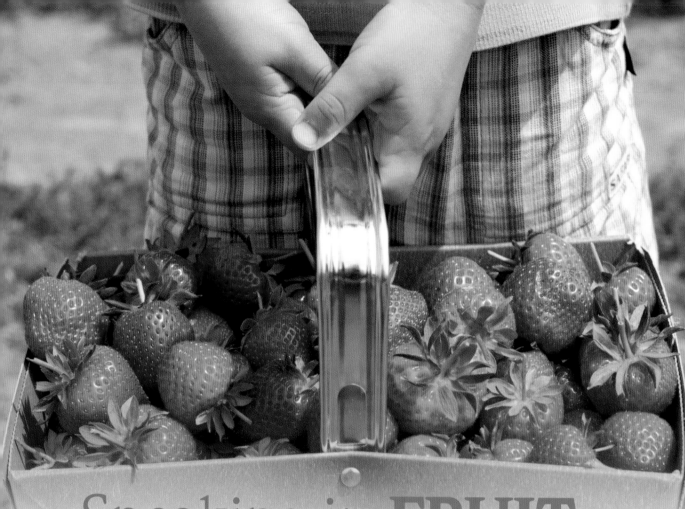

Sneaking in **FRUIT**

You've no doubt heard talk of the global economy. Well, you need look no farther than your local supermarket to see it in action. There, grapes from South America meet kiwis from New Zealand and pineapples from Hawaii – in February. But because of concerns about the carbon footprint of these items, we are being urged increasingly to buy locally sourced fresh food, which makes sense for good health and for the environment.

You know the drill by now – for optimal health you should be aiming for three to four to five servings of fruit a day. It's not difficult, especially with these clever tips.

21 WAYS TO GET ALL YOU NEED

Make it a rule: every breakfast includes a piece of fruit. It's the ideal morning food, filled with natural, complex sugars for slow-release energy, fibre and nutrients galore. Cantaloupe, an orange, berries – all are perfect with whole-wheat toast, cereal or an egg.

Make another rule: eat fruit for dessert at least three nights a week. A slice of watermelon, a peach, a bowl of blueberries – they're a delicious ending to a meal, and are so much healthier than cookies or cake. Like more sophisticated desserts? How does chocolate-covered strawberries, poached pears in red wine or frozen fresh raspberry yogourt sound? They count too.

Start each week with a fruit slushie. Add 160 g of fresh fruit, 1/2 cup (125 ml) of fruit juice and two or three ice cubes to a blender and liquefy. That gives you two servings of fruit before 8 a.m. For a creamier smoothie, add 175 g of plain fat-free yogourt.

Substitute fruit sorbet for ice cream. One scoop contains up to one serving of fruit.

Keep a fruit bowl filled wherever you spend the most time. This could be at work, near your home computer or even in the television room. And keep five to eight pieces of fresh fruit in it at all times, such as bananas, oranges, apples, grapes or plums. Most fruit is fine left at room temperature for three or four days. But if it's out and staring at you, it's not likely to last that long.

Carry dried fruits with you. Dried fruits are very portable and have a long shelf life. Take them to work, on shopping trips or even on vacation. Raisins and prunes are classic choices. Also try dried cranberries and blueberries, which are extremely high in phytonutrients, or dried apricots, which are chock-full of beta carotene. Other options include dates and dried figs, peaches, pears and bananas.

Take fruit with you whenever you are driving for more than an hour. Once you're on the highway and cruising along, an apple or a nectarine tastes great and helps to break the tedium.

Keep an apple in your pocket whenever you go for long walks. It will be your reward for getting to the midpoint of your chosen route.

Make Monday red day. And eat only red fruits. Tuesday could be orange day and so on. Here's how your weekdays might work to give you maximum fruit variety (you could make weekends a fruit free-for-all):
Monday. Red: apples, cherries, cranberries, red grapes, plums, strawberries.
Tuesday. Orange: apricots, cantaloupe, kumquats, nectarines, oranges, papaya, peaches.

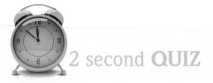

2 second QUIZ

Strawberries or blueberries?
ANSWER: **BLUEBERRIES.**

Of course, both are great for you, so try to eat lots of these two fruits. But when you compare the nutrients in an equal amount of each, blueberries have a slight edge. Blueberries are particularly rich in fibre – four times that of strawberries – as well as containing more natural sugars, much more vitamin E and some unique micronutrients that are good for memory.

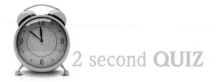

Fresh fruit or dried?
ANSWER: **FRESH.**

The higher water content (most fresh fruits are more than 80 per cent water) means a larger volume, making the fruit more filling and satisfying with fewer calories. But for convenience and shelf life, use dried fruit as your back-up plan.

Wednesday. Yellow or white: bananas, yellow apples, grapefruit, mango, pineapple.
Thursday. Blue or violet: blackberries, blueberries, grapes, plums, figs.
Friday. Green: limes, pears, green apples, kiwis.

Mix fruits in with your salad. A sprinkling of raisins, some chopped strawberries, a diced apple, some fresh or dried mango or some sliced kiwi all make tasty additions to the typical tossed salad.

Purée fresh or canned fruits (peaches, pear, mangoes, apricots, etc.) and use as a delicious and healthy ice cream or pancake topping.

Add frozen berries to cereal, salads or ice cream. They also work well stirred into yogourt or muffin mix.

Freeze banana slices or grapes for a refreshing summer snack. Simply pop the banana slices and/or grapes into a sealable bag, freeze, then eat as desired.

Every time you want a chocolate bar, eat a small box of raisins instead. Raisins are sweet and healthy, and small boxes contain just the right amount to fulfill the need for a sweet treat.

Get your fruit from bread and cake once a week. How about apple cake, banana bread, strawberry, apple or blueberry tart? Pineapple upside-down cake, anyone?

Spice up store-bought salsas with fruit. Or make your own fruit-based salsas with pineapple, mango or papaya. Mix with onions, ginger, a bit of garlic, some mint and/or cilantro, sprinkle on a few hot pepper flakes for a bit of a kick, and enjoy.

Add diced kiwi, sliced grapes or chopped apple to chicken, tuna and turkey salads.

Keep cubed or sliced melon in a container in the fridge. Use as a first course before dinner; wrap with prosciutto for a starter; mix with cottage cheese for breakfast; have a small bowl for a snack; even consider puréeing it for a quick sauce over fish.

Grate fruit over plain yogourt. Use the larger holes of a box-type grater for a quick and tasty topping.

Mash bananas and spread them on toast and bagels for a treat that brings back childhood. Or freeze whole bananas for a delicious, healthy summer snack.

Every week, buy one exotic fruit you've never tried. It could be something as relatively common as a mango, or as unusual as a cherimoya. Here are some tips on some exotic fruits and how to enjoy them:
● **Asian pear.** Also called a Chinese, salad or apple pear, this firm pear is meant to be eaten immediately when it's hard. It's sweet, crunchy and amazingly juicy.

- **Cherimoya.** Also called a custard apple, this large tropical fruit tastes like a combination of pineapple, papaya and banana. Purchase fruit that's firm, heavy for its size and without skin blemishes or brown splotches. Let it soften at room temperature, then refrigerate it, wrapped, for up to four days. To serve, cut it in half, remove the seeds and spoon the fruit from the shell.
- **Guava.** Sweet and fragrant with bright pink, white, yellow or red flesh. Buy when it is just soft enough to press, and refrigerate it for up to a week in a plastic or paper bag. To use, cut in half and scoop out the flesh for salads, or peel and slice. Try cooking and puréeing slightly underripe guava as a sauce for meat or fish.
- **Kiwi.** This fruit didn't take off until its name was changed from Chinese gooseberry to kiwi. Now it's one of the most popular of the exotic fruits. With a flavour that's a cross between strawberries and melon, kiwis are ready to eat when they're slightly soft to the touch. Peel and chop, or cut in half and scoop out the flesh with a grapefruit spoon.
- **Lychee.** Once, lychee trees were found only in southern China, but the popularity of this tropical fruit has caused its spread. The lychee fruit is about 4 cm (2 in.) in size, oval, with a bumpy red skin. Peel off the inedible skin and you get a white, translucent flesh similar to a grape, but sweeter, surrounding a cherry-like pit. Eat them like large grapes, one after another. They're available for only a few months of the year, but buy a bag in spring and you'll discover why Asian people call lychees the king of fruits.
- **Mango.** One of the most commonly eaten fruits, along with bananas, the mango is often included in fruit salads, and is used to add flavour to a variety

In PERSPECTIVE

Deconstructing antioxidants

The reason that fruits (and vegetables) are so important to your overall health is that they are major purveyors of antioxidants. Antioxidant molecules are like the missile-defence system of your body, preventing damage from molecular bombs called free radicals. It works like this: in order to breathe, move or eat, your body's cells convert food and oxygen into energy. This chemical reaction releases harmful by-products, the free radicals. Basically, they are highly reactive forms of oxygen that are missing an electron. Desperate for that missing electron, they steal them from normal cells, damaging the healthy cell and its DNA in the process. This damage eventually contributes to any number of major health problems, including heart disease, memory loss and cancer.

Antioxidants, however, interfere with this process by giving free radicals one of their own electrons to stabilize them. Or they combine with free radicals to form different, more stable compounds. There are also antioxidant enzymes that help free radicals to react with other chemicals to produce safe, instead of toxic, substances. Antioxidants, for instance, help to prevent "bad" LDL cholesterol from becoming stickier and forming artery-clogging plaque.

This is why the health establishment is so insistent on people eating more fresh produce: it provides round-the-clock defences against free-radical damage to your arteries.

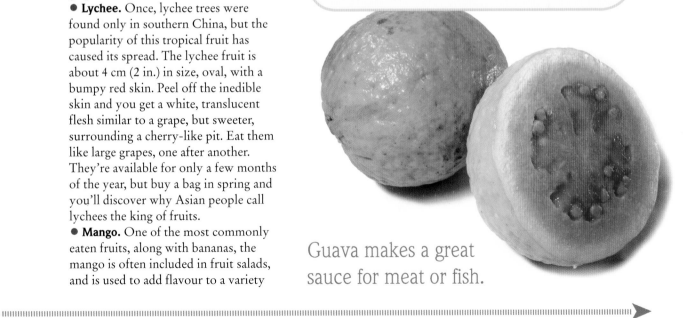

Guava makes a great sauce for meat or fish.

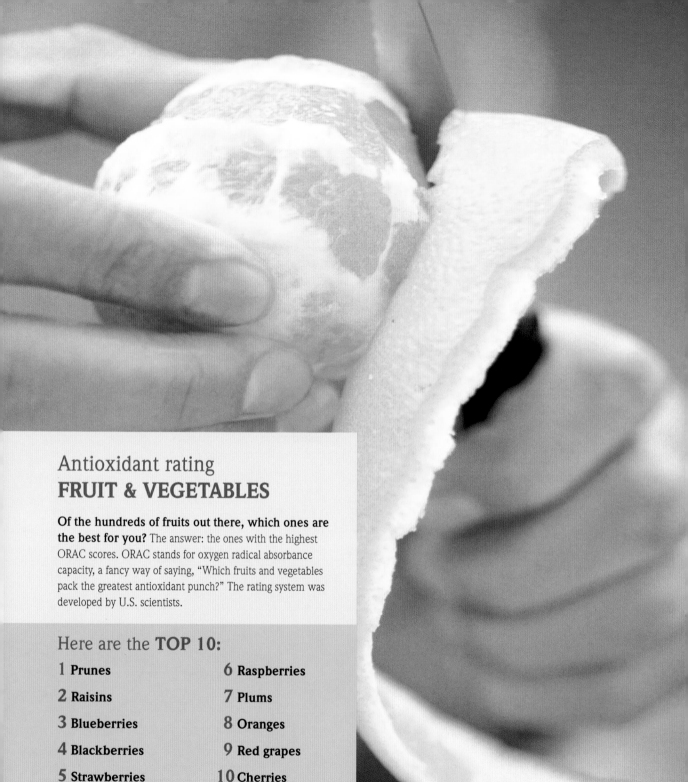

Antioxidant rating
FRUIT & VEGETABLES

Of the hundreds of fruits out there, which ones are the best for you? The answer: the ones with the highest ORAC scores. ORAC stands for oxygen radical absorbance capacity, a fancy way of saying, "Which fruits and vegetables pack the greatest antioxidant punch?" The rating system was developed by U.S. scientists.

Here are the TOP 10:

1 **Prunes**
2 **Raisins**
3 **Blueberries**
4 **Blackberries**
5 **Strawberries**

6 **Raspberries**
7 **Plums**
8 **Oranges**
9 **Red grapes**
10 **Cherries**

of fish. The flavour is a combination of peach and pineapple, but spicier and more fragrant (it is sometimes called the tropical peach).

- **Papaya.** Soft, juicy and silky-smooth flesh with a delicate, sweet flavour. The centre of the papaya is filled with small, round, black, pepper-tasting seeds, which can be eaten but aren't usually. Peel, then slice into wedges or cut into chunks, or slice in half, remove seeds and scoop out the flesh with a spoon. Unripe papayas can be peeled, seeded and cooked as a vegetable, and you can grind the seeds like pepper for adding to sauces or salads.
- **Passion fruit.** Passion fruit has golden flesh with tiny, edible black seeds and a sweet-tart taste. When ripe, it has wrinkled, dimpled, deep purple skin. To serve, cut in half and scoop out the pulp with a spoon.
- **Persimmon.** Delicate in flavour and firm in texture, the persimmon, sometimes called the Sharon fruit, can be eaten like an apple, sliced and peeled, and is great in salads.
- **Pomegranate.** Available in the autumn, it's the seeds of this crimson fruit that you eat. Each tiny, edible seed is surrounded by translucent, brilliant-red pulp that has a sparkling sweet-tart flavour. Choose fruit that feels heavy for its size with a bright colour and blemish-free skin. Pomegranates can be refrigerated for up to a month, while the seeds can be frozen for three months. To serve, cut the fruit in half and pry out the seeds. Use them to top ice cream, sprinkle into salads or eat simply as a snack.
- **Quince.** Tastes like a cross between an apple and a pear, with a dry, hard, yellowish-white flesh that has a tart

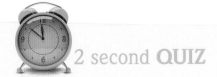

flavour. Better cooked than raw. Quinces keep for up to two months wrapped and refrigerated, and are primarily used for jams, jellies and preserves.

- **Star fruit.** Slice crossways for perfect five-pointed star-shaped sections as a garnish or as an ingredient in fruit salads. The star fruit's flavour combines the best of plums, pineapples and lemons.
- **Tamarillo.** This subtropical fruit is sometimes called a tree tomato, but the comparison ends there. Native to South America, this egg-shaped fruit has a glossy outer skin that hides crimson fruit which turns golden when cooked or heated. The orange-yellow flesh, studded with a swirl of edible dark-red seeds, has the texture of a plum and is slightly tart. To peel tamarillos, plunge into boiling water for about 30 seconds, then slip off the skins. Cut crossways into slices.

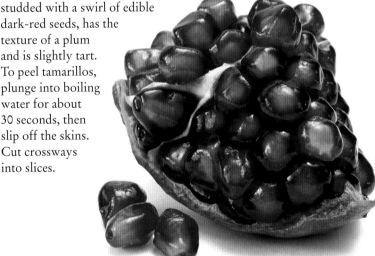

Pomegranates are packed with jewel-like seeds bursting with flavour.

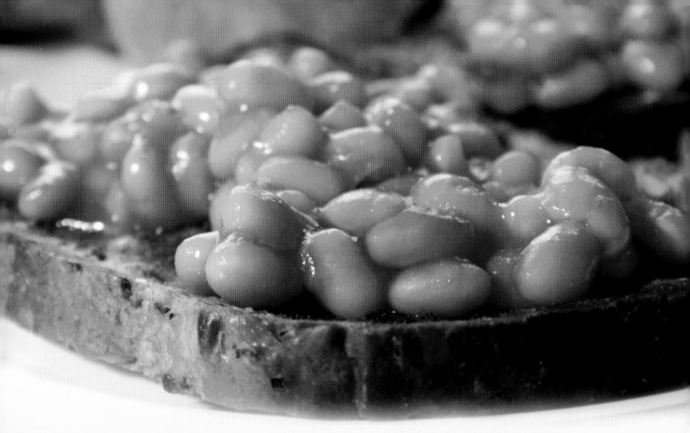

Sneaking in **FIBRE**

The term "good" carbs refers to complex carbohydrates. These are foods, such as whole grains and beans, which are composed largely of complex sugar molecules that require lots of time and energy to digest them into the simple sugars your body needs for fuel. One of the biggest benefits of these foods is that they also contain large amounts of fibre – the indigestible parts of plant foods. Fibre protects you from heart disease, cancer and digestive problems. Depending on the type of fibre, it also lowers cholesterol, helps with weight control and regulates blood sugar. This is one nutrient you don't want to miss. Yet the average Canadian consumes far too little fibre. In the next two chapters, we'll talk about how to remove "bad" carbs from your diet and up your "good" carbs – two of the best things you can do for your health.

25 WAYS TO GET MORE "GOOD" CARBS INTO YOUR DIET'

● **Enjoy cereal every day for breakfast.** Ideally, aim for a whole-grain, unsweetened cereal with at least 3 g of fibre a serving. Just eating any cereal might be enough, though. A University of California study found that cereal eaters tend to eat more fibre and less fat than non-cereal eaters.

● **Eat two apples every day.** Not just to keep the doctor away, but because apples are a good source of pectin, a soluble fibre that contributes to a feeling of fullness and which is also digested slowly. A 1997 study published in the *Journal of the American College of Nutrition* found that 5 g of pectin was enough to leave people feeling satisfied for up to 4 hours.

▮▮▮▶ **Designate one day a week to have a yogourt mix for breakfast.** Take 175 g of yogourt and mix in ¹/₃ cup (75 ml) of All-Bran cereal, 1 tablespoon of ground flaxseeds and 5 large, diced strawberries for a whopping amount of fibre.

☺ **Mix your usual cereal with the high-fibre stuff.** You might not want to face an entire bowl of All-Bran in the morning. Mix it with an equal amount of your usual cereal and you'll barely know it's there.

● **Dip baby carrots and broccoli florets into low-fat yogourt dip or salsa** for your afternoon snack three days a week. You'll fill up the empty afternoon space in your stomach while getting about 5 g of fibre from each 150 g of veggies.

● **Make sure that the first ingredient in whole-grain products has the word "whole" in it,** as in "whole wheat" or "whole grain." If it says multigrain, seven-grain, nutragrain, cracked wheat, stone-ground wheat, unbromated wheat or

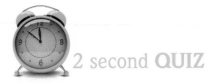

2 second **QUIZ**

Broccoli or cauliflower?
ANSWER: **BROCCOLI.**

At 2.6 g of fibre per 100 g, broccoli has twice the fibre oomph of cauliflower.

enriched wheat, it's not whole wheat, and is thus lacking some of the vitamins and minerals, not to mention fibre, of whole grains.

● **Keep a snack container in your car and office for the munchies.** Mix together peanuts, a high-fibre cereal such as All-Bran and some chocolate-covered raisins. Allow yourself one handful for a sweet, yet high-fibre, snack.

● **Switch to whole-grain crackers.** You'd never think a tiny cracker could make a difference, but one regular whole-grain cracker contains 500 mg of fibre. Ten crackers give you 5 g of fibre. So next time, try spreading some peanut butter on whole-grain crackers instead of bread.

● **Add kidney beans to your next salad.** Adding kidney beans, or other legumes, is a great way to add fibre to your diet.

▮▮▮▶ **Every week, try one "exotic" grain.** How about amaranth, bulgur or wheatberries? Most are as simple to prepare as rice, yet are packed with fibre and flavour. Mix in some steamed carrots and broccoli, toss with olive oil and a bit of Parmesan or feta cheese, maybe throw in a can of tuna or 50 g or so of sliced chicken,

Eat two apples a day. And not just to keep the doctor away.

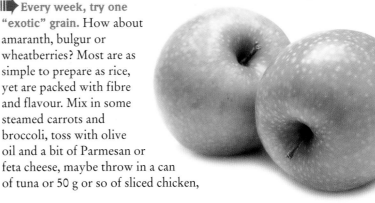

The weight-loss wars

For a while now, there has been a war among both consumers and doctors regarding the best approach to weight loss: a low-carbohydrate diet or a low-fat diet. In terms of popularity, the winner is clear: low-carb diets such as Atkins have won the hearts of many weight-conscious people. But the medical establishment remains vehement about the low-fat message. So why can't they all just agree?

As is often the case, research has caught up with all the claims, and proved that there are strengths and weaknesses in both approaches. The message is that excess animal fat in your diet is indeed bad for your health and your weight. But certain fats, particularly plant-based fats such as olive oil, are necessary for good health and nutrition. Likewise, excessive amounts of simple carbohydrates are bad for your health too. They are converted too easily into blood sugar, and cause all types of metabolic havoc when you eat them regularly. Much better are unrefined, whole-grain foods that take longer to digest and contain more nutrients and fibre.

Put it all together and you get a sensible diet rich in complex carbohydrates and lean, healthy meats and seafood. Plus loads and loads of vegetables.

At the end of the day, weight loss is about eating moderate amounts of healthy foods. What had been confirmed most recently is that simple carbs are more unhealthy than was once thought. Respond sensibly to that finding, and you are on your way to a lifetime of healthier eating.

and you've got dinner. Or serve as a side dish to chicken or fish. Make sure all the grains you try are whole grains.

● **Once a week, make pearl barley** (no soaking before cooking required) as a side dish. A 100 g serving of cooked pearl barley contains 3.8 g of fibre.

☺ **Sneak in oatmeal.** Use basic oatmeal in place of breadcrumbs for meatballs, sprinkle it on top of casseroles and ice cream, bake it into cookies and muffins, and add it to homemade bread and cakes.

☺ **Use whole-wheat bread to make your lunchtime sandwich every day.** Even sandwich store chains offer whole-wheat options for lunchtime munching. If you want to break into the whole-wheat club gradually, use whole-wheat bread as the bottom slice of your sandwich and white bread as the top layer. Eventually, make the move to all whole wheat.

● **Every week, switch from a white food to a brown food.** So instead of instant white rice, you switch to instant brown rice. Instead of your usual pasta, choose whole-wheat pasta. Similarly, go for whole-wheat pitas and whole-wheat couscous. Within two months, you should be eating only whole grains, and you should have increased your daily fibre intake by an easy 10 g without radically changing your diet.

● **Spread your sandwich with hummus.** Add 2 heaping tablespoons of hummus and you've got 2 g of tasty fibre. Add some spinach leaves and a tomato slice for another couple of grams.

● **Make beans a part of at least one meal a day.** They're packed with fibre. Just rinse first to remove excess salt. Here are some health-boosting tips for getting your beans:
● Purée a can of cannellini beans for a tasty dip. Add 2 cloves of garlic and a tablespoon each of lemon juice and olive oil to the blender. Use as a dip for veggies and whole-grain crackers.
● Fry a couple of tablespoons of mixed beans with some onion and chicken in a little oil and use to fill a soft flour tortilla.
● Mix black-eyed beans with finely chopped onion, chili, garlic and tomatoes to make a salsa.
● Make a bean salad with canned black-eyed beans, fresh or frozen corn, chopped

cilantro, chopped onion and chopped tomato. Drizzle with olive oil and a dash of vinegar, salt and pepper.

• Make your own special chili pizza. Top a prepared (whole-wheat) pizza base with some kidney beans, grated cheese and ground turkey cooked with chili.

• Start serving edamame (soy beans) as a side dish. You'll get 5 g of fibre from 100 g of edamame, not to mention the cancer-fighting phytonutrients that soy contains.

● **Add puréed cauliflower to mashed potatoes.** You won't taste much of a difference, but you'll get some extra fibre.

● **Have a beet salad for dinner.** These bright red veggies have virtually no fat, no cholesterol, no sodium, quite a bit of potassium and 2 g of fibre. Try roasting whole, peeled beets for 45 minutes, chilling, then dicing into a summer salad.

● **Make rice pudding for dessert tonight.** Only, instead of white rice, use brown to kick it up a notch.

● **Switch to whole-wheat flour when baking.** You can start by going half and half, eventually using only whole-wheat for all your cooking needs. Adding a little baking powder helps to lighten foods made from whole-wheat flour (note that you may have to add a little more liquid if using whole-wheat flour).

||||▶ **Add some flaxseeds, wheat germ** or other high-fibre ingredients to batter. They add crunch to your cookies, muffins and breads – and loads of fibre.

● **Eat the skin of your baked and sweet potatoes.** Eating baked potatoes with the skin on ups the fibre by at least 3 g (depending on the size of the potato).

Do **THREE** things…

The three best ways to get more fibre into your diet:

1 Eat more fruit and vegetables. They're the healthiest fibre sources around.

2 Start each day with a bowl of whole-grain cereal.

3 Switch to a whole-grain bread.

● **Start every dinner with a mixed green salad.** Not only will it add fibre, but, with a low-calorie dressing, it will partially fill you up with very few calories, and thus offers great weight-loss benefits.

● **Use beans or lentils as the main protein source** for dinner once or twice a week. A classic dish such as pasta e fagioli (pasta with beans) works well.

● **Drink your fibre.** Make your own smoothies by blending whole fruits (take out the large pips or seeds). If all the fruit goes into your glass, you'll get all the fibre – often missing from fruit juice.

DON'T FORGET to …

Drink plenty of water. You need water to help the fibre pass through your digestive system without getting stuck. So as you're increasing the fibre in your diet, also increase your intake of water or other unsweetened drinks. And don't up your fibre intake all at once. That's just going to overwhelm your system, leading to gas, bloating and constipation. Instead, start slowly. Try one tip a week for the first couple of weeks, then two, then three. By week four or five, you should be up to the full 24 g – or more.

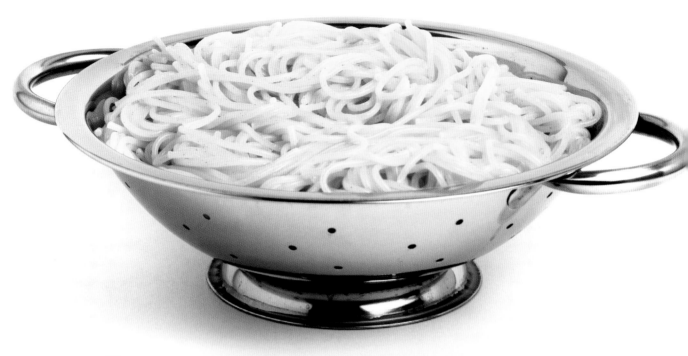

Cutting back on
"BAD" CARBS

Thanks to the popularity of low-carb diets, many of us are now watching the amount of carbohydrates we eat. The last chapter detailed the benefits of "good" carbs. Now it's time to explain what a "bad" carb is. Put simply, it's white flour, refined sugar and white rice. More broadly, it's any carb that has been processed to strip out ingredients which hinder quick and easy cooking. Why are refined carbs a problem? Easy: they are digested so quickly that they cause blood sugar surges, leading to weight gain and other health troubles. The next chapter shows you ways to reduce the amount of sugar you eat. For now, read on for other ways to avoid troublesome carbs while still getting enough fuel for good health.

10 WAYS TO AVOID THE WORST CULPRITS

● **Say no to the bread basket.** At almost every restaurant, the first thing a waiter brings is a basket of rolls and bread made from white flour. If it's not put on the table, you won't eat any. Or, if you really need something to nibble on, ask if they have whole-wheat varieties.

● **Choose brown rice, not white,** and limit how much you eat to 180 g. Brown rice hasn't been processed and it still has its high-fibre nutrients.

☺ **Wrap your food in lettuce leaves.** Yes, skip the rolls, tortillas and bread slices and instead make a sandwich inside lettuce leaves. Go Mexican with a sprinkle of Cheddar cheese, salsa and chicken; or Chinese with sesame seeds, peanuts, bean sprouts, sliced green beans and shrimp with a touch of soy sauce; or deli style with turkey, cheese and mustard.

● **Buy your snacks in child-sized bags.** The truth is, potato chips, tortilla chips and cookies are mostly bad carbs, made primarily from refined flour, sugar, salt and/or oil. You want to remove as many of these foods from your daily eating as you can. But if you can't live without them, buy them in small bags – 30 g is a typical "lunch box" size – and limit yourself to one bag a day.

▐▐▐▶ **Cure yourself of your old spaghetti habits.** Almost everyone loves a big bowl of pasta, topped with a rich tomato sauce. The tomato sauce couldn't be better for you; the spaghetti, however, is pure carbohydrate. While spaghetti is fine to eat every now and then, for those sensitive to carbs or wishing to cut back on their pasta intake, here are some alternatives to the usual spaghetti dinner:
● Here's the easiest choice: switch to whole-wheat pasta. It's denser than

traditional pasta, with a firm, al dente texture similar to what you'd get in Italy.
● Grill vegetables such as eggplant, zucchini, peppers and onions and slice into long, thin pieces. Mix up and pour your spaghetti sauce over the vegetables for a tasty and immensely healthy meal.
● Try healthy whole grains as a replacement for pasta. Spaghetti sauce goes better than you'd expect on brown rice, barley, chickpeas and so on.

Cutting the carbs without **HITTING YOUR WALLET**

Specialist low-carb diets can be expensive. For easy ways to stay low-carb without breaking the bank, follow these recommendations:
● Replace salmon and other more expensive fish with chicken breast or tofu.
● Always buy frozen fish rather than fresh (much fresh fish has been previously frozen anyway). There is little nutritional or taste difference, but you will see savings in price.
● Buy frozen berries, including blueberries, strawberries and raspberries. They're almost always less expensive than fresh (except maybe during peak growing season for your area).
● Replace mixed green salads with any dark leafy green (mustard, kale, spinach). Buy whole heads of greens rather than bagged and washed greens, which could cost up to 20 per cent more.
● Replace extra virgin olive oil on salads and in recipes with lower grade olive oil or canola oil.

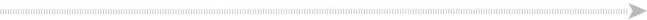

In PERSPECTIVE

Glycemic index vs. glycemic load

The glycemic index (GI) is a measure of how much, and how fast, the sugar in a food raises the level of sugar in your blood. A high or fast rise in blood sugar leads to high blood insulin levels, contributing to weight-control problems and possibly even increasing your risk of diabetes over time. So, in theory, a high glycemic index is a bad thing.

But the measure has important limitations. For one thing, it compares foods directly to one another to determine which raises blood sugar more. These comparisons are based on an equivalent "dose" of sugar in each food in an effort to be fair. To make the dose of sugar in carrots equivalent to the dose of sugar in ice cream, however, calls for the comparison of a tiny bowl of ice cream to a bushel of carrots. Of course, the carrots will have the higher glycemic index. It's also based on the effects of just one food, eaten alone. In real life, the foods we eat interact with each other to determine blood sugar levels. High-fibre cereal at breakfast, say, will blunt the rise in blood sugar from eating high GI foods at lunch.

A newer measure, the glycemic load, accounts for both how fast the sugar in a food is converted to blood sugar and the dose of sugar in the food. Whereas the glycemic index of a soft drink is similar to that of carrots, the glycemic load of the soft drink is ten times higher than that of carrots.

Should you worry about the glycemic index or load of the foods you eat? That's one for your doctor to answer. If you have diabetes or are prone to blood sugar swings and weight gain, being aware of the impact of food on your blood sugar is important. But for most of us, a healthy diet probably precludes the need to track these measurements.

● **Cut up 30 g portions of cheese** and measure out 30 g portions of nuts, then put one of each into snack bags. Now you have a handy snack at the ready.

● **Eat potatoes boiled with the skin still on.** The effect of potatoes on blood sugar depends on how the potatoes are prepared. There's no need to avoid them completely, but keep your portion size modest. Also, new potatoes tend to have fewer simple carbs than other types of potatoes.

▮▮▶ **Never let yourself get too hungry.** Eat every 3 to 5 waking hours, and only until you're satisfied but not stuffed. You should never reach the point where you feel ravenous. Not only is that a recipe for overeating, but your body will want sugary, quick-to-digest "bad" carbs to satiate your need for fuel quickly.

● **Instead of eggs and bacon, try a bowl of oatmeal.** Sweeten it with sugar-free sweetener or sugar-free granola.

● **At the movie theatre, skip the popcorn.** Popcorn isn't a bad food – it contains useful fibre, for example. But it does happen to be a simple carb with little other nutritional value and, when bought at the theatre, it's often drowning in salt and fat. Better snacks are small bags of nuts or seeds and fresh or dried fruit. Just take them into the theatre with you.

Oatmeal is a tasty high-fibre way to start the day.

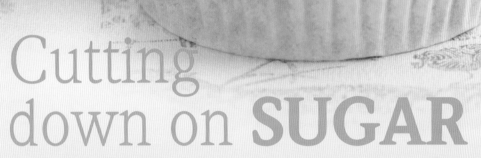

Cutting down on SUGAR

Canada is drowning in sugar. And it is getting worse. Although not all of us take sugar in our coffee, and we sprinkle less on our cereals, we are actually consuming more, hidden away in processed foods, leading to weight problems and obesity. Even worse, as sugary foods often replace more healthy foods, nutrition experts say the influx of sweets indirectly contributes to diseases such as osteoporosis, heart disease and cancer – all of which are directly affected by what we eat. In this third chapter on carbohydrates, there's advice on getting your sugar consumption down to healthy levels.

20 WAYS TO GET RID OF THE SWEET STUFF

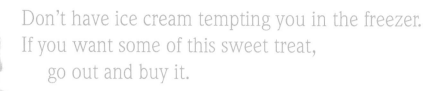

Don't have ice cream tempting you in the freezer.
If you want some of this sweet treat,
go out and buy it.

● **Cut down slowly.** Forget going cold turkey. Therein lies failure. Instead, if you normally have two chocolate bars a day, cut down to one. Then, next week, have one every other day. The following week, have one every three days, until you're down to just one a week. If you normally take 2 teaspoons of sugar in your coffee, use the same routine, cutting down gradually to $1/2$ teaspoon. Eventually, get to the point where you're using artificial sweetener if you still need the sweet taste. The more sugar you eat, the more you'll crave. So cutting down slowly is the best way to tame a sweet tooth gone wild.

● **Choose sugar-free and reduced-sugar alternatives** to foods such as baked beans, ketchup and cereals, when available.

● **Go half and half.** Mix half standard soft drink with half diet version; half sweetened yogourt with half plain yogourt; half a glass of juice with half a glass of soda water. Do this for two weeks, then cut back to a quarter sweetened to three-quarters unsweetened. Continue until you're taking only the unsweetened version.

● **Grant yourself a daily sugar "quota,"** and use it on the foods where it matters most. For the majority of us, that means desserts. Don't waste it on dressings, spreads, breakfast cereals and soft drinks. Not only will this reduce your sugar intake in a day, but it will help you to lose your sweet tooth. The more sugar you eat, the less sensitive your taste buds seem to become, so you want more. Train your taste buds to become accustomed to less and you'll be satisfied with less.

▐▐▐➤**Establish rules about dessert.** For instance, have dessert only after dinner, never after lunch. Or eat dessert only on odd days of the month, or just at weekends or in restaurants. If you have a long tradition of daily desserts, then make it your rule to have raw fruit at least half of the time.

● **Similarly, establish rules about ice cream.** A tub of ice cream in the freezer is temptation defined. A recommended rule: no ice cream kept at home. Ice cream should always be a treat worth travelling for.

▐▐▐➤**Remember these code words found on ingredient lists.** The only way to know if the processed food you're buying contains sugar is to know its many aliases or other forms. Here are the common ones: brown sugar, corn syrup, dextrin,

2 second QUIZ

An apple or sugar-free apple sauce?
ANSWER: **AN APPLE.**

You'll get all the nutrients of the apple sauce, but you'll also get the added fibre kick from the skin of the apple, which is removed before the apple sauce is made.

dextrose, fructose, fruit juice concentrate, high-fructose corn syrup, galactose, glucose, honey, hydrogenated starch, invert sugar, maltose, lactose, mannitol, maple syrup, molasses, polyols, raw sugar, sorghum, sucrose, turbinado sugar.

● **Try xylitol.** Xylitol is a natural sweetener as well as a sugar substitute, which is found in fruits such as strawberries, pears and plums. It is very like sugar in appearance, so is often added by manufacturers to candies and chewing gums, as well as to medicated syrups and some mouthwashes and toothpastes. It's safe for those with diabetes and it actually improves the quality of your teeth, as well as having fibre-like health benefits. Beware, though: eating large quantities of xylitol may have a laxative effect.

● **Look for hidden sources of sugar.** Cough syrups, chewing gum, mints, tomato sauce, baked beans and cold meats often contain sugar. Even some prescription medicines contain sugar. For a week, be particularly vigilant and scan every possible food label. Make a mental note of what you discover.

● **If you must eat candies, eat them with meals.** The other foods will help to increase salivary flow, thus clearing the sugary foods from your mouth faster and helping prevent cavities. Of course, this does nothing for the calories you're imbibing and won't affect your weight, but at least you'll have a healthier mouth.

● **Seek out substitutes.** With saccharin, aspartame, acesulfame potassium and sucralose all commercially available, you can still get the sweetness of sugar without the calories. These sweeteners can be particularly useful as part of a diabetic diet.

In PERSPECTIVE

Corn syrup
Ask people what they think of when they hear the word "sweet," and chances are they'll reply "sugar." But since its arrival in the marketplace in 1966, the real story in the sweetness world has been corn syrup, to the point that some newspapers and magazines are now declaring this alternative sweetener to be the number one evil in our diets. High-fructose corn syrup is generally cheaper and easier to refine than granulated sugar. So, increasingly, processed-food companies have been switching to corn syrup to add sweetness to their products, especially in soft drinks and juices. That would have been the end of the story, except for recent research results which suggest that the human body processes corn syrup differently from sugar.

According to the studies, when the body processes sugar, it triggers the production of a chemical that signals fullness to your brain, and also prevents the release of a chemical that indicates hunger. But when scientists monitored how the body processes corn syrup, the worst-case scenario seemed to have occurred: the hunger chemical wasn't affected, and the fullness chemical was suppressed. In short, corn syrup, in theory, makes you hungrier.

Is this true? Doctors are debating the point. Many believe that the issue is merely that calories consumed as liquid are less filling than calories from solid food, independent of the form of the calories.

Whatever the case, corn syrup is a big issue for anyone trying to eat healthily. It is a huge source of empty calories that mess with your body's chemistry. So fight back, starting with any drinks that you buy. If corn syrup is one of the main ingredients in a drink, put it back.

● **Substitute apple sauce or puréed prunes for half the sugar in recipes.** You can also use them in place of the fat in the recipe.

☺ **Choose the right breakfast cereal.** Many are full of sugar. You want one with less than 8 g of sugar per serving or, preferably, one that is unsweetened altogether. Use diced fruit instead to sweeten your cereal.

Dip fresh strawberries in a low-fat chocolate sauce for a decadent treat.

cases, it's just not needed. Try the recipe without the sugar first. If you think it needs sugar after tasting, you can always add it, but don't do it automatically.

● **Get your chocolate in small doses.** Dip fresh strawberries into low-fat chocolate sauce, scatter chocolate sprinkles over your plain yogourt or eat a mini-piece of dark chocolate – freeze it so that it lasts longer in your mouth. Think rich and decadent but in tiny portions.

● **Watch out for mixed alcoholic drinks.** Have you ever stopped to think about the sugar quotient of a cosmopolitan? How about a margarita or mai tai? Drink mixers and many alcoholic beverages are absolutely thick with sugar. Stick with beer, wine or, if you prefer spirits, mix them only with unsweetened soda water or drink them straight. Of course, a glass of soda water with lime will also do just fine.

☆ **Go for a walk when you crave sweetness.** Studies find that athletes' preference for sweetened foods declines after exercise. Instead, they then prefer salty foods.

● **Choose fat-free if you must have sweet foods.** Studies find that many sweet foods, such as doughnuts, muffins, ice cream and so on, are also high in fat, more than doubling the calorie load. When you do indulge in sweet foods, choose fat-free options, so you get the full flavour of a favourite food with none of the calories from the added fat.

● **If you're having a hard time cutting back on soft drinks or juices,** try having a glass of iced water or soda water every other time you reach for a drink.

● **Don't skip meals.** Are you too busy to eat? When you go without breakfast, lunch or dinner, your blood sugar levels drop, and that propels you towards high-sugar (often convenience) foods to quell your cravings.

● **Don't add sugar to foods.** Many everyday recipes – including some for vegetables, soups, casseroles and sauces – call for sugar to add sweetness. In most

2 second QUIZ

Brown sugar or white sugar?
ANSWER: **NEITHER.**

They're both sugar. Neither has any nutritional benefit or is any better than the other. Here's a case where the brown colour does not imply a healthier version.

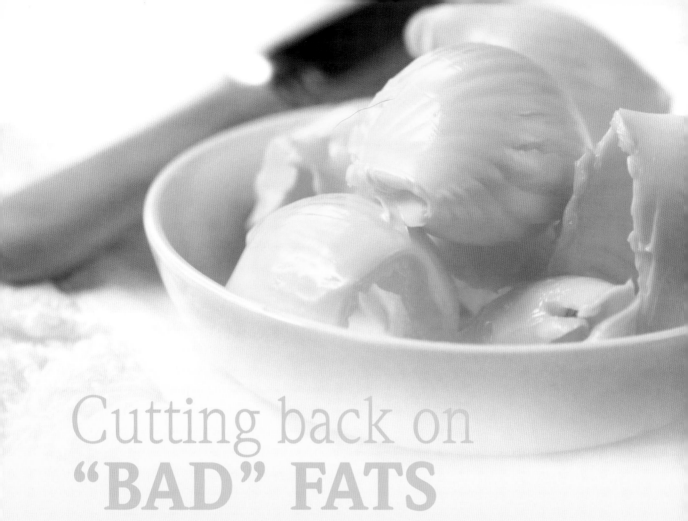

Cutting back on "BAD" FATS

We've come a long way from the days when all fat was bad. Today, researchers have identified "good" fats (monounsaturated and polyunsaturated) and "bad" fats (saturated and trans fats). So we can now eat certain fats and still be perfectly healthy. The down side? You have to be conscious of four types of fats. But there's an easy way to work it out: basically, if a fat is solid at room temperature – animal fats, butter, lard – chances are it's a bad fat. The good fats are usually found in fish and plant oils, but even they have their limits. All fats provide your body with 9 calories per gram, more than twice as much as proteins or carbohydrates. For good health, keep your total fat intake to 30 per cent of calories or less and your saturated fats to less than 10 per cent. Trans fats? Keep them to zero.

27 WAYS TO GET LEAN THE RIGHT WAY

Get a taste for 2% milk before moving onto skim.

✩ **Here's the easiest first: choose reduced-fat and low-fat products rather than standard.** Do not accept the argument that reduced-fat and low-fat versions don't taste as good. It's not true. Low-fat versions may lack some of the flavour you or your family are used to, but after a week or two, you'll stop noticing the subtle decline in richness. Here are the places to start:

● Milk: you needn't jump all the way to skimmed; use 2% as a stepping stone from whole milk, but don't stop there – 35 per cent of the calories still come from fat in 2% milk.

● Ice cream: most "light" versions taste as rich and creamy as the full-fat versions.

● Yogourt: given that most people eat their yogourt flavoured, it's hard to notice the difference between standard and low-fat or fat-free versions.

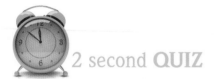

2 second QUIZ

Burger King Tendergrill BLT Salad or Original Chicken Sandwich?
ANSWER: **TENDERGRILL BLT SALAD.**

The Tendergrill BLT Salad has 23 g of fat, with 10 g of saturated fat. The Original Chicken Sandwich has 43 g of fat, with 8 g of saturated fat. What's more alarming is that adding balsamic vinaigrette to the salad accounts for another 17 g of fat. Ordering the sandwich without mayonnaise will removes 23 g of fat. So while neither is particularly healthy, avoid the mayonnaise with the Original Chicken Sandwich, and the balsamic vinaigrette with the Tendergrill BLT Salad.

● Ground beef: don't think that buying fatty ground beef and pouring off the grease makes it healthy. Much of the fat is bound in with the meat. Buy extra-lean ground – but bear in mind, even that can contain up to 10 per cent fat, so keep portions modest and bulk it out with vegetables or beans.

● Cheese: choose reduced-fat or low-fat, particularly with mozzarella cheese for pizza. Low-fat versions still have all the taste and texture you could want.

● **Keep your spreads soft.** Choose soft margarines and leave your butter out of the fridge. The softer the spread, the less you'll use on your bread or toast, which means you'll be eating less fat.

● **Choose spreads wisely.** One typically thinks that a spread will be tasty only if it is of the full-fat variety. But there are many low-fat options that are bursting with flavour, and as is always the case when one changes one food for another, it sometimes takes a few tries before one grows accustomed to the slightly different taste. Tasty options include low-fat cream cheese or hummus.

▶ Buy a pretty bottle, fill it with olive oil, then top it with a pourer. Now keep it in plain view and use it for everything except frying (as olive oil burns at lower temperatures than other oils; for frying canola oil is a healthy alternative). Olive oil is the best oil to use because it contains high amounts of monounsaturated fats and low amounts of saturated fats (all oils contain a mixture of the three: mono, poly and saturated; the key is the ratio). Buy the deepest green, extra virgin olive oil you can find – the darker the colour, the greater the amount of phytonutrients, potent little plant-based cancer fighters.

● If you can't go without your butter, mix it with olive oil. Let a thick slice of butter (about 100 g) soften at room temperature, then beat the butter smooth, before slowly beating in between 3 and 7 Tbsp (50 and 100 ml) of olive oil. This cuts the amount of saturated fat significantly while adding plenty of healthy monounsaturated fat.

● Eat the right meats. Of course, meat is one of the primary forms of saturated fat. But meat – whether red or white – is also an excellent source of protein and trace minerals such as zinc and iron. The key is choosing lean cuts of meat and trimming off visible fat before cooking.

● Don't be taken in by the "other white meat" slogan. Put simply, lean chicken is much less fatty than lean pork. A 100 g serving of broiled chicken breast (no skin) provides 140 calories, 27 from fat, and only one-third of that fat is saturated. The same serving of roasted

Healthy INVESTMENT

A non-stick pan
In the old days, you needed lots of butter and oil in order to keep your meats and veggies from sticking to the pan. A non-stick pan eliminates all that. Hint: make sure the pan is hot before adding the oil. This creates a barrier between the pan and the food, eliminating any possibility of sticking. Another great option: invest in a panini maker for grilled sandwiches (see page 59).

lean pork loin delivers 275 calories, 189 of them from fat, half of which is saturated. To top it off, the chicken has 6 more grams of protein than the pork.

☺ Cook steak with other ingredients. The goal is to stop eating great slabs of steak. Instead, slice the raw beef and sauté it with peppers and onions, fajita-style. Or cook strips of steak in a wok with plenty of vegetables. Or top a crunchy, large salad with steak slices. Or make shish kebab with steak cubes and chunks of vegetable. Why? Because you almost always eat less meat when you've prepared it as part of a nicely integrated dish. Keep the whole steak just for very special occasions.

● Eat an exotic meat occasionally. How about emu, venison, wild boar or ostrich? All have less than 1 g of saturated fat per 100 g serving, are super-rich in protein and taste extremely good.

● Substitute tofu for meat once a week. Tofu is high in protein, but has little fat.

● Be wary of recipes that allow starches and veggies to absorb fat. Many classic winter dishes have potatoes, carrots, turnips and other vegetables roasting slowly with chicken, beef, lamb or pork.

In PERSPECTIVE

The ins and outs of fat

Confused about fat? Don't be. It's really quite simple. There are three naturally occurring types of fat: monounsaturated, polyunsaturated and saturated. A fourth type of fat – "trans fats" – is largely man-made. Here's what you need to know about each one, minus all the science.

● **Monounsaturated fat.** This should take the lead in your diet (at least, as far as fat is concerned). These fats star in the so-called Mediterranean diet, proven to lower cholesterol and reduce heart-disease risk. A primary source is olive oil. Other good sources include canola oil, seeds, nuts and avocados.

● **Polyunsaturated fat.** This form of fat is prevalent in vegetable oils, nuts, fish and some leafy green vegetables. There are two main types: omega-6s, which we tend to get plenty of through vegetable oils, and omega-3s, found primarily in fish and certain seeds, which we rarely get enough of. Focus on increasing the amount of omega-3 fatty acids in your diet while reducing the amount of omega-6s.

● **Saturated fat.** This form of fat is found in the highest amounts in animal products, and in palm and coconut oil. Saturated fat raises levels of "bad" LDL cholesterol, and can increase your heart-disease risk. In fact, swapping just 5 per cent of your overall calories from saturated to unsaturated fats could slash your risk of a fatal heart attack by 42 per cent.

● **Trans fats.** Trans fats are created when polyunsaturated fats are whipped with hydrogen to make them solid at room temperature. They not only increase LDL levels, but can decrease HDL levels, plus they've been implicated in heart disease and breast cancer. When it comes to trans fat, no level is safe, yet they're everywhere you find processed foods. But you can now find many trans fat-free options; look for key words on labels (see page 109) to know what to avoid.

Delicious, yes. But all those veggies are soaking up a whole lot of fat that's dripped off the meat. Either find ways to cook the vegetables separately, or wait until you've skimmed the fat from the meat juices before adding in the veg.

● **Use skimmed evaporated milk** in place of cream for cream-based soups and other recipes.

☺ **Follow a simple rule:** if you can plainly see fat on your food, remove it. So:
● If there's fat on the meat, trim it off.
● If there's skin on the chicken, remove it.
● If there's oil pooling on the top of the pizza, soak it up with a paper towel.
● If there's leftover dressing at the bottom of your salad, pour it off.
● If there's a pool of fatty juice under a piece of cooked meat, drain it.
● If there's fat at the top of a bowl of stew or soup, skim it off.

● **Cook flavour into breads, batters, cakes, buns and other carb-based foods** so you don't need to add butter. For example, add herbs to breads; blueberries to pancakes; nuts and bananas to buns and cakes. Grain-filled foods are often the ones you want to butter, but if you make them more flavourful, you avoid the urge.

● **Put salsa on your baked potato, not butter or sour cream.** You not only skip the fat, but add in a healthy, low-cal serving of vegetables.

● **Mist your fat.** Use an olive oil spray to coat pans and foods. You'll use much less, and still get the great taste.

☆ **Sauté foods in broth, wine or even juice.** These are just a few of the alternatives to filling the bottom of your cookware with calorie-dense oils.

● **Watch out for trans fats in unexpected places.** Start with peanut butter, cookies, energy bars, frozen pizza and cereal. Even foods you might think of as health foods – such as granola – often carry large amounts of trans fats.

● **Put soups and stews in the fridge overnight.** Voilà! The next morning you can skim the congealed fat off the top before reheating the dish.

● **Grate your cheese.** You'll use less on pasta dishes, sandwiches, etc., if it's grated rather than sliced.

● **Order pizza without the fat.** Sausage and pepperoni are very high in fats, as is full-fat mozzarella. The answer? As mentioned, soak up the excess grease on the top of the pizza, order vegetables on top, ask for low-fat cheese and sometimes order a cheeseless tomato pizza. Never tried one? You are in for a surprise. A vegetable pizza can have 25 per cent fewer calories and about 50 per cent less fat and saturated fat than a meat pizza.

● **Stick to mustard, ketchup and other non-creamy condiments** in place of mayonnaise and tartar sauce. Mayonnaise is particularly dense with fat. Aim to have it only in small doses.

● **Purée a cooked potato and an onion** to thicken soups instead of cream. This also adds extra flavour.

● **Use avocados in place of butter and cream.** There's a reason these green fruits are called butterfruit in Mexico – they mash up into the same creamy texture as butter. Try them in soups as a thickening agent, and in mashed potatoes to provide a creamier texture. Interestingly, avocados and olives are the only two fruits high in fat – yet both are rich in heart-healthy monounsaturated fat.

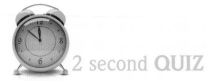

2 second **QUIZ**

Green olives or black olives
ANSWER: **GREEN OLIVES.**

Green olives haven't ripened fully, so they contain roughly half the fat levels that they would have achieved had they ripened and blackened.

⭐ **Eat a high-fibre cereal for breakfast.** Fibre fills you up and seems to reduce your interest in fatty foods. American researchers found that men who ate two daily servings of cereal, each containing 7 g of fibre, reduced their average total fat intake from 91 to 82 g a day, and their saturated fat intake to less than 10 per cent of calories.

● **Try soy milk on your cereal.** Be sure to look for brands with added calcium. You can also substitute soy milk in baking and other recipes.

● **Look for the key words on labels.** Note the serving size, grams of fat and how much of it is saturated.

▶ **Be fast-food savvy.** The amount of fat in a fast-food meal can be stunning. The fries, the burgers, the "special sauces," even the salads swimming in dressings may be your worst dietary enemy. Go to the website of each fast-food chain you frequent, and look at the nutritional information on the foods you prefer. After the shock wears off, make a commitment to healthier choices.

Liven up your foods with mustard or ketchup, not mayonnaise or tartar sauce.

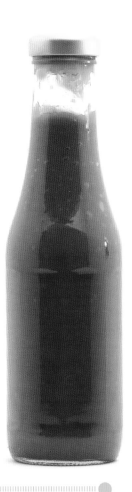

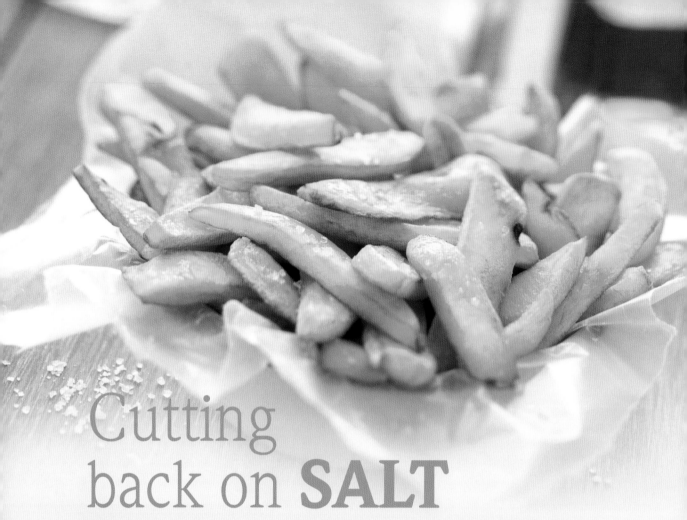

Cutting back on **SALT**

Ask anyone about salt and they'll tell you that too much is bad for you. They're right. Salt is one part sodium and one part chloride, and although our bodies don't produce sodium, it is an essential nutrient that regulates blood pressure and nerve function. Health Canada advises an adequate daily intake of 1,500 mg for adults and a tolerable upper limit of 2,300 mg. Unfortunately the average Canadian consumes more than 3,100 mg of sodium daily, which can lead to hypertension. Not only that, a high-salt diet can have other adverse effects such as osteoporosis, stomach cancer and obesity, as well as exacerbating asthma symptoms. So try these tips to make food taste great without all that shaking going on.

17 WAYS TO EAT WELL WITHOUT IT

● **Invest in a pepper mill.** Use freshly ground black pepper instead of salt, or look out for lemon pepper, a seasoning that adds wonderful flavour, not salt, to foods.

● **Mix low-salt foods with standard foods** to start you on the path to reducing your salt intake. For instance, mix unsalted peanuts with salted. Slowly increase the amount of the salt-free product as you decrease the amount of the salted until you're eating only the salt-free version.

● **Say no to sports drinks.** Research does indicate that endurance athletes need higher levels of salt and far more to drink than everyday folk. Sports drinks deliver both – they are rich in salt, which not only provides the necessary sodium but also stokes continued thirst. For the rest of us, the extra salt provides no benefit at all. Even if you exercise regularly, unless you are testing your body's physical limits for extended periods, water should be fine to quench your thirst.

● **Keep your table salt in a small bowl,** and use a tiny spoon or a pinch of your fingers to season your food. You'll find that you use far less of it. Cover it with a snug lid or some plastic wrap to keep it dry (and make it less accessible).

● **Put a big X on your calendar for six weeks from today.** Unlike our preference for sugar, which we're born with, salt is an acquired taste, learned from habit. So it takes time to "unlearn" your preference – about six weeks, to be exact. Slowly reduce your intake of salt between now and then, focusing on food categories where the salt will be missed the least, such as cereals, breads and dessert items. As long as you know you aren't going to stop wanting salty food overnight, you won't get discouraged.

READING LABELS

Food manufacturers are obligated by law to indicate the amount of sodium in prepackaged foods sold in Canada. Listed on the nutrition facts label is the number of milligrams of sodium in the product, or in a serving of the product. The label also provides a percentage of the daily value for sodium. This makes it easy to quickly determine if a product (or a serving of it) has a small amount of sodium – or too much.

FREE, LOW AND REDUCED

Apart from reading the nutrition facts label, another quick and easy method to determine how much sodium is in a food product, is to take note of ones labelled "salt-free," "low in sodium" or "reduced in sodium."
● **Salt-free** is less than 5 mg of sodium per serving.
● **Low in sodium** is 140 mg or less of sodium per serving.
● **Reduced in sodium** is at least 25 per cent less sodium than the regular product.

Most of us don't need the higher levels of salt found in sports drinks. Water is the best thirst-quencher.

Know your GARLIC

The hot, strong taste of fresh garlic gives food a zing no amount of salt can equal. Buy cloves in bulk and store in a cool, dark place. To get the most health benefits out of your garlic:
- Always peel it first. Otherwise, some of the disease-preventing compounds might not form.
- Give it a break after cutting or crushing it. Leave it there on the cutting board for about 10 minutes to allow the health-promoting compounds to form.
- To get rid of garlic breath, chew on fresh parsley, mint or lemon or orange peel, and use lemon juice to get the odour off your hands.

● **Look out for non-salt sources of sodium.** Here's what to beware of on food labels: sodium, Na, monosodium glutamate or MSG, sodium citrate, baking soda and baking powder. They're all forms of – that's right, you guessed it – sodium.

● **Replace salt in the salt shaker with a salt-free mixture.** This way you can still use the shaker, but eliminate the salt. Mix garlic powder, black pepper, onion powder and oregano together. Grind the mix fine enough for it to come out of the shaker's holes, or buy a Parmesan cheese shaker from a kitchen-supply store. Another tasty mixture is garlic, onion and chili powder, cumin, dried oregano and a touch of red pepper flakes.

● **Choose no-added-sugar-and-salt cans of veggies and beans.** Look for varieties that contain no additional sugar and salt when picking canned foods such as kidney beans, chickpeas and corn. If you can't find beans packed in water, rinsing them thoroughly before use will help to remove some of the salt.

● **Watch out for salty condiments and nibbles.** Capers, pickles and olives are packed with salt. In fact, the pickling and brining processes used to make foods such as these primarily involve soaking them in a solution dense with salt.

☆ **Skip meat that's been dried or cured.** This includes salami, corned beef, prosciutto, ham and dried sausages. Each is laden with salt, which is used to draw out the liquid and preserve the meat. At lunchtime, pick turkey instead.

● **Brush off visible salt.** For instance, on salted bagels or chips.

☺ **Use the calories-to-salt formula.** To meet, or at least approximate, the recommended salt intake requires taking in no more milligrams of sodium than calories. So if a food has fewer milligrams of sodium per serving than calories, you'll hit the target. If it has more sodium than calories, you'll find it much harder to remain within recommended daily limits.

● **Substitute citrus juice such as orange, lemon or lime for salt in salad dressings.** That way your dressing will have extra zing without the salt.

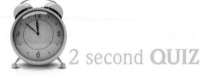

2 second QUIZ

Tomatoes or a V8?
ANSWER: **TOMATOES.**

A 340 ml can of V8 contains a rich assortment of healthy vegetables, including carrots, celery, beets, spinach and watercress. But it also boasts 710 mg of sodium. A fresh tomato has between 1 and 14 mg.

● **Watch out for cereals.** Much of the salt that we eat comes from cereal and cereal products (including bread). To reduce your intake:

● If toast is for breakfast, choose breads with a small amount of sodium (check the nutritional facts label).

● Pick breakfast cereals with no added salt, for example, oatmeal, Shredded Wheat, puffed-wheat cereals and granola with no added salt.

● **Check your medicines for salt.** You might not think that you'd find salt in your drugs, but you could be wrong. Particular culprits in your medicine cabinet include soluble tablets, antacids, cough medicines, pain relievers and laxatives. If you find high salt levels, talk to your doctor about alternatives.

● **Make your own salt-free salad dressing.** Mix $^3/_4$ cup (200 ml) of olive oil, $^1/_3$ cup (75 ml) of balsamic vinegar,

Healthy INVESTMENT

Garlic peeler and garlic crusher

These two gadgets make using fresh garlic so much easier. A garlic peeler – really, a small plastic tube – takes the work and mess out of peeling garlic. Just put a whole garlic clove inside the tube and roll it back and forth, pressing firmly. Voilà! A naked clove, ready for your garlic crusher.

1 pinch of sugar and 2 crushed garlic cloves in a bowl. Blend until emulsified. This delicious dressing keeps in the refrigerator for a month. Just remove it an hour before serving so that it can liquefy.

● **Go for chips rather than pretzels –** if salt is your main concern. Pretzels can have four times the salt of potato chips or tortilla chips. That's because chips get much of their flavour from being cooked in oil, making them fattier and higher in calories. Baked pretzels contain far less fat, so much of the flavour comes from salt.

The problem with PROCESSED

Manufacturers of processed foods pile on the salt to help create big, attractive flavours. Here are examples of what happens to "real" food once manufacturers get their hands on it:

NATURAL FOOD	SODIUM	PROCESSED FOOD	SODIUM
Baked potato	8 mg	Potato chips, about 110 g	600 mg
		Large order of fries	350 mg
		Instant mashed potatoes	770 mg
		Potatoes au gratin	355 mg
Fresh corn-on-the-cob	15 mg	Corn chips, 200 g bag	630 mg
		Cornflakes	230 mg
Fresh broccoli	27 mg	Frozen broccoli and cheese sauce	330 mg
		Canned cream of broccoli soup	770 mg
Brown rice	120 mg	Rice and sauce	900 mg

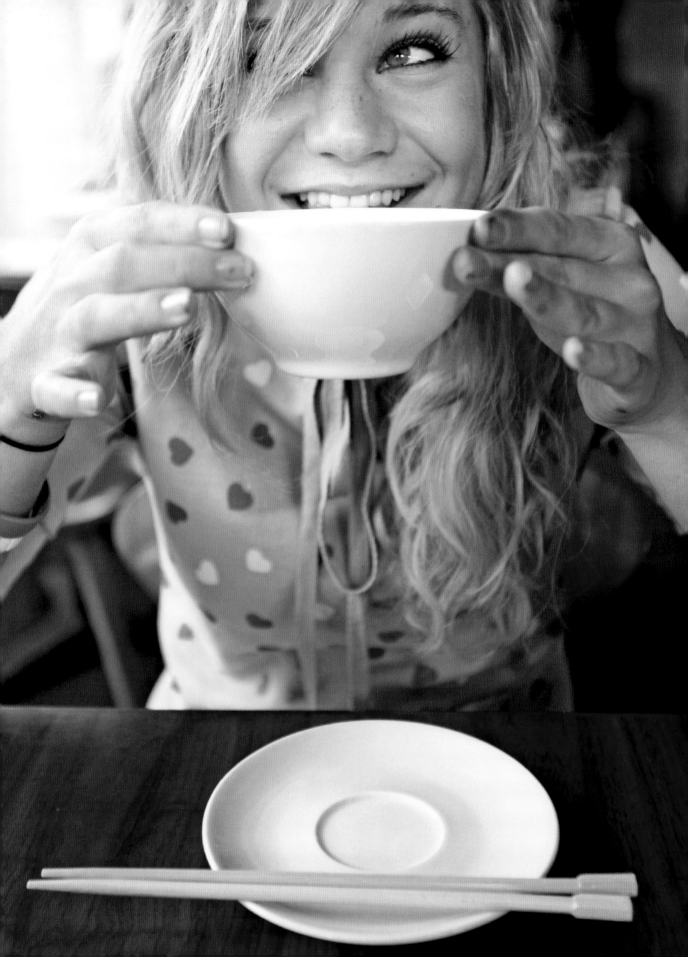

part 3

STEALTH HEALTHY DINING OUT

Eating healthily at home is an excellent first step. But for all-round healthy eating, you need to control what you eat when you're not at home. Here's the best advice.

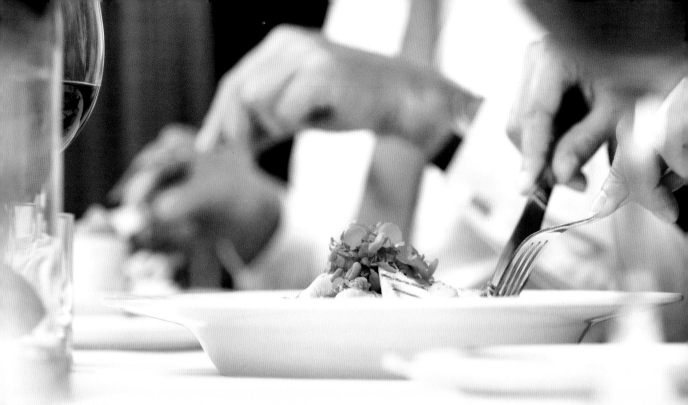

Eating in
RESTAURANTS

Suddenly it seems that chain restaurants such as Subway, Tim Hortons and Burger King are everywhere you look. In fact, there are thousands of restaurants in Canada today, and the number continues to grow. But as we eat out more often, many of us would welcome clear nutritional information about what we're eating. The good news: things are starting to change for the healthier. And whether you're dining out at a major national chain or a locally owned family restaurant, following a few of these health-boosting tips will guarantee you a pleasant meal while keeping your health goals firmly in view.

25 IDEAS FOR EATING WELL
WHEN EATING OUT

Above all else, be assertive. Dining out is no time to be meek. Assert yourself by requesting changes to what's on the menu. For instance, if an item is fried, ask to have it grilled. If it comes with fries, request a side order of veggies instead. Ask for a smaller portion of the meat and a larger portion of the salad; for salad instead of coleslaw; a baked potato instead of fried. Just assume you can have the food prepared the way you want it. Very often, the restaurant will cooperate. In the tips that follow, you'll find more specific requests.

Ask your waiter to "triple the vegetables, please." Often a side order of vegetables in a restaurant is really just a garnish – a carrot and a forkful of peas. If that's the case where you're eating, ask for three or four times the normal serving of veggies, and offer to pay extra. This is a good way to get full, not fat.

Ask how the food was prepared; don't go by the menu. For instance, cholesterol-free does not mean fat-free; the dish could still be filled with calorie-dense oil. Neither does "light" necessarily mean no calories or fat.

Why not double up on starters? If there is a healthy selection of seafood and vegetable-based starters, consider skipping the main course and having two starters for your meal. Another tip: before you order, look around to see what other people are eating – if portion sizes look huge, going for two starters is a sensible option. Often, that is more than enough food to fill you up. And it will probably save you money.

Try to be the first to order. Studies show that people are often unduly influenced by their companions' choices

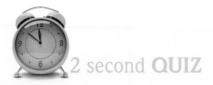

2 second **QUIZ**

Sirloin steak or rib-eye?
ANSWER: **SIRLOIN.**

A 300 g sirloin steak contains 325 calories and 13 g of fat, 6 of them saturated, compared to the 423 calories and 23 g of fat (12 of them saturated) found in the same size of rib-eye steak served in many restaurants.

when they eat out. If you order first you're not as likely to be tempted by the less healthy options on the menu.

Order a salad before choosing anything else on the menu. American scientists found that volunteers who ate a big salad packed with vegetables before the main course ate fewer calories overall than those who didn't have a first-course salad.

But remember: salads shouldn't be fatty. This is a vegetable course – keep it tasty but healthy. That means avoiding anything in a creamy sauce (coleslaw, pasta salads and potato salads), and skipping the bacon bits. Instead, fill up on the raw vegetables, treat yourself to a few well-drained marinated vegetables (artichoke hearts, red peppers or mushrooms) and, for a change, add in some fruit or nuts. Indeed, fruits such as mango, kiwi, cantaloupe and pear are often central to top-notch salads.

Watch the extras on vegetable salads. Even salads that include mostly raw vegetables are a problem if they're also full of cheese and meat. Take the typical Caesar salad in most restaurants – it usually comes with lots of cheese and mayonnaise in the dressing. Add in the fried croutons, and it can contain more

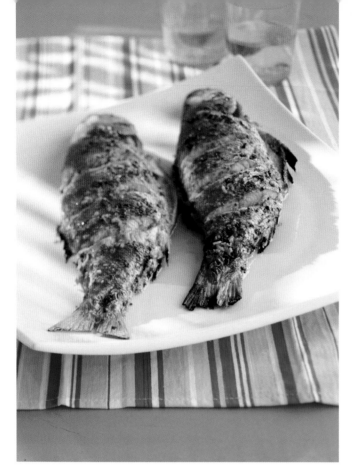

Have your fish any way but fried.

than 500 calories, with more than 35 g of fat. Italian antipasto salads are also a health challenge, with all their salami, spicy ham and cheese. Get the salad, but ask for vegetables only.

Do the fork dip. The best way to combine salad dressing with salad? Get your dressing on the side, in a small bowl. Dip your empty fork into the dressing, then skewer a forkful of salad. You'll be surprised at how this tastes just right, and how little dressing you'll use.

Top a baked potato with veggies from the salad bar. Or ask if you can have salsa – the ultimate potato topper, both in terms of flavour and health. Just avoid the butter and sour cream.

Check out the menu before you leave home. Most chain restaurants post their menus on their websites. You can decide before you even open the door what you're going to order. Conversely, if you don't see anything that's healthy, pick another restaurant.

Read between the lines. Any menu description that uses the words creamy, breaded, crisp, sauced or stuffed is likely to be full of hidden fats – much of it comprising saturated or even trans fats. Other words to beware of include: buttery, sautéed, pan-fried, au gratin, thermidor, Parmesan, cheese sauce, scalloped, as well as au lait and au fromage (with milk and with cheese).

Don't assume that ordering vegetarian will be the lower-calorie choice. It isn't always the case – avoid dishes containing lots of nuts and cheese, for example.

Ask the waiter to skip the bread basket. If you must have something to munch on while you wait for your meal, ask for a plate of raw vegetables or some breadsticks.

Avoid the fancy drinks. If you insist on ordering an alcoholic drink, forget the margaritas, piña coladas and other exotic mixed drinks. They include sugary additions that pile on the calories. Opt instead for a glass of wine, a light beer, a vodka and tonic or a simple martini.

Order fish. But make sure it's not fried. Fish is a good low-fat, low-salt option. Plus, you can order seafood cooked so many different ways – steamed, baked, barbecued, sautéed, blackened or grilled. Avoid any sauce, or ask for it on the side.

Drink water throughout the meal. It slows you down, helps you to enjoy the food more, and gets the message to your brain that you're full – before your plate is empty. If it doesn't come automatically, ask for a jug of water as you sit down.

Keep an eye on your wine glass refills. If you're drinking wine, don't allow the waiter to fill up your wine glass before it's empty. If your glass is constantly being topped up, it's impossible to keep track of how much you've had to drink.

Always dress up to go out, even if it's to an ordinary family restaurant. If you view eating out as an event or a treat, rather than as a way to get an everyday dinner, you won't eat out as often. And that's good from both a health and a cost point of view.

Skip the dessert. You can always have some sorbet or even a small piece of chocolate at home. That is much more healthy than a rich chocolate Black Forest cake or a mountain of ice cream topped by a second mountain of whipped cream. Plus, it will save you money.

Cuisine-specific advice

A perk of modern living is having so many restaurants to choose from. But with choice comes confusion. To help, here are tips for sensible eating at some of the most popular restaurant types.

Stealth healthy Chinese dining means you:
- Order fewer dishes than there are people at the table. Chinese starters are usually designed for sharing, not just for one person.
- Avoid the fried noodles. If the waiter plops them down on the table, ask him to take them away. If you get a packet with your soup, hand them back.
- Start with soup to fill you up.
- Avoid fried starters. So no spring rolls. And have dumplings steamed, not fried.
- Also opt for steamed rice, not fried. If the restaurant serves brown rice, go for it.
- Use the 2:1 ratio. Eat twice as much rice as main dish.
- Avoid menu items described as crispy, golden-brown or sweet-and-sour. They're all deep-fried.
- Choose dishes rich in vegetables and order at least one vegetarian starter.
- Always ask for the sauce on the side. Chinese restaurant chefs often stir-fry the main ingredients, then mix them together and ladle on the sauce. Get the sauce on the side and you'll be guaranteed to use far less.
- Eat with chopsticks. You'll get less of the high-calorie, high-salt sauce that way.

DEADLY SECRETS
of the restaurant trade

How do restaurants make their food taste so good? Here is the unhealthy truth:

- **BUTTER** In the soup. In the sauce. On the meat. On the vegetables. Butter is the easiest, quickest way to make dishes taste rich and wonderful.

- **OIL AND FAT** Another way to make foods taste richer is to use lots of oil (remember, oil is a fat). This is why fried foods taste good: they're sponges for the oil in which they're cooked. Then there's animal fat. Want to make anything taste better? Add bacon or other forms of pork fat – to vegetables, soups and mashed potatoes.

- **SALT** When you cook at home, you may shake in a little salt as you go. At a restaurant, it's poured in to give maximum flavour.

- **SWEETENERS** Ever have vegetables that tasted sweeter than a dessert? That's because the cook added lots of sugar.

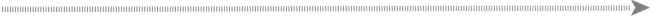

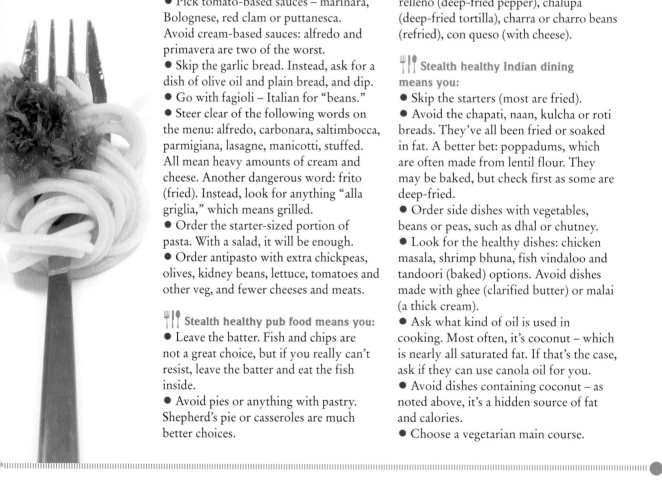

Stealth healthy Italian dining means you:

- Split and share. One order of pasta is usually enough for two people, especially if you also have a salad.
- Dine on pasta rather than pizza. Pizza dough is calorie-dense – about 275 calories per 100 g (without the cheese, sausage and pepperoni). A much better choice is pasta. A linguini puttanesca (olives, mushrooms, tomato sauce and fresh basil), arrabbiata (spicy tomato sauce) or vongole (clams with marinara sauce) takes you down to 600 or 700 calories per 450 g. You can increase the health benefits by ordering a side dish of fresh veggies or spinach and mixing it in with your pasta dish.
- Pick tomato-based sauces – marinara, Bolognese, red clam or puttanesca. Avoid cream-based sauces: alfredo and primavera are two of the worst.
- Skip the garlic bread. Instead, ask for a dish of olive oil and plain bread, and dip.
- Go with fagioli – Italian for "beans."
- Steer clear of the following words on the menu: alfredo, carbonara, saltimbocca, parmigiana, lasagne, manicotti, stuffed. All mean heavy amounts of cream and cheese. Another dangerous word: frito (fried). Instead, look for anything "alla griglia," which means grilled.
- Order the starter-sized portion of pasta. With a salad, it will be enough.
- Order antipasto with extra chickpeas, olives, kidney beans, lettuce, tomatoes and other veg, and fewer cheeses and meats.

Stealth healthy pub food means you:

- Leave the batter. Fish and chips are not a great choice, but if you really can't resist, leave the batter and eat the fish inside.
- Avoid pies or anything with pastry. Shepherd's pie or casseroles are much better choices.

Stealth healthy Mexican dining means you:

- Keep away from the fried tortilla chips. Instead, ask for a few soft tortillas to scoop up the healthy salsa and help you to get a couple of vegetable servings under your belt straight away.
- Pick beans to fill your burritos instead of beef or cheese.
- Choose fajitas. Not only can you fill up on the vegetables, but you can pick and choose how much cheese to add.
- Ask for black or pinto beans, not refried.
- Avoid the sour cream.
- Go for soft tacos, not hard tacos. Hard taco shells are fried; soft shells are baked.
- Avoid dishes with the following words in their names: chimichanga (fried burrito), relleno (deep-fried pepper), chalupa (deep-fried tortilla), charra or charro beans (refried), con queso (with cheese).

Stealth healthy Indian dining means you:

- Skip the starters (most are fried).
- Avoid the chapati, naan, kulcha or roti breads. They've all been fried or soaked in fat. A better bet: poppadums, which are often made from lentil flour. They may be baked, but check first as some are deep-fried.
- Order side dishes with vegetables, beans or peas, such as dhal or chutney.
- Look for the healthy dishes: chicken masala, shrimp bhuna, fish vindaloo and tandoori (baked) options. Avoid dishes made with ghee (clarified butter) or malai (a thick cream).
- Ask what kind of oil is used in cooking. Most often, it's coconut – which is nearly all saturated fat. If that's the case, ask if they can use canola oil for you.
- Avoid dishes containing coconut – as noted above, it's a hidden source of fat and calories.
- Choose a vegetarian main course.

Dine on pasta rather than pizza.

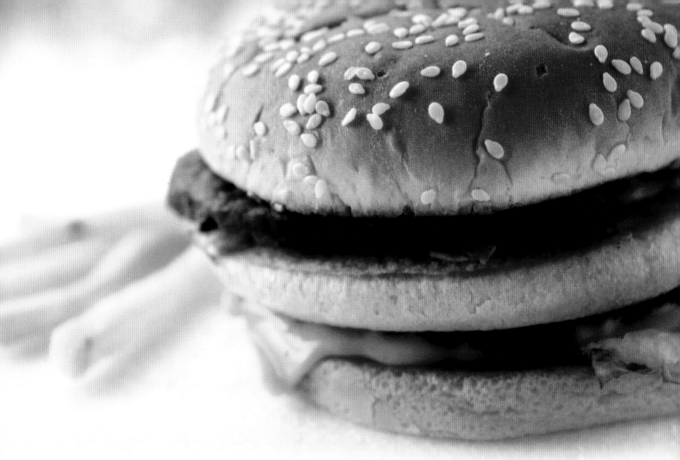

FAST food

Here in Canada we often eat fast food and takeout meals. Some are healthy, others less so; if you stick to double cheeseburgers, large fries and soft drinks, you could see your waistline expand rapidly and your cholesterol levels soar. But something has been happening to fast-food restaurants. As we have become more concerned about what we eat, the KFCs, McDonald's, Burger Kings and many others have taken notice. They've added salads that actually fill you up, reduced serving sizes and introduced more healthy dishes. Here's how to take advantage of these changes, and how to choose the best dishes from some of Canada's many fast-food restaurants.

17 WAYS TO MAKE THE RIGHT CHOICE

● **Go for the salad, minus the fried toppings.** Although most fast-food restaurants offer decent-sized salads these days, if you top them with fried chicken, cheese and all of the dressing, you will end up with as much artery-clogging saturated fat and calories as if you'd had the double-cheeseburger and fries. Instead, choose grilled or roasted chicken as your protein source, skip the croutons and ask for the low-fat dressing – then use only half.

● **Skip the cheese.** Craving a burger? That's OK – just get a plain burger without the cheese. For instance, at McDonald's that saves you 50 calories, 40 of them from fat, and 2.5 g of saturated fat.

☺ **Ask for extra onions, lettuce and tomato.** Whatever sandwich you choose, it'll now be healthier, crunchier and more filling. And it ticks off one more serving of vegetables from your day's quota.

● **Order water.** Or if you must have a soft drink, choose the diet version. A large coke contains 320 calories. Making this one change might save you the same number of calories as the meal you're about to eat.

☆ **Always say no to the "special" sauce.** Many are just dressed-up mayonnaise,

A tasty, filling potato, in its jacket, is a great fibre provider.

and thus overflowing with fat and calories. The best topping for your chicken, fish or burger? Mustard (few calories, lots of flavour). The second best? Ketchup (no fat, but a fair amount of sweetener). Other good choices: olive oil and vinegar (in moderation), spicy sauces, red pepper sauce.

● **Do not supersize.** Ever. The regular meals are large enough, and high enough in calories and fat that you should never add more. If possible, fill up on some veggies before hitting the restaurant. You will likely find that your desire for the massive burger is not quite what it was.

● **In fact, order a child's meal.** A small burger, a small fries and an orange juice is a surprisingly filling meal for most adults, and has many fewer calories than the adult version. Plus, you get a free toy!

☺ **Give sweet-and-sour dishes a wide berth.** These meals should be a rare treat – one portion may contain as much as 8 teaspoons of sugar. That includes lemon chicken and some spicy beef dishes. Chicken with cashew nuts or peppers, stir-fried noodles and seafood dishes are all healthier, especially if you have boiled rice or noodles rather than egg fried rice.

● **Look for ways to sneak in fibre.** That means a baked potato (with skin on) and chili (no cheese), bean burritos and tacos instead of meat (a bean burrito has 12 g of fibre – roughly half your daily needs met) and baked beans and corn on the cob (without butter) as side (or main) dishes.

● **Stay away from coconut milk.** Some cuisines, such as Thai, use a lot of coconut milk as a base, which is high in saturated fat. You'll leave the restaurant healthier if you opt to start with a soup such as tom yam, beef or chicken satay or Thai fish cakes, and follow up with a chicken, pork or fish-based noodle dish. Thai menus often feature lots of delicious vegetarian dishes too, as well as salads.

● **Try a drier style of curry.** Some of the drier Indian dishes, such as tandoori, tikka and bhuna, are usually the lower-fat options on the menu. Other healthier choices include vegetable and shellfish-based curry dishes such as sag aloo (spinach and potato) and mutter paneer (peas with cheese) and baltis. It goes without saying, avoid anything deep-fried.

☺ **Go for skinless chicken,** particularly when you're eating at KFC. Ditch the skin on a chicken thigh and you'll save 160 calories and 12 g of fat.

☆ **Choose chicken, not lamb.** Research showed that of nine types of takeout foods tested, a lamb kebab was the outright loser. These kebabs were found to contain far more trans fats than any other takeout meal. If you want a kebab, choose chicken instead, and pile on the salad.

● **Look for the words "grilled," "baked" or "chargrilled."** If something's cooked that way, it's not fried – and you'll automatically be reaping some savings in terms of fat and calories.

Healthy **INVESTMENT**

A box of cereal bars
Try the crunchy type – more substantial and pleasing to eat – and splash out on a whole box, which could cost the same as a large combo meal at a fast-food restaurant. Keep them in the car as a preventive measure against impulse visits to fast-food places. Next time your stomach growls when you're driving down a takeout-filled street, have a granola bar instead. Then have a healthy meal at home.

● **Have an apple, banana or fat-free yogourt,** or some other healthy snack an hour before you go for your meal. That way you won't arrive starving.

☺ **Make a supermarket your fast-food restaurant.** Run in, grab a piece or two of fruit, some yogourt, an energy bar, a salad at the salad bar, a turkey sandwich at the deli counter, and you'll be out via the express check-out with breakfast, lunch and snacks in 10 minutes.

● **Avoid processed or cured meats.** That includes hot dogs, salami and ham. These heavily processed meats are often full of fat, salt, chemical additives and, in some cases, sugar. At a deli or a sandwich shop, go for turkey breast, chicken breast or roast beef instead.

Reminder

 Fast results
These are tips that deliver benefits particularly quickly – in some cases, immediately.

 Easy gains
These are health boosters that offer the best value for the least amount of effort.

 Super-effective
This is advice that scientific research or widespread usage by experts has shown to be especially effective.

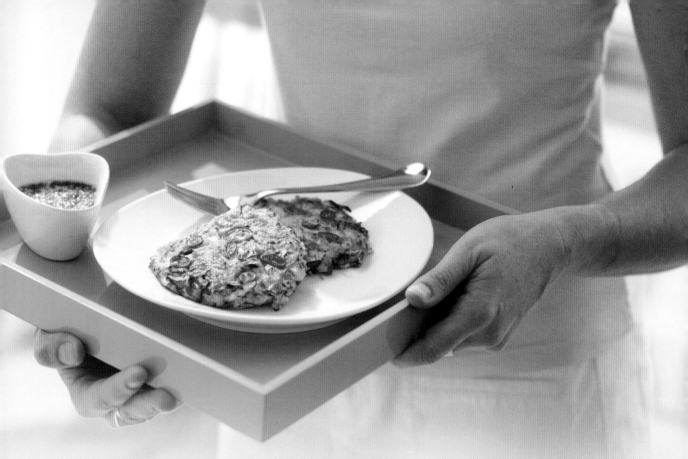

PREPARED meals

These days, many of us stop at the supermarket on our way home, not
for raw ingredients for dinner but for "home-cooked" meals that just need to be slipped
into the microwave for a few minutes. They're called "prepared meals," and more and
more supermarkets are turning over large sections of floor space to them, as well as to
frozen foods. If you're willing to spend the money, you may never need to cook or eat at
home again. As with everything in life, though, what you choose helps to determine your
health. Here are a few basic guidelines for shopping wisely for food, wherever you are.

12 WAYS TO MAKE THEM AS HEALTHY AS HOME COOKING

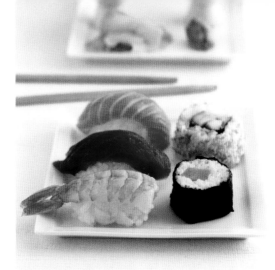

- **If you buy prepared food to save time,** buy only those things you don't have time to make. The less you buy premade, the more control you have over what you're eating. So choose a rotisserie chicken, by all means, but also go to the fresh food department for a potato to microwave instead of buying fried or roast potatoes, and add some broccoli that you can quickly steam or some colourful fresh salad ingredients.

- ☺ **Always think vegetables.** How are you going to get vegetables into your meal? If you don't want to cook, fill a salad bar container with raw veg, but stay away from too many marinated veggies. And, of course, those pre-washed mixed greens make salad preparation about as complicated as finding a bowl. But remember that it's always better and tastier to prepare your own from fresh.

- ☺ **Get two meals at a time.** Again, you're trying to save time. So that whole roasted chicken you got for tonight can double as a chicken Caesar salad tomorrow night. If you're making a bowl of couscous to go with your takeout dinner tonight, double the amount and pick up some extra vegetables and feta cheese at the salad bar for a Mediterranean salad the following night. Or perhaps for lunch tomorrow.

- **Go for sushi.** Low in fat, sushi is one of your best bets when running into your supermarket for dinner, and many stores now stock a good selection. Can't stand the thought of raw fish? Lots of stores offer cooked-fish sushi or even veggie-only sushi.

- **Grab a can of beans before you pay for your food.** Then add the beans to the salad bar selection you've just bought.

Be good to yourself: choose fresh sushi from your supermarket.

You'll save money (because beans are so filling) while still adding valuable fibre and other nutrients to the salad.

Have an indoor picnic for dinner. For a fresh take on healthy eating, buy a loaf of whole-grain bread, a basket of strawberries, a favourite low-fat cheese, some thinly sliced roast beef or turkey, some olives, pre-cooked shrimp, cherry

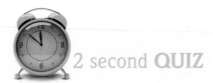

2 second **QUIZ**

Soup or salad?
ANSWER: **SALAD.**

Of course, some soups are far healthier than some salads. But, in general, you're better off with a salad of mixed greens and raw vegetables, coupled with a light, healthy dressing. You'll get more fibre and thus more filling for your calories, not to mention the healthy dose of disease-fighting antioxidants found in raw vegetables. Many soups are very healthy, but the cooking process can diminish some of the ingredients' nutritional value.

Stealth healthy **PIZZA**

Canadians order millions of pizzas every year.
Although it's not the healthiest food you could choose, there's no reason to cut pizza out of your life – it offers a quick, easy, tasty way to get loads of vegetables, fruit, fibre and even fish. But pizza, like any other takeout food, has its own pitfalls. When American scientists evaluated pizza slices from the top chains, it discovered fat levels approaching – and sometimes surpassing – a fast-food cheeseburger. The main culprit: far too much cheese. Add to that fatty meat such as sausage and pepperoni, and you are in the unhealthiest reaches of the food world. Here's how to make pizza a healthy delight:

- Order half-fat cheese or no cheese.
- Ask for extra veggies.
- Steer clear of stuffed-crust pizzas. You don't need the extra cheese.
- Avoid anything called Meat Lover's, All the Meat or Super Supreme. In fact, order your toppings individually.
- The best toppings: after veggies and fruit (ever tried pineapple-topped pizza?) come chicken, ham, shrimp and anchovies. These offer the greatest nutritional punch with the lowest saturated fat.

tomatoes, pre-sliced green or red peppers and bite-size carrots. When you get home, throw it all on the table and – after properly cleaning any fruit or veg – declare that dinner is served. This type of "grazing" dinner is fun, easy and a pleasant change. Make it a twice-monthly ritual.

● **Order sandwiches or rolls with turkey or chicken,** lots of vegetable fillings such as tomato, lettuce, peppers and cucumber and just a little spread. Ask for whole-grain bread.

● **Order twice as much** of the prepared vegetables as you do of the main course.

● **If you can see that there's mayonnaise** pooling around the chicken, tuna, seafood or pasta salads, skip them. Mayonnaise is a combination of eggs and oil – primarily fat.

● **Pick up a rotisserie chicken ...** Add a salad, a box of instant brown rice and some sliced tomatoes and you've got a healthy, easy, barely-have-to-cook-it meal.

● **... But remove the skin.** Much of the internal fat from a rotisserie chicken drips out in the cooking, but the skin still holds lots of the stuff.

● **Choose prepared soups made with veggies** in place of meat, such as black-bean soup, lentil soup or minestrone. Little fat is added to these varieties. However, avoid creamy or cheesy soups such as broccoli and cheese or cream of asparagus. If you're not sure, check the composition of the soup stock. The best soup base is vegetable broth, followed by chicken broth, then beef stock and, finally, cream.

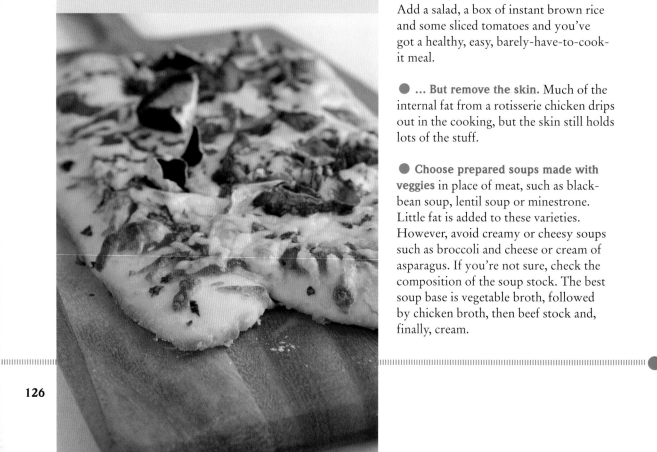

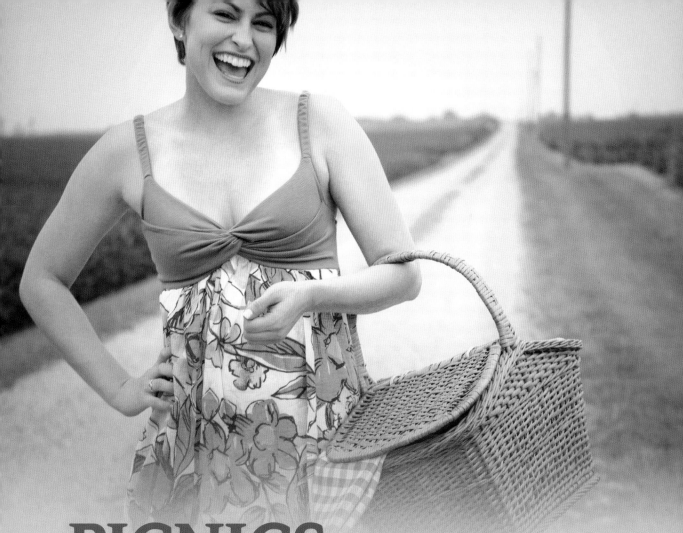

PICNICS

Eating outside in the sun, with the crash of waves on the beach or the wind through the trees as your musical accompaniment, makes any meal taste better. That's why picnics should feature in your healthy-eating master plan. If the word "picnic" is synonymous in your mind with overstuffed sandwiches, potato salad and chips, this is for you. Here are 13 stealth healthy ways to ensure that dining al fresco doesn't translate as dining al fatso!

13 WAYS TO GO BEYOND SANDWICHES AND POTATO SALAD

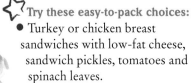

Get a healthy crunch from celery and peanut butter.

⭐ **Try these easy-to-pack choices:**
- Turkey or chicken breast sandwiches with low-fat cheese, sandwich pickles, tomatoes and spinach leaves.
- Hummus stuffed into whole-wheat pita bread with bean sprouts, diced tomatoes and sliced grapes.
- A green salad topped with grilled chicken. Pack the dressing separately.
- Whole-wheat wraps with smoked salmon, capers, tomato, avocado, hummus, spinach and grated carrots.
- Cumin, black-eyed bean and corn salad. Rinse and drain a can of black-eyed beans and a can of corn. Mix together with a drizzle of olive oil, 1 tablespoon of balsamic vinegar and a pinch of cumin.
- Ricotta, spinach and Parmesan whole-wheat wrap. Place about 120 g of loosely packed raw spinach leaves in a food processor and grind. Mix in 125 g or so of low-fat ricotta and 1 tablespoon of Parmesan cheese, and wrap the mix in a whole-wheat flour tortilla.
- Mediterranean tomato salad in whole-wheat pita. Dice fresh tomato and cucumber, mix with a thinly sliced red onion and black olives, drizzle with a little olive oil, red wine vinegar, salt and pepper and stuff into a pita pocket.

● **Stuff celery with low-fat cream cheese,** peanut butter or goat's cheese for a delicious starter. Or try baked corn tortilla chips with salsa, tzatziki or a low-fat yogourt dip.

● **Substitute this for fried chicken.** Brush boneless, skinless chicken thighs with olive oil and sprinkle with rosemary, salt and pepper. Bake (350°F/180°C) until the juices run clear – about 45 to 60 minutes. Prepare the day before your picnic and chill overnight. For something as deliciously messy as fried chicken, mix the juice of a lemon with 1 tablespoon of Dijon mustard, $1/3$ cup (85 ml) of honey, a pinch of curry powder and a pinch of salt. Coat skinless chicken drumsticks in the mixture and bake until done (350°F/180°C) – about 45 to 60 minutes.

● **Instead of coleslaw drenched in mayonnaise,** buy a bag of shredded vegetables used to make coleslaw and drizzle on fat-free Italian dressing when you're ready to eat.

● **Make a lower-fat alternative to mayonnaise for summer salads.** Simply mix equal quantities of mayonnaise with fat-free Greek yogourt.

● **Go Mediterranean.** Microwave two boxes of whole-wheat couscous (put boiling water in a heat resistant measuring

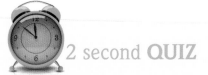

2 second QUIZ

Charcoal or propane
ANSWER: **PROPANE.**

Of course, grilling aficionados will debate this point for hours. But from a safety point of view, there are more reported deaths and injuries due to carbon monoxide poisoning from charcoal grills than there are burns due to propane-grill fires. In terms of cooking, propane cooks more evenly, so you have fewer cases of food that's raw at one end and well-done at the other. Plus, the smoke from charcoal is unhealthy for you, whether breathed in while cooking or eaten via the grilled food.

cup, add the couscous, cover with a plate and let it steam) and add fresh or roasted vegetables, a can of chickpeas, a sprinkling of feta cheese and sliced black olives and a drizzle of olive oil. Now you've got a gorgeous Mediterranean salad that's great for a picnic.

● **Pack crudités for dipping.** Strips of vegetables (peppers, cauliflower, carrots, radishes and cucumber, for example) are delicious served with a low-fat dip or salsa.

● **Instead of soft drinks or fruit juices, bring soda water mixed with all-natural fruit juice;** unsweetened, flavoured iced tea; or plain bottles of water. Freeze the plain bottled water the night before to use as cold packs to keep food chilled. When you're ready to eat, you'll have an icy bottle of water ready to drink.

● **Pack frozen mango cubes.** They provide a sweet, healthy accompaniment to any picnic. Or mix several bags of frozen fruit in a container. By the time you're ready to eat, you'll have a sorbet-like treat.

☆ **Make your own salsa.** Drain a 398 ml can of diced tomatoes with green chilies and add a handful of fresh cilantro leaves and a pinch or two of cumin and salt to taste. Put through the food processor or mini chopper and voilà! Salsa. Serve with baked tortilla chips or add to black-eyed beans for a cold salad that's perfect for picnicking.

● **Try making a sweet potato salad.** In a great variation on the original that's chock-full of valuable antioxidants and beta carotene, peel and boil a few sweet potatoes, then let them cool. Cut them into chunks and toss with enough orange

HEALTHY FOOD storage

To keep unwanted guests such as *Salmonella* and *E. coli* from your picnic, follow this basic advice:

● Keep hot foods hot and cold foods cold. Anything perishable should be kept at room temperature for no more than 2 hours.

● Bring along antibacterial wipes or hand-washing liquid to clean your hands before laying out (and eating) the food.

● Bring two coolers: one for food and one for drinks. Since you'll probably open the drinks cooler more often than the food cooler, this prevents warm air from reaching your perishables.

● Avoid bringing anything made with fresh eggs, which can become a breeding ground for bacteria.

● Avoid bringing meat, fish, potatoes and pasta mixed with mayonnaise. These foods can reduce the acidity of the mayonnaise (which keeps bacteria at bay), encouraging the growth of bacteria. Instead, bring your salad ingredients in separate containers and mix when you're ready to serve.

● Keep your cooler in an air-conditioned car.

● Thaw meat before grilling so it cooks evenly. Cook to an internal temperature of 160°F (71°C). Poultry should cook to 180°F (82°C).

● Keep raw meat, fish and poultry (and the containers on which they sit) separate from cooked foods.

● Wash the outer surface of fruits, including melons, well before cutting.

juice to cover, a pinch of cinnamon and your favourite dried fruit (cranberries work well). Serve cold.

● **Turn your pasta salad into a main meal.** Before the picnic, try grilling skinless chicken breasts, cutting them into strips and adding them to pasta salad. Toss in some fresh broccoli, peppers and tomatoes, mix in some low-fat dressing and you've got an easy and healthy main course.

☺ **Bring a whole watermelon or a cantaloupe or honeydew melon** and slice it open on the spot. Nature's packing works beautifully to keep fresh fruit cool and fresh.

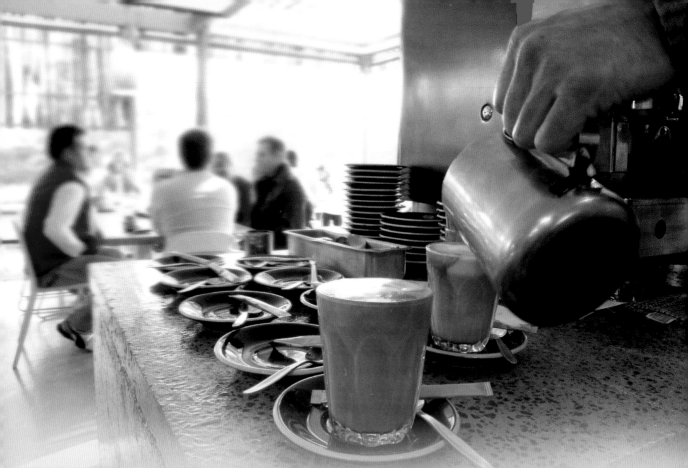

COFFEE shops

What would the world be like without Starbucks and other coffee shops? Somewhat thinner, perhaps. These havens for coffee lovers, specializing in sweet drinks to wash down irresistible pastries and cakes, have become a staple in Canada and elsewhere – there are 15,000 Starbucks around the world. What's worrying is that they're a major, often hidden, source of fat and calories. Did you know that a large Starbucks Java Chip Frappuccino made with whole milk and whipped cream has more calories and saturated fat than a McDonald's Quarter Pounder with cheese? Read on to find out how to make coffee shop visits healthier.

9 WAYS TO GET OUT HEALTHY

Classify doughnuts as treats, not breakfast. A doughnut as an occasional treat is fine, but as a breakfast it's disastrous. Not only will the simple carbohydrates and high sugar leave you drooping and hungry an hour later, but you get little to no nutritional benefit from the fat and calories. If you must eat on the run at your coffee shop, order a whole-wheat bagel.

Classify specialty coffee drinks as dessert, not coffee. Fancy-flavoured, whipped-cream, hard-to-pronounce coffee drinks can be worse for you than a big slice of cake. For example, a medium Java Chip Frappuccino with whipped cream at Starbucks has 460 calories, 19 g of fat and 55 g of sugar. Of the various cakes, muffins and pastries Starbucks lists on its website, most have fewer calories per serving than the drink. If you must have a fancy coffee drink, treat it like a banana split – a rare indulgence, to be had by itself and not as a mere beverage.

Choose biscotti. These twice-baked Italian delicacies are perfect for dunking; at Starbucks they carry just 110 calories and 5 g of fat.

Order plain coffee and add the extras yourself. Not only are many of the specialty coffee drinks at coffee shops loaded with fat and calories, but some items are made from mixes, some of which may contain large amounts of trans fats. The solution: get a black coffee and add in healthy amounts of skimmed milk, sugar or sugar substitute and, if you wish, top with separate flavourings such as ground chocolate or cinnamon.

If you must order specialty beverages, order those made with milk, such as cappuccino or latte. And ask that

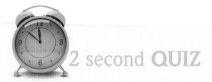
they be made with skimmed milk. You'll get a good amount of calcium but without the saturated fat.

Forget the whipped cream topping. You'll instantly save 100 calories and 10 g of fat.

Share a muffin with a friend. As with a doughnut, think "treat" rather than breakfast when you order a muffin at a coffee shop. Muffins – even bran muffins – tend to be more about good-to-taste than good nutrition.

Go for a flavoured bagel. If you're ordering blueberry, cinnamon and raisin or some other tasty flavour, you won't need the extra cream cheese, butter or other spreads. Better still, go for whole-wheat, multigrain or oat-bran varieties – you can eat your bagel and have some good nutrition too.

Pick the low-fat option. Many coffee shops and bakeries do offer low-fat versions of their tasty treats. This is still a long way from health food, but it's a stealth healthy step closer.

Fruit bagels are tasty without the spreads.

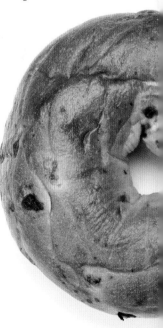

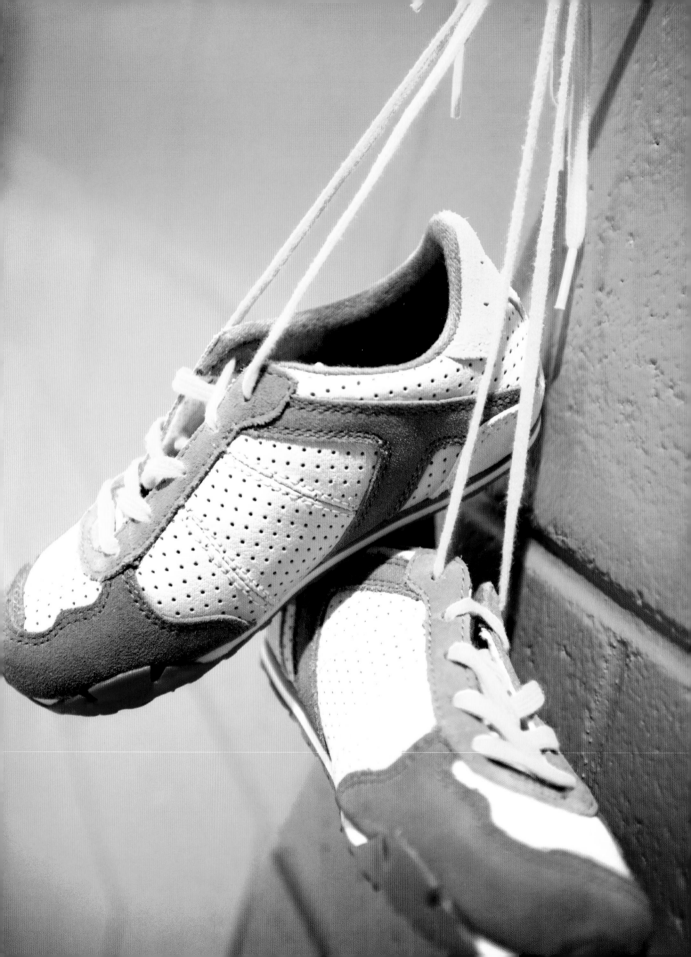

part 4

STEALTH HEALTHY EXERCISE

After tackling food, there's no better way to improve your health than by getting up and moving. Here's how to work extra movement into your days without hassle or sweat.

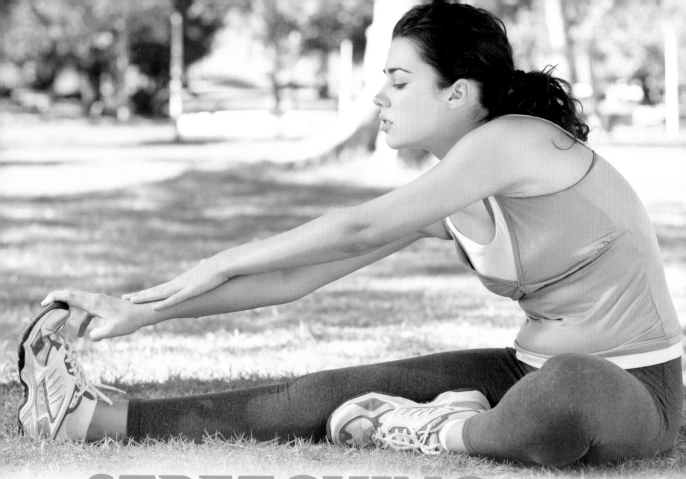

STRETCHING

The human body was engineered for standing and moving. Sitting down for hours – like at a desk or in front of the TV – is unnatural, and takes its toll on our well-being. To survive the daily office-job marathon without eventually suffering some form of chronic pain or injury, it's important to stretch regularly. Of course, stretching is good for more than just that. One of the most common complaints about aging, for example, is stiffness and joint pain. Stretching regularly helps to keep you lithe, active and injury-resistant. And a regular stretching routine may even improve your sleep. The following 14 tips will show you how to sneak some stretches into your day.

14 WAYS TO SNEAK IN SOME LIMBERING UP

EARLY MORNING routine

● **Every morning, roll out of bed and do these stretches.**
Can you get away with just three stretches for your
entire body? "Yes, if your main goal is overall
body health," says Claire Small, a specialist
musculoskeletal physiotherapist. Small suggests
the following gentle mini-routine first thing in
the morning just after getting out of bed. It's safe
to perform even with cold muscles.

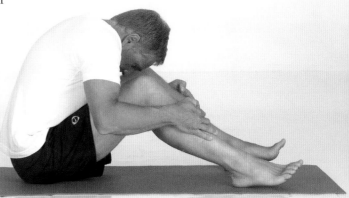

1 TRUNK EXTENSOR STRETCH Prepare your
back for the challenge of sitting at a desk all day long
with this stretch. Repeat it periodically during the day to
release tension in your lower back. Sit on the floor with
your knees bent and feet flat on the floor. Lift your toes

until only your heels touch the floor. Sit tall with your back
straight and spine long and extended. Place your hands on
your shins. Tuck your chin into your chest, bend forward
from the hips, and pull your torso as far down as you can.
Hold for 2 seconds then release. Repeat ten times.

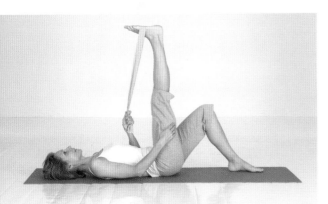

2 HAMSTRING STRETCH This will help to
lengthen your hamstrings first thing in the morning.

Lie on your back with your knees bent and your feet on
the floor. Lift your right knee in towards your chest and
loop a rope (or a tie or towel) round the arch of your
right foot. Hold the ends of the rope with your left hand.
Extend your leg towards the ceiling. Place your right palm
against your right thigh and press into it as you use the
rope to increase the stretch. Hold for 30 seconds, release
and repeat three times. Switch legs and repeat.

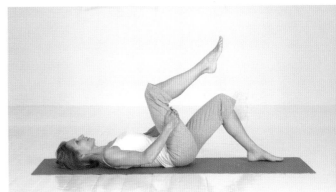

3 PELVIC TILT Doing this stretch helps to increase
blood flow to your midsection, relaxes your back muscles
and helps to realign your sacrum, one of the large, flat
bones that form your pelvis.

Lie on your back with your knees bent and feet on the
floor. Lift your right thigh towards your chest, grasping the
back of your thigh with both hands. Bring your knee as
close to your chest as you can. Hold for 2 seconds, release,
then repeat ten times. Switch legs and repeat.

● **Stretch during your shower.** The perfect time of day to squeeze in a little stretching is right after – or during – a warm shower in the morning. Experts say that it's ideal because your muscles are being warmed by the water. It'll also help energize you for the rest of the day. Here is an example of a good morning shower routine:

● While in the shower, raise your arms above your head, clasp your hands and reach upwards to stretch your shoulders and back.

● With the water spray hitting the back of your neck, slowly turn your head to the right until your chin is over your shoulder. Pause, then slowly turn your head all the way to the left. Repeat five times in each direction.

● Dry off with one foot on the edge of the bath or shower tray, lean forward and stretch your hamstring.

● While drying your hair, hold a calf stretch by extending one leg 0.5 to 1 metre (1$\frac{1}{2}$ to 3 feet) behind the other.

● **And get in some stretching with each bite of breakfast.** Do this sitting down. As you eat, roll your ankles in clockwise and counterclockwise circles. Then draw large, imaginary letters with your big toes, spelling your first, middle and last name with each foot.

⫸ Better still, do a more thorough 3 minute stretching routine every morning. This routine works for two reasons: first, it comprises very simple, natural moves; second, it is particularly good for anyone with stiff joints or mild arthritis. It gently warms your muscles and moves your shoulders, knees, elbows, wrists and neck through a full range of motion, stimulating the release of synovial fluid, a thick secretion that lubricates and cushions your joints. Complete the following stretches from a standing position, starting with whatever range of motion you find comfortable and gradually increasing it as your joints warm up. Complete 10 to 12 slow repetitions of each stretch, moving clockwise and counterclockwise, pausing for a moment at the full extension on each stretch.

Neck roll. Bring your chin to your chest, then move your chin in a half-circle, bringing your left ear over your left shoulder, then your right ear over your right shoulder.

Shoulder shrug. Lift your shoulders to your ears, then slowly drop them.

Shoulder circle. Slowly roll your shoulders in circles.

Arm circle. Extend your arms straight out to your sides, so they are parallel to the ground. Slowly whirl them in circles as if they were propellers on an airplane.

Hip circle. With your knees slightly bent and your feet placed slightly wider than your hips, circle your hips in one direction and then the other, as if you were balancing a hula hoop.

● **Do finger stretches regularly to keep your hands nimble and strong.** Do one hand at a time for best effect.

Finger stretch. Place a hand on a tabletop or thigh, with your palm facing down. Spread your fingers as far as you can and hold for 20 to 30 seconds.

Thumb touch. Place your hand, palm up, on a table with your fingers open and relaxed. In a smooth movement, touch the tips of your thumb and index finger together. Hold this for a second, then return to the starting position. Then touch the tip of your thumb to all of your other fingertips.

Spider walk. Place your hand palm-down on a tabletop. Use your fingers to pull your palm across the table as far as you can reach.

Good stretching TECHNIQUE

Follow these tips to increase the effectiveness of your stretching routine:

● **Feel the muscle you are targeting.** As you slowly proceed through the movement, you should feel a stretching sensation in your muscle as it lengthens and relaxes. If you feel a sharp pain in a joint, such as your knee, you have either gone too far or your technique is off. If you feel nothing at all, you have either not gone far enough or, again, are using the wrong technique.

● **Relax.** Many people tense up as they stretch, for example, hunching their shoulders towards their ears. Don't. Notice whether you are clenching any other muscles and gently allow them to release as you exhale.

● **Breathe into it.** If you breathe slowly and deeply as you stretch, you'll increase blood flow and make your stretching more effective. Always exhale as you move into the stretch. As you hold, inhale by expanding the abdomen, ribcage and chest, then exhale as you visualize your breath flowing through the tension you feel in your muscle.

● **Stretch each and every day.** When it comes to flexibility, what you don't use, you lose – and quickly. The lesson: it is much better to stretch a little every day than to do a long stretching routine once or twice a week.

● **Hold a stretch on the tighter side of your body twice as long as on the more flexible side.** Prevent muscle imbalances by training the major muscle groups equally. If you are tighter on one side of your body, stretch that muscle for twice as long or repeat a stretch on that side to even things out.

● **Use proper body alignment.** It's easy to cheat when you stretch, but then you fail to get the stretch you need. The most typical "cheating" is rounding your back. In 95 per cent of all stretches, you want to keep your spine long and flat. Before bending forward into any stretch, first inhale and extend upwards, creating as much space as you can between each vertebra in your spine. When you bend forward into a stretch, bend from the hips, not the waist. As you bend forward, your pubic bone should move forward while your coccyx (tail bone) moves back and up.

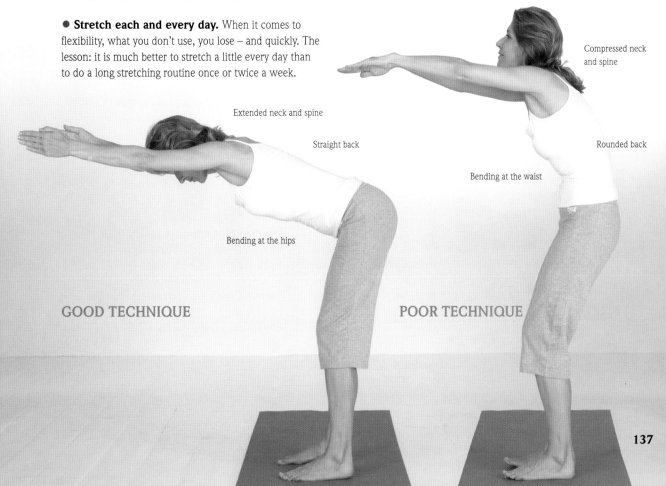

Extended neck and spine

Straight back

Bending at the hips

Compressed neck and spine

Rounded back

Bending at the waist

GOOD TECHNIQUE

POOR TECHNIQUE

● **Stretch after every walk, run, bike ride, aerobic class or any other cardiovascular activity.** Your muscles are at their most flexible and pliable after your workout, making your stretching more effective. After any activity designed to increase your heart rate, spend about 5 to 10 minutes cooling down and bringing your heart rate back to normal. Then do the full sequence of stretches outlined on page 135.

● **Hang.** Grab a chin-up bar and just hang from it – no pulling or swinging – for a minute or two. It's surprisingly refreshing and can do a lot of good for your spine, as well as your arm, shoulder and chest muscles. A great place to do it is on the monkey bars at a children's playground. However, if you haven't exercised for a while, or have a history of shoulder problems, ask your doctor first about this one, since you require your hands and shoulders to hold your entire body weight.

☆ **Dance your way to flexibility once a week in a dance class.** A Swedish study published in the *Journal of Strength Conditioning Research* tested 20 cross-country skiers for flexibility. Half the skiers took a dance class, and the other half served as a control group. Within three months, the skiers who took the weekly dance class improved the flexibility of their spines and consequently also increased their agility and ski speed on a slalom and hurdle test.

● **Stretch every time you get out of the car.** Even short periods of driving can cause back pain if you don't periodically stretch it out. When you get out of the car, lean backwards. Stand with your feet shoulder-width apart, put your hand in the small of your back and lean backwards using your hand to support your lower back. Then bend forward and place your hands on your knees. Exhale as you round your back and tuck in your chin. Then flatten your back, inhaling as you go. Hold each position for a count of two, repeating in both directions ten times.

● **Stretch your legs as you wait in a line.** If you're stuck in a line, stand on your toes, as high as you can, for as long as you can. Then, with your feet back on the ground, lift the toes of your right foot as high as they can go without lifting your heel, and hold for 20 seconds. Do the same with your left foot. These simple moves are good for any other occasion when you are on your feet for a long time.

● **Release your neck whenever you're on hold during a call.** Get a speakerphone or a headset. The next time someone puts you on hold, do some neck rolls or, if you're at home, get down on the floor and start doing your stretching routine.

☺ **Stretch during TV time.** Sprawl out on the floor and again go through your stretching routine, doing the three stretches described on page 135. If you feel good, do them a second and third time. If you do these stretches later in the day, your muscles will be warmed up from your daily activities. If nothing else, make a point of stretching during the commercials.

● **Rest your legs up a wall before going to bed every night.** Sit with one hip as close to the wall as you can get it. Then lie on your back and extend your legs up the wall, so that your bottom, the backs of your thighs and your heels touch the wall. You'll feel a mild stretch in your legs as gravity encourages fluids to drain out of your legs, back up to your heart. Hold the position for 5 minutes.

AFTERNOON routine

● **Near the end of your working day, do another 2 minute stretch routine.** Because your muscles are relatively warm and pliable from walking around all day, now is the perfect time to do the following static stretches. Some research suggests that flexibility peaks between 2:30 p.m. and 4 p.m., due to the body's natural circadian rhythms. So although you'll achieve some benefit no matter what time of day you stretch, an afternoon routine may help you to gain more flexibility

1 **LATERAL SIDE STRETCH** Sit on the edge of your office chair with your feet on the floor. Place your left palm against the seat of the chair. Reach your right arm overhead. Extend upwards through your spine, then bend sideways to the left. Hold for 20 seconds, release, then repeat on the other side.

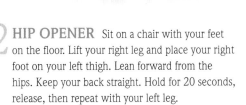

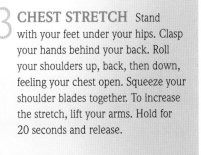

2 **HIP OPENER** Sit on a chair with your feet on the floor. Lift your right leg and place your right foot on your left thigh. Lean forward from the hips. Keep your back straight. Hold for 20 seconds, release, then repeat with your left leg.

3 **CHEST STRETCH** Stand with your feet under your hips. Clasp your hands behind your back. Roll your shoulders up, back, then down, feeling your chest open. Squeeze your shoulder blades together. To increase the stretch, lift your arms. Hold for 20 seconds and release.

4 **SEATED HAMSTRING STRETCH** Sit on the floor with your left leg extended. Place your right foot against your left thigh. Lengthen your spine and bend forward from the hips. Don't let your back arch. Hold for 20 seconds. Repeat with your right leg extended.

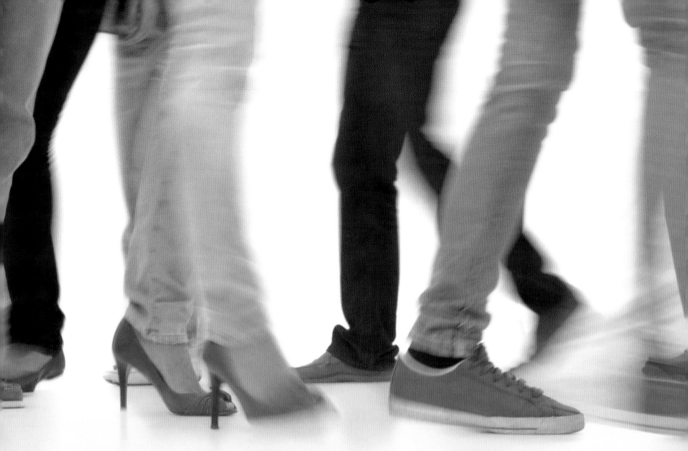

WALKING

It's so simple and convenient it couldn't possibly count as exercise, right? Wrong. Study after study shows that regular moderate walking can help you to lose weight and reduce your risk of heart disease. In a study published in *Diabetes Research in Clinical Practice*, Japanese researchers tested obese men before and after they joined a one-year modest walking plan. All they did was increase the number of steps they took during their daily activities. The result: their blood pressure and cholesterol levels improved and the amount of body fat around their abdomen – the dangerous kind that leads to higher rates of heart disease and diabetes – significantly decreased. Here are some ways both to get more walking into your life and to reap the most benefits from every step.

29 WAYS TO DO IT BETTER AND MORE FREQUENTLY

Learn the basics. Before you take your next step outdoors, you need to know how much walking to do, and how often. Here are the facts:

● For it to be exercise, walk at a pace that has you breathing heavily, but still able to talk.

● Your goal, first and foremost, is to walk five days a week, 30 minutes a walk. Do that, and you are getting the base-level amount of exercise that research says should maintain your health and vigour.

● Don't assume you can reach that goal quickly. Walking hard for 30 minutes can be difficult at first. Walk for as long as feels comfortable during the first week, even if it's just to the mailbox and back. Each subsequent week, increase that amount by no more than 10 per cent.

● Start every walk with 5 minutes of easy-paced walking, about the same pace at which you'd do your grocery shopping, to get your body warmed up. Then, cool down at the end of each walk with another 5 minutes of easy-paced walking. This allows your heart rate to speed up and slow down gradually.

● When you reach your target of 30 minutes a day, five days a week, set a new target. Either you should up your walking habit by increasing your time, or you might be ready for new forms of exercise, such as strength-building exercises twice a week.

● **Walk for entertainment one day a week.** Instead of walking around your local area, walk through a park, an art gallery or a shopping centre. First circle the perimeter of your location at your usual brisk pace. Then wander through again more slowly to take in the sights.

● **Walk with a friend.** If you have a friend expecting you, you're more likely to get out of bed on cold winter mornings or skip the cafeteria for a lunchtime walk. If one of you backs out for any reason, put $1 in a kitty. If you manage to build up a substantial sum, donate it to charity.

● **Pick a charity and pledge to contribute a small sum for every kilometre that you walk.** You'll take pride in the fact that you are walking for something beyond yourself, which will motivate you to walk faster and for longer. After every walk, mark the amount you owe on a chart then, when you reach your target amount, send off a cheque.

Use a pedometer. These nifty gadgets measure how far you've walked in steps and miles or kilometres. They provide motivation by spurring you to meet a particular goal and showing you if you've met it. And research shows that they work. In one U.S. study of 510 people, those who wore a pedometer automatically increased the amount of steps they took in a day. Often, pedometers hook onto your belt and are small and easy to use.

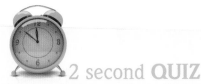

2 second QUIZ

Walk or run?
ANSWER: **WALK.**

Although runners and other high-energy athletes may scoff at walking, saying that it doesn't burn enough calories to result in real weight loss, research has shown time and time again that a regular walking program, mile for mile, has just as beneficial an effect on your waistline. And as is clearly documented, people are far more likely to stick with a walking rather than a running regimen.

Walk your way to health with a pedometer.

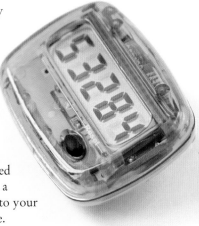

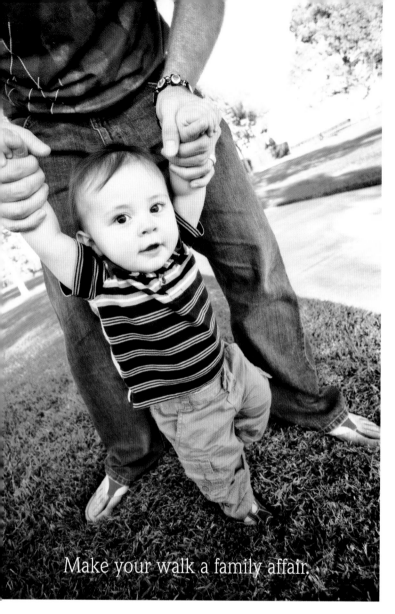

Make your walk a family affair.

active." Using a pedometer, find your baseline of how many steps you normally take in a day. Then, increase that amount by at least 200 steps a day until you reach 10,000 to 12,500 daily steps.

● **Take the entire family on your daily walks.** Not only will you be exhibiting good fitness habits for your children, but you'll also be able to supervise them while you walk rather than getting a babysitter. If your children walk too slowly, ask them to ride their bikes or roller skate beside you. To keep everyone entertained, play your usual repertoire of long car-trip games such as I Spy. You can also try a treasure hunt, where you start out with a list of items to check off during your walk.

● **Improve your walking posture.** Proper posture will reduce discomfort as you walk and help you to burn more fat and calories. So when you go on your next walk, adjust yourself as follows:
● Stand tall with your spine elongated and breastbone lifted. This allows room for your lungs to expand fully.
● Keep your head straight with your eyes focused forward and shoulders relaxed. Avoid slumping your shoulders forward or hunching them towards your ears.
● Roll your feet from heel to toe. As you speed up, take smaller, more frequent steps. This protects your knees and gives your butt a good workout.
● Allow your arms to swing freely.
● Firm your stomach and flatten your back as you walk to prevent lower back pain. Hold in your lower stomach around your waistband. Make sure you continue to breathe normally.

● **Once a week, complete your errands on foot.** If you live within a kilometre or two of downtown or the supermarket,

● **Aim for 10,000 steps a day.** Don't let that amount scare you. Most people walk about 5,500 to 7,500 steps during an average day as they amble to and from meetings, to the water cooler, to the mailbox. In fact, researchers in the field consider 5,000 steps a day a "sedentary lifestyle." Studies have found that you should be able to cover 7,499 steps a day without participating in formal sports or exercise. If you reach 10,000 steps a day, you're considered "active," while 12,500 steps a day earns you the title of "highly start from your house. If you live out in the middle of nowhere, drive to within walking distance of your destination and walk the rest of the way there and back. You'll be surprised how much you can accomplish on foot and, even better, how many people you'll meet along the way.

● **Breathe deeply as you walk to a count of 1-2-3.** Many people unintentionally hold their breath when they exercise, then suddenly feel breathless and tired. Oxygen is invigorating, and muscles need it to create energy. So as you inhale, bring the air to the deepest part of your lungs by expanding your ribs outwards and your stomach forward and inhale for a count of three. Then exhale fully through your mouth, also to a count of three.

Periodically increase the pace. Boredom can quickly bring a walk to a premature end. Keep your mind and your body engaged by increasing the pace or challenging yourself by trudging up a hill from time to time. Every 10 to 15 minutes, complete a 2 to 3 minute surge. During your surge, try to catch a real or imaginary walker ahead of you.

● **Take your dog with you (or get a dog).** Once your dog gets used to your walks, he or she will look forward to them and give you a gentle nudge (or annoying whine) on the days you try to get out of it. There's nothing more effective than a set of puppy-dog eyes to get you up off the couch and out the door. In addition to walking locally, consider signing up for a dog agility class (see the local vet or visit the Canadian Kennel Club's website at www.ckc.ca for more information). During the class, you and your dog will circumvent a course with see-saws, hurdles, tunnels and other obstacles. (Your dog tackles the obstacles.

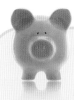

Healthy INVESTMENT

Walking shoes
Why? A good pair of walking shoes will help you to travel farther and faster with more comfort. Go to a respected sports store so that a skilled salesperson can measure your feet and find the best shoe for your foot shape and size. Tell the salesperson what type of terrain you'll be walking on and how many kilometres on average you plan to walk a week.

If you have an old pair of runners, bring them to the store with you. The salesperson can look at the wear pattern on your shoes to determine your foot type. For example, if the inner heel is more worn than the outer heel, your foot probably turns in excessively as you walk. In this case, you'll want some extra arch support and a shoe designed for "motion control."

Try on your shoes and walk around the store. Make sure the shoe hugs your heel; your heel should not slide up and down as you walk. The shoe should also have a firm arch support and the forefoot of the shoe should bend with the natural bend in your foot. Most important, the shoes should feel comfortable when you walk. A good walking shoe lasts about 563 kilometres (350 miles). If you walk 16 kilometres (10 miles) a week, that's about eight months.

You run or walk alongside and shout the appropriate command.) Both you and your dog will get a great workout and you'll end up with a better-behaved and calmer dog as a result. If you don't have a dog, offer to walk a neighbour's dog twice a week. The commitment will keep you motivated.

● **Explore on your walks.** You can walk anywhere at any time, from your neighbourhood to your local stores to a local nature trail. You can even walk laps around your office building. But rather than walking the same old tired route day in and day out, use your walks as a way to experience and explore the great outdoors. Varying your route and terrain will do more than keep you mentally engaged. It will also help you to target different leg muscles.

Healthy INVESTMENT

Walking poles

Why? These lightweight walking poles sold at many sports stores can help you feel more steady and safe when walking on rough ground. The poles encourage you to bend your elbows and use your arms as you walk, which will prevent swelling in your hands. The movement also provides a great upper-body and lower-body workout, which burns more calories as well as strengthening your muscles. Finally, the poles take stress off your knees.

● **Pump up the volume.** In a study published in the journal *Chest*, people with severe respiratory disease who listened to music while walking covered 6 more kilometres during the eight-week study than a similar group who walked without listening to music. Researchers speculate that the music made the participants less aware of any shortness of breath and distracted them from possible boredom and fatigue. It's something everyone can enjoy. Bring along an iPod and play your favourite tunes, or invest in a portable radio.

● **Sign up for a stroller walk.** If you're a new mom, you know only too well how hard it is to fit in time for fitness – not to mention time for other basics such as taking a shower. The good news is you can take your infant on your walk. A growing number of community groups and fitness centres offer group stroller walks for new mothers. Check your local community centre, children's hospital or YMCA to see what's available in your area.

● **When you feel like cancelling your walk, promise yourself you'll do just 10 minutes.** Too tired? Go out for a shorter walk. Once you've warmed up, the hardest part's already done so you'll probably just keep going. Even if you don't take the longer walk, the 10 minutes you did are better than no walk at all.

● **Five times a day, climb up and down a flight of stairs for 2 minutes.** You'll get the same heart rate-enhancing results in those 10 minutes as you would get from 36 minutes of walking on a level surface.

☺ **Roll out of bed, get dressed, put on your shoes and go.** It's easy to get caught up in your day-to-day activities and tell yourself that you don't have time for a walk. If you exercise first thing in the morning, however, you have no excuse. Research shows that people who plan to exercise in the morning are more likely to fit in their workouts than people who plan to exercise later in the day. Exercising in the morning may offer a side benefit: you'll sleep better at night. When American researchers compared morning and evening exercise, people who exercised for at least 225 minutes a week in the morning had an easier time falling asleep at night than those who completed the same amount of exercise in the evening.

☺ **Or, walk in the evening.** That U.S. sleep study aside, there's still a good case for after-dinner walks. They get you away from the television, they keep you from eating too much at supper, they give you a chance to chat to your neighbours and it's often a lovely time of day. Don't let bad weather stop you, though – that's what jackets, boots and umbrellas were invented for. There's something childlike and fun about a walk in the rain or snow.

● **Learn your k.p.h.** That's kilometres per hour, of course. Knowing your walking speed isn't that useful, but if, like many people, you love statistics, monitoring your speed will help to keep you motivated. A leisurely pace is 3.2 kilometres per hour, a healthy, brisk pace is 5.6 k.p.h., and going over 6.5 k.p.h. is fast. A pedometer will measure this for you, but if you don't have one, you can simply count your steps during various 15 second periods. For a normal adult stride, if you walk 15 steps in 15 seconds, you're walking at a leisurely pace of 3.2 kilometres per hour. At 23 steps, you're walking at a moderate pace of 5 k.p.h., and at 30 steps, you're walking at about 6.5 k.p.h.

● **Walk in the nicest part of town.** It just might encourage you to walk more often. When researchers from the University of Wollongong in New South Wales, Australia, questioned walkers about their walking habits, they found that men who perceived their neighbourhood as "aesthetic" were much more likely to walk around their locale. Other research finds that neighbourhoods with well-maintained sidewalks and safe, well-lit walking areas encouraged more walking than neighbourhoods that were ill-maintained and poorly lit. In fact, one study found that people who live in so-called walkable neighbourhoods walk an average of 70 more minutes each week than people in less walk-friendly surroundings.

● **If you're over 60, walk on soft surfaces.** As you age, the fat padding in your feet deteriorates. The absence of this natural shock absorber can make walking on sidewalks and other hard surfaces feel like foot torture. Flat grass and dirt paths will provide more cushioning for your feet than roads or sidewalks. Or, alternatively, buy some shock-absorbing insoles, which help with shock absorption. They are readily available at most pharmacies.

● **Shop in person instead of online.** Walking around the mall can burn about 200 calories an hour, much more than the calories you'll burn sitting down surfing the Internet for great deals.

● **Train for an event.** It's a great motivator. Check your local sports store for details of walks being held in your area. Generally, fun runs and sponsored walks raise money for good causes. Two examples are the Run for the Cure (www.cibcrunforthecure.com) and The Weekend to End Women's Cancers (www.endcancer.ca).

▐▐▐▶ **Split it up.** When you're too busy to go for your usual 30 to 60 minute walk, divide it up and get out there for 5 or 10 minutes at a time. That may be as

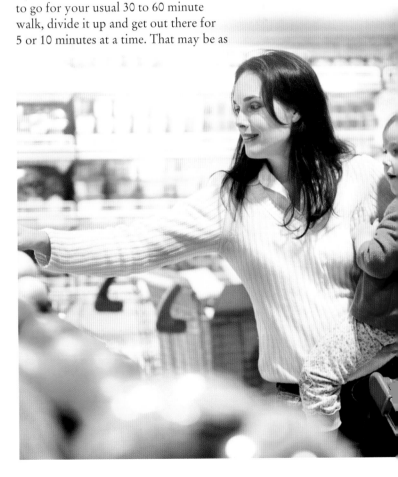

Burn calories by shopping in person.

simple as taking a 5 minute walk break around the building after completing a big project at work. Such short walking breaks will refresh your mind, so you can return to work with more vigour. In fact, research shows that most people can focus at top capacity for only 30 minutes at a time. After that, concentration begins to drop off. So your intermittent walk breaks may actually make you more productive.

● **Walk and talk.** Use a cordless phone and walk around the house or up and down the stairs as you chat with friends or conduct your business. This is also a good way to make use of those long times spent on hold. You get some heart-healthy exercise, and that exercise will help you to maintain your mental cool. Use your pedometer to count your steps and you'll get the added bonus of feeling as if you have accomplished something rather than wasting time.

● **Apply some Vaseline.** If you're a long-distance walker or somewhat overweight, chafing clothes can make you want to call it quits. You can solve the problem by wearing skin-hugging

Avoid chafing with Vaseline.

clothing and applying Vaseline to your sensitive areas. The Vaseline acts like a barrier to protect your skin.

● **Walk faster earlier in your walk.** If you want to increase the amount of fat you burn, add some bursts of faster walking near the beginning of your walk, rather than going for a final spurt. A study in the *European Journal of Applied Physiology* found that people exercising burned more fat and felt less tired when they inserted their faster segments towards the beginning of a workout. You'll speed up your heart rate early and keep it elevated for the rest of your walk.

● **Take light weights (1 kg to 2 kg) on your walks.** Periodically work in arm exercises as you walk. This does more than increase the benefit of the workout. Carrying weights also builds muscle, and each kilogram of muscle burns about 65 to 110 calories more a day. Build a kilogram of muscle in your arms alone and you'll burn an extra 100 calories a day – even while you're channel surfing. Or try isometric exercises of the arms, chest and abdominal muscles. For instance, as you walk, go through the action of throwing a punch in slow motion. As you extend your arm, tense the muscles along it and do the same as you retract it. You should feel tension in your triceps, biceps, deltoids and pectoral muscles. Then repeat with your arms going straight up and down, or out to the side. You can also tense your chest muscles by bringing your hands together in front of your body and contracting across the chest and shoulders. Do this rhythmically to match your gait. Also try doing curls with no weights. Simply curl your arms alternately, in rhythm with your gait. Each time you curl your forearms, tense your biceps.

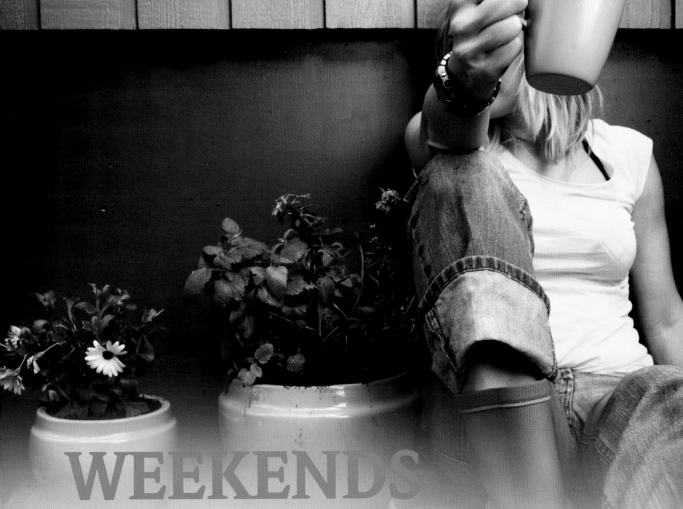

WEEKENDS

If you were to believe some of the commercials on TV, you'd think that most of us spend our weekends cycling, rock climbing, playing games on the beach and generally being active. But a look at the shopping centre parking lot on a Saturday afternoon paints a different picture. The weekend has become a time of errands, shopping and finishing up the work we didn't get to during the week. For too many of us, our spirit of adventure is being satisfied by the thought of finding a great bargain. And for parents, any thrill-seeking is being fulfilled through our children, as we shuttle them to and from parties and classes, watching from the sidelines. It's time to reclaim your weekends – or at least, a good chunk of them. Here are suggestions for squeezing in some weekend activity.

20 IDEAS FOR MORE ACTIVE DAYS OFF

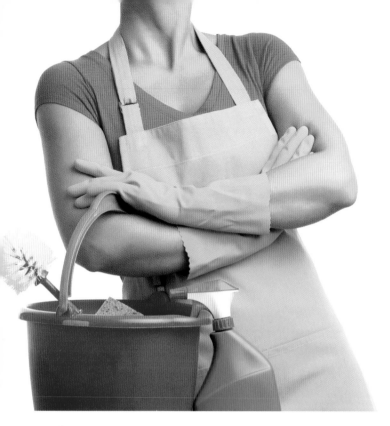

Cut out some extras and you may
be able to hire a cleaner.

then rather than sitting in front of the TV.
That way, you'll have free days to do as
you wish on the weekend.

● **Designate each Thursday evening
as the weekend planning time.** Start by
getting the weather forecast. Next, detail
your must-do stuff, such as hiking in
the park or taking your child to a class.
Then, be creative and bold by filling in
the blank spaces with interesting and
new activities. Get on the phone – make
reservations, call friends or family to
arrange get-togethers. Too many of us
enter the weekend without solid plans,
which is why we end up watching TV.

● **If you *must* work, get it out of the
way early.** A good way to reclaim your
weekend from your work is to get up an
hour earlier than normal, set the alarm for
2 to 3 hours, stay focused, then, when the
alarm rings, turn off the computer. The rest
of the weekend is yours – with no guilt.

● **To determine the scope of your
weekend hassles, keep a log of your
activities.** Jot them down in a notebook
this weekend. Then, on Sunday night,
take stock of the weekend that passed
you by. Where did you spend your time?
How can you cut back on those activities
to make time for fun and fitness? You'll
probably find that working, shopping,
cleaning, cooking and driving are
dominating your weekend. Once you
document what's eating up your time, it
gets easier to come up with a solution.

☺ **Shift weekend duties to weekday
evening duties.** There's no need to
wait until the weekend to go to the
supermarket, clean the house or mow the
lawn. Make, say, Tuesday and Thursday
evenings your "weekend duty" evenings
and get the housework out of the way

● **Save enough money to hire a
cleaner.** That way, you won't spend
your weekends cleaning. Want to know
how to fund it? Easy. Just cut out the
little extras that add up. For example,
borrow DVDs from the library instead
of renting or buying them. Brew your
own coffee instead of going to Starbucks.
Make packed lunches, dye your own hair,
cook your own gourmet dinner instead
of going to a restaurant. The sacrifices
will be worth it when you walk into your
home and see (and smell!) the cleanliness
and have time to enjoy your weekend.

☆ **Get out of bed at the same time
as during the week.** You may often
have great intentions to be active at the
weekend – that is, until you sleep in
until noon. When you spend half the day
under the covers, it's hard to find time for

fun and exercise. Make it a habit to get out of bed at the same time on weekends as during the week. In addition to freeing up more time for your weekend fitness forays, you'll also regulate your body clock better. Once your body gets used to a regular wake and sleep schedule, you'll fall asleep faster, feel more refreshed when you wake up, and avoid that Monday morning "hungover" feeling.

● **Go for a walk first thing in the morning.** Get out the door first thing, before you become too engrossed in the Sunday newspaper and your breakfast. Walking first thing in the morning ensures you fit in your workout. Once you return, you'll feel invigorated and be more likely to be active during the rest of the day.

● **Make nature part of your weekend routine.** For many of us, the great outdoors has a way of sparking our love of life, making us feel more spiritual. So add a weekly family walk through the park or woods to your weekend. It will lift your heart, as well as exercise it.

▐▐▐▶**Always commit one day to fun.** Never, ever let errands and work spread to both Saturday and Sunday. Pick one of those days and visit a park, go hiking or spend the day playing tennis, badminton or other games you enjoy with friends and family. You and your companions will soon look forward to this day, devoted not to formal exercise but to fun activities you can do together.

▐▐▐▶**Spend as much time playing sports as watching sports.** Many people have become addicted to watching sports on television. So take up this challenge: for every hour that you watch sport on TV, commit to 30 minutes of doing a sport or some other exercise. Gradually increase

2 second QUIZ

Movie theatre or rental?
ANSWER: **MOVIE THEATRE.**

Assuming cost is not an issue, going to a movie theatre provides more fun, activity and social interaction – all of which are good for your health – than sitting in front of your television at home. Just don't snack too much when you're there.

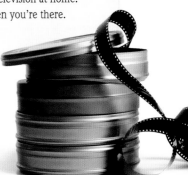

the ratio to one-to-one; that is, an hour watching, an hour doing. The fact is, nothing compares to taking part yourself.

● **Spruce up the yard – manually.** Many types of yard work, from leaf raking to digging and mowing, build upper-body strength and burn excess calories. In fact, one major study found that yard work was the best physical activity for preventing osteoporosis. But don't make it too convenient for yourself. Rake the leaves rather than using a leaf blower. Use a lawnmower that you have to push rather than one that is self-propelled. The more you use your own body, the more calories you burn.

● **If you cycle, go for a long ride.** During the week you probably can't ride much, but weekends allow you the luxury of riding for half the day or more, if you're so inclined. Scout out a local route or put the bike in your car and drive to a great cycling location. Don't forget to take along plenty of healthy food and some cash, in case you want to make a pit stop.

● **Join a club.** Many outdoors organizations arrange group hikes and other outings on the weekend. In fact, there are surprisingly large numbers of

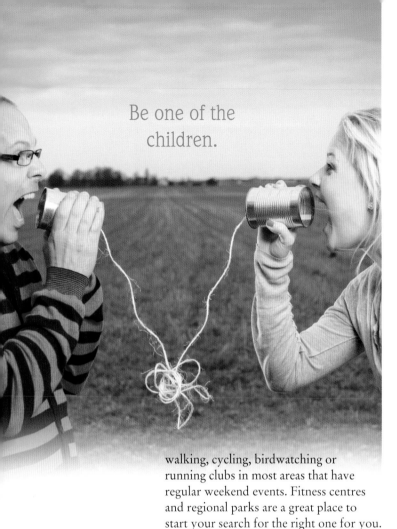

Be one of the
children.

Make a list of weekend fitness activities and choose one activity from the list every week. The more varied your weekend fitness routine, the more likely you'll be to stay active on the weekend. On your list, you might write hiking, canoeing, walking, cycling, birdwatching and other activities.

Keep a fitness kit in your car. Stock your car with a bat and ball, soccer ball, Frisbee or other favourite gear. Be sure to include a pair of sneakers. You never know when you'll find yourself away from home with a little free time. If your fitness kit is stocked and ready, you'll have everything you need for fun.

Train for a race. Whether you walk, run, cycle or do some other sport, signing up for a race will give you the incentive to train on the weekend. Suddenly fitness becomes the top priority in your life. Plus, this is what serious athletes do – complete their longer workout sessions on the weekend, when they have time away from work.

walking, cycling, birdwatching or running clubs in most areas that have regular weekend events. Fitness centres and regional parks are a great place to start your search for the right one for you.

▶ **Be one of the children.** Don't just push them out the door and spend the afternoon inside reading or cleaning. Join them. Find a tree and climb it with them. Spend the day skating or cycling or playing tag. After all, even those of us with aging bodies have some childishness still inside us, just aching to get out. See page 154, "Family Fun," for more ways to stay fit with your family.

Take the family camping. There's nothing quite like the great outdoors to put your body in a calorie-burning state, or to create happy, memorable times for your children. After you've set up your site, you can look into other activities such as swimming, canoeing and hiking.

Take calisthenics breaks. If you find yourself working at the office (or at home) over the weekend, take a 10 minute break every hour and do star jumps, lunges, push-ups and crunches. Over the course of the day, you'll have exercised for more than 60 minutes.

Combine physically active work with pure indulgence. For instance, chop some logs or gather firewood as the physically active part of your day, then sit in front of the fire with someone special for the pure indulgence part. Or work in your backyard by day, then have a barbecue that evening. Or take a long walk, knowing you have a well-stocked picnic basket waiting for you in the car.

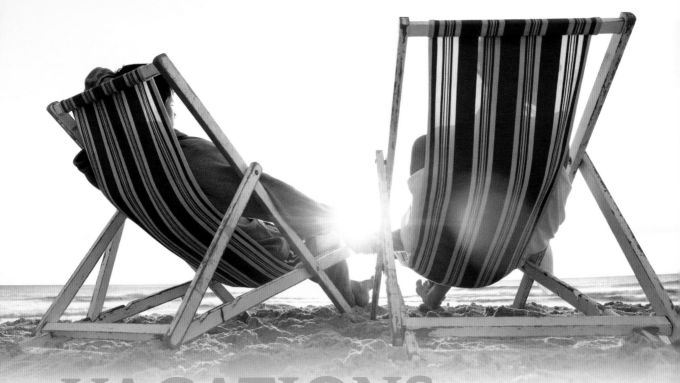

VACATIONS

When we take a vacation, what many of us want most is simply to relax. And so we spend long, lazy days on a deckchair and socialize the night away drinking and indulging in calorific desserts. Too often, we return home flabbier than we've been since, well, our last vacation. It doesn't have to be this way. Active vacations can often be the most relaxing of all. Yes, really. It's all about defining what an active vacation is. The idea is to try to spend 2 to 4 hours a day doing things. Walking the city streets. Exploring a nature reserve. Going to a zoo. These kinds of activities improve your physical and mental health and make vacations memorable. Here are some fresh ideas to make your trips away as pleasurable as they are active and healthy.

13 TIPS FOR ACTIVELY INDULGENT TRAVEL

☀ **Make morning time your activity time.** The weather will probably be friendlier, your energy levels higher and your agenda emptier than later in the day.

☀ **Reacquaint yourself with sunrises and sunsets.** A walk at dawn or dusk is rejuvenation defined. Try to make this a daily ritual of life away from home, and you will guarantee yourself both physical and spiritual replenishment.

☺ **Get into the water as much as you can.** Don't allow yourself to spend all your time sitting in front of the water. Whether it is the ocean, a swimming pool or a tree-lined lake, make sure you get into the water for swimming or games or even walking. Merely standing in waist-high water is a good workout, thanks to the action of the water.

☀ **Get on the water as much as you can.** Paddle boats are fun. Canoeing is a joy. Row boats are romantic. Powerboats exhilarating. Sailboats serene. Kayaks pure adventure. Even standing at the rail of a steamboat is exciting. Boats make you feel young, and whether you are propelling them or not, being on a boat burns calories and engages your muscles more than being on dry land.

☀ **Choose a cruise.** It's amazing how active you can be while stuck on a boat in the middle of the ocean. Most cruise ships offer numerous options for seaworthy exercise. Many have pools, golf simulators, climbing walls, fitness centres, jogging and walking areas and instructor-led fitness classes – and that's just what's on board. During any ocean and land excursions you can burn calories as you snorkel, hike, scuba-dive and horse ride.

☺ **Get out of the car every 2 hours.** Many of us spend a large part of our vacations on the road, either getting to and from our destinations, or using the car for sightseeing. But no matter how beautiful the scenery is, great, memorable trips don't happen in a car seat. Don't wait for exhaustion or the call of nature to get you to pull over. Get out frequently and stretch, walk, picnic, shop, visit and have fun. It's important for your health and energy, and it makes travelling a lot more interesting.

▮▮▮▶ **Play active games.** When most people think of outdoor games, they think of team sports such as hockey, baseball or soccer, all of which can be both intimidating and excessively strenuous for adults who stopped playing such sports a long time ago. Opt instead for gentler games – badminton, table tennis, lawn bowling. Your goal: to play an outdoor game every day while on vacation.

Play an outdoor game every day while you're on vacation.

152

Create a silly tournament. Particularly if there are children on the trip, it can be a riot to create your own mini-Olympics. For example, if you use the swimming pool every day, have a daily competition, such as holding your breath underwater, swimming between people's legs or having a big splash contest. Or maybe a week-long badminton competition. "Silly" is the operative word – don't make it a serious competition, just a chance to have active fun.

Play miniature golf. You burn more calories sitting rather than lying, standing than sitting, and walking than standing. Although miniature golf won't incinerate fat, it will burn more calories than lying in a hammock. Plus, your children will have a great time. You probably will too.

Beware the food obsession. Let's be honest: for many of us, vacations are about eating splurges. That means fresh seafood by the ocean, amazing restaurants in great cities, unlimited buffets at the hotel. This is the stuff of great vacations and you shouldn't deny yourself these pleasures. Instead, limit yourself to one such indulgence a day. Any more and the uniqueness of the splurges fades away. And you'll spend too much time sitting in restaurants – then sitting some more, recuperating from the overindulgence.

Explore on foot. Of course, you can rely on your travel agent, travel guides, maps or a tour bus to get you acquainted with a new location. But only by getting out and walking can you truly get the feel for a place. Spend the first few hours at your vacation destination walking around the area. If you're in a city, pick a few restaurants to try to make your reservations in person. Locate the parks, museums and shopping areas.

Fly a stunt kite. If there's a good wind blowing, buy a stunt kite and take it to the beach or other large open space. These kites can be easily assembled, then taken apart, making them perfect for travelling. You'll give your upper body a great workout as you struggle to control the kite. You may also have to run or walk to keep the kite in the air – or chase it down once it plummets to the earth.

Schedule an activity-based vacation. Plan your entire vacation around an activity, such as sailing, hiking, cycling or swimming. No expertise is necessary – just a willingness to take on a new challenge. There are any number of vacation packages targeted at novices to experts, adolescents to older people, singles to whole families. A skiing vacation with lessons for different ages and ability levels is perfect.

Reminder

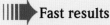 **Fast results**
These are tips that deliver benefits particularly quickly – in some cases, immediately.

 Easy gains
These are health boosters that offer the best value for the least amount of effort.

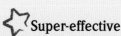 **Super-effective**
This is advice that scientific research or widespread usage by experts has shown to be especially effective.

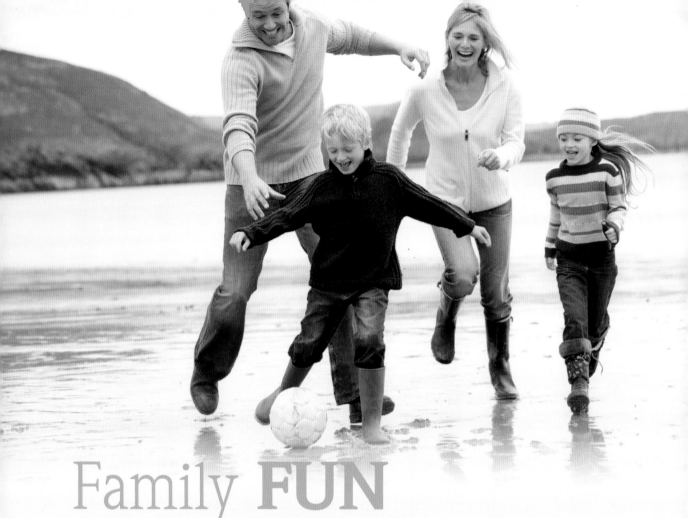

Family FUN

If you have children living at home, this chapter is for you. It's also for grandparents, and for all the uncles and aunts who love to spend time with their nieces and nephews, and all of the babysitters, day-care and after-school workers, neighbours and school volunteers. In short, it's for any adult who spends time with children. The message of this chapter is twofold: first, that you have a wonderful opportunity to get some fun, high-quality exercise by playing with children; second, that you have a responsibility to teach them about the joys and importance of exercise. Engaging your children in a health-promoting lifestyle should be a priority for every loving parent. But if you want trim and healthy kids, you have to get trim and healthy yourself. This is how to do it.

39 WAYS TO USE THE ULTIMATE EXERCISE MACHINES – CHILDREN

● **Go on a treasure hunt.** Here's a great way to keep the family fit and teach your children about trust, teamwork and problem solving at the same time. Take them to a local park and set an expedition course on a map, circling various "checkpoints." Take turns navigating to each point on the map and leading the team to each destination. "Start out with an easy course in an open park, then progress to a trail system," suggests musculoskeletal physiotherapist Claire Small. "Stay together and explore terrain features, study map clues, and look for the secret treasure." Sound too complicated? Then merely go hunting for insects, animals or flowers. You can't entertain a young child much better than finding a slumbering beetle under a log or rock.

☆ **Plan 10 minute spurts of activity followed by 5 minute rest periods.** Don't force your adult exercise program on your children. That's a recipe for disaster. Studies published in the journal *Medicine & Science in Sports & Exercise* show that forcing children to participate in structured exercise turns them off exercise later in life. Instead, take advantage of their natural tendency to participate in intermittent and sporadic play and exercise bouts. A game of tag is a perfect example. Children's bodies are designed to sprint and rest, sprint and rest. Because they are easily distracted and incapable of long periods of focused activity, they will resist long exercise sessions that don't include rest periods.

● **Hold a sports party.** Rather than the typical pin-the-tail-on-the-donkey birthday party, hold your child's birthday party in an active location, such as a roller skating or ice-skating rink, a ski or climbing centre, or an indoor "soft

A SERIOUS message

Childhood obesity experts in Canada are warning that more and more children in this country are overweight or obese. Not only that, many under-12s already show signs of high blood pressure, high cholesterol and liver disease. This has serious implications:

● Children are now subject to an epidemic of Type 2 diabetes, a disease that once occurred exclusively at or beyond middle age in adults.

● The obesity epidemic holds more harm for today's children than exposure to tobacco, drugs and alcohol combined.

● If they don't mend their ways, today's children may well have a shorter life expectancy than their parents, as they eat themselves into an early grave.

Studies show that the family environment is one of the strongest predictors of childhood obesity. In one study, children of sedentary parents (so-called couch potatoes) were more likely to gain weight and become overweight than the children of active parents.

One important fact for parents and carers to remember: you and your child burn more calories standing than sitting, walking than standing. The more you move, the more you burn. And it doesn't really matter what type of activity you choose: if you are moving and having fun, you're burning calories and getting in shape. It's that simple.

play" area. You don't have to limit this to parties. A growing number of indoor playgrounds offer structured games every week. Or you can have your own "no particular reason" party. Children might not think of what they're doing as exercise – but it is.

● **Play "chase my shadow."** The children have to jump and run to catch your shadow, then vice versa.

● **Play follow-the-leader with one or more children.** Line up in single file and weave your way through the house or backyard. Every few steps, hop, skip, jump or do some other movement that your followers must imitate. Once the children get the hang of the game, let them take turns as leader. Their naturally creative minds will come up with all sorts of fun movements for the followers to imitate. You'll be out of breath before you know it.

● **Purchase some family-friendly aerobics tapes for cold or rainy days.** Choose tapes that describe the workout as "low intensity" or "low impact." These types of aerobic exercise are better for children's developing bodies.

● **Give your child a head start – and race around the house.** You can do the same with other exercises, such as stretches or star jumps. You do ten, and your child does five. See who can complete them first.

☺ **Spend an hour doing yard work together.** Raking leaves, pulling weeds and spreading out mulch all help to build strength and endurance. Plus, when your children help, it doesn't take as long or seem as much of a chore (depending on

the age of the child, of course). There are numerous ways to make yard work more fun for children. For instance, when you finish raking a pile of leaves, you get to jump in them.

● **Wash the car together.** The scrubbing is good exercise, but everyone getting wet and soapy is the fun part for children.

● **Give your children a list of indoor chores – then join them.** Younger children often like to feel helpful and will enjoy helping you with household chores. Ask them to help you to make the beds, join in with the dusting, fold the laundry and put it away and set the table – all are physical activities that can help to get your heart rate up, stretch your body and build your muscles.

▐▐▐▶ **Take a hike at least twice a month.** Get together your backpack, plenty of water (everyone should aim to drink 1 cup [250 ml] every half-hour) and a light lunch and head to a local trail for a hiking expedition. Wear hiking boots for rocky terrain or running shoes for smoother paths, and pack sunscreen and insect repellent. To make it more fun, get children to focus on something else, such as looking for a particular animal, climbing to see a lake or pond or seeing how many rocks you can scamper over without touching the ground. Children like hiking much better when they don't realize it's about hiking! Bring a picnic; this is a great opportunity to share a delicious but healthy meal.

● **Dance during commercial breaks.** Make it a rule that whenever you watch television, you have to stand up and dance around during the commercials. This goes for everyone in the room. Whoever gets caught sitting on the couch during a

Healthy INVESTMENT

A mini-trampoline

Your children will probably turn up their noses at most adult types of fitness equipment such as a treadmill or hand weights. A mini-trampoline, however, is another story. You can set one up in your living room and line it with pillows. When you feel tempted to babysit your child with the TV, suggest he or she jumps on the trampoline for 15 minutes. That will burn about 100 calories rather than the mere 10 calories burned during 15 minutes of watching television. Buy a trampoline designed for indoor use that contains handles for safety and make sure it's far away from any hard or sharp objects in case of falls.

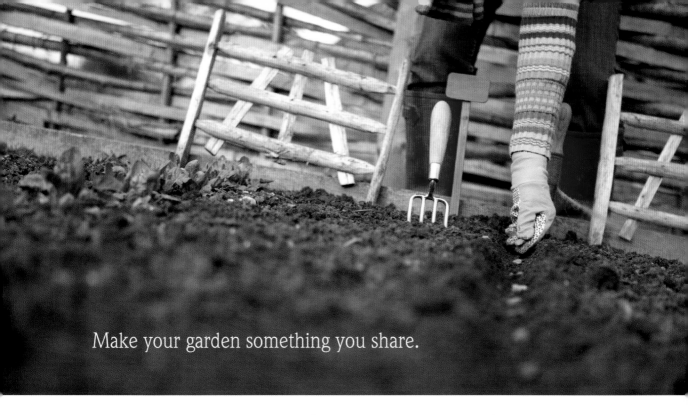

Make your garden something you share.

commercial must perform his or her least-liked chore for a week.

● **Sign up for a race.** Check your local paper for a list of 5 K and 10 K walks or runs in your area. Many of these events also raise money for charity, which can inspire your children to train with you. You will contribute to your family's health, and to research to help find cures for many diseases. Don't worry about finishing; the motivation involved in training for it is enough on its own.

● **Play volleyball once a week in warm weather.** Set up a net, get a ball and invite other children and their parents over for a game. For even greater fitness, add these rules:
● When the opposing team scores a point, the other team must do ten additional moves, such as star jumps, push-ups or crunches.
● Whoever is responsible for fumbling a shot must walk, dance, skip or jog around the court.

● **Plan a garden together.** As you dig holes, plant seeds and pull weeds, you'll build your child's and your own upper-body strength. As an added bonus, research shows that children are more likely to eat the vegetables they help to grow, which means your gardening forays will help your child to follow a more nutritious diet.

● **Try a family-friendly game of "flag football."** Buy some table napkins in two colours. Divide your family into two teams and ask everyone to tuck one of the coloured napkins into his or her waistband. When an opposing team member pulls a napkin from the ball-carrier's waistband and places it on the ground, the play has ended. Allow only 20 seconds to prepare for the next kick-off. Switch positions every 15 minutes to keep the entire family active. Not only will you get in some family fitness time, but you'll also be teaching your children valuable lessons about practice, perseverance, cooperation and teamwork.

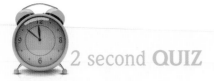

2 second QUIZ

Organized sports or fun in the backyard?
ANSWER: FUN IN THE BACKYARD.

It's controversial, but the best choice is old-fashioned fun, peppered with lots of silliness, made-up games, chasing each other and ball games. At their best, organized team sports let those with good sporting skills hone their game and learn competition, teamwork and mental toughness. The problem is that many children get turned off to exercise and competition – or they start to think that exercise can happen only in formal, rigorous situations. Simply having fun in the backyard is easier to fit into your hectic schedule, doesn't depend on scheduled practices and games and knows no seasons. It's an approach to exercise that lasts for life.

Dance, dance, dance. Put on your favourite music and dance with your children. Vigorous dancing burns just as many calories as brisk walking. And children love it – particularly when the adults pick them up and swing them around every now and then. And don't just leave dancing to chance, or when you happen to be in the mood – make sure you have one or even two family dance sessions a week. Here's an idea: perhaps a Friday night dance can become a family tradition. Let everyone take turns to choose some music, and let yourself go.

Act like a child. Remember duck-duck-goose or hopscotch? You probably thought of these games as just that, children's games. But they also require movement and count as exercise. Teach them to your children and play along. As you laugh, you'll burn extra calories.

Move like an animal. If you have young children aged three to eight, organize an animal race. Let everyone in the family pick an animal, such as a snake, monkey, horse or crab. Then race across the room as you imitate how that animal might move. For example, if you choose a monkey, race using your hands and feet, but not your knees or torso. If you are imitating a snake, slither across the room. Add some animal noises for real fun.

Walk around the world. Place a city, country or world map somewhere prominent in your home. Work with your children to arrive at a certain destination. Then, based on your daily family walks, plot your progress on the map using drawing pins. There are about 1,300 steps in a kilometre, so you can plot your progress using a pedometer. To add some incentive, why not promise to take a trip to your actual destination once you complete the number of steps it takes to get there?

Start a ball fight. "A large, air-filled exercise ball can provide you and your children with plenty of fun, laughter and a great workout," says Liz Applegate, author of *Bounce Your Body Beautiful*. She suggests the following ball exercises:
● Stand facing your child with the ball between you. You should both grasp the ball at about chest level. This may mean you need to get on your knees depending on the height of your child. Then fight over the ball, rotating it from side to side for 15 to 20 seconds at a time.
● Stand holding the ball at chest level with your arms extended. Ask your child to try to knock the ball out of your hands by tapping different parts of it from different directions. To really up the ante, try it with your eyes closed.

● **Walk your children to and from school.** By walking with them, you not only get peace of mind that they're safe, but you also get to hear about their upcoming day on the way there, and how their day went on the way home.

● **Throw a ball or a Frisbee to one another.** It seems more like relaxation than structured exercise, but you'll get your heart rate up every time you have to run or leap for an errant ball or Frisbee. Plus, you'll both improve your hand–eye coordination.

● **Hold a night of active family games every week.** Organize a night of three-legged races, wheelbarrow races and so on, and challenge another family from your street to a friendly competition.

● **Place small children on the floor at least once a day** – and let them crawl, move and toddle. "Children are inherently active when given the opportunity to move," says Melinda S. Sothern, author of *Trim Kids*. Yet we often confine children and prevent the very exercise they need. For example, have you ever placed your baby in a swing to give yourself some free time? Ever settled your children in front of the DVD player or television when you needed a break? Instead of automatically finding a stationary activity for your children when you need your own personal time-out, encourage more activity. For toddlers and crawlers, find a safe space on the floor where they can move. Suggest that older children play in the sandbox or climb your backyard tree as you keep an eye open nearby.

● **Waltz with your baby.** If your baby is crying for attention, don't just stick a pacifier in his or her mouth or go for a

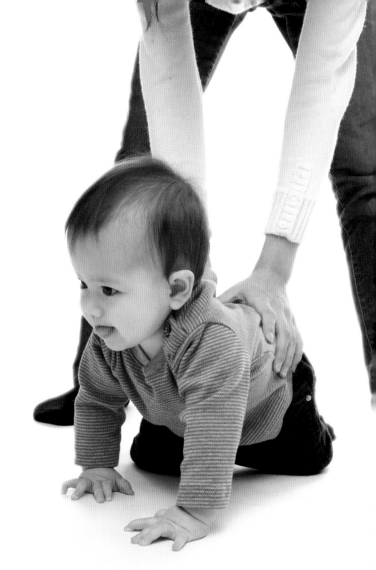

Place young children on the floor at least once a day.

Healthy **INVESTMENT**

Water bottles with carrying straps
Get one for every member of the family, strap them on, and head out for a five-kilometre hike/walk. They're handy – not to mention cost effective, as you avoid having to buy bottles of water to carry with you.

Setting limits on
TELEVISION TIME

One study of children aged 2 to 18 found that they spend an average of 5 hours and 29 minutes a day watching television, playing video games and using various other types of electronic media. You can increase your children's physical activity and decrease their sedentary behaviour with the following simple actions.

- Remove TVs and computers from children's bedrooms. According to research done at Johns Hopkins University, a child's weight increases with the number of hours he or she watches television.
- Place active toys such as skipping ropes, mini-trampolines and hula hoops within easy access in children's bedrooms or playrooms.
- Encourage your children to exercise during commercial breaks on TV.
- Put a curfew on electronics. For instance, nothing that requires batteries or electricity may be used until 5 p.m. on school days.
- Set a tit-for-tat rule. For every 30 minutes of television watching or Internet surfing, your child must do 30 minutes of physical activity.

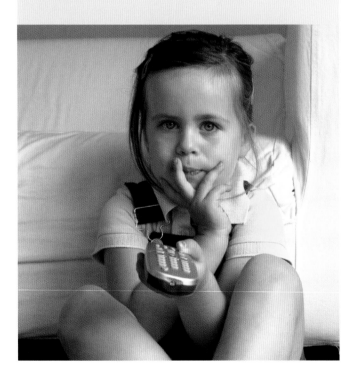

drive. Instead, take your baby in your arms and waltz around the room. The more exaggerated and smooth your movements, the better. The waltzing will give your baby new sights to focus on, soothing the crying. You'll burn extra calories and tone your arm muscles.

☺ **Design your backyard for activity.** What you put in your backyard helps to determine how fit your children become. If they see it, they will play. If they don't, they will watch TV. Older children enjoy climbing on ropes or ladders and playing in forts. If you can, get a trampoline, a swing, slide or monkey bars, a net for practising netball or basketball, and other outdoor sporting equipment.

● **Play active computer games.** Although most computer games exercise only the muscles in the fingers and eyes, a few can produce a decent workout. At the video arcade, challenge your child to one of the dance-mat games where you step on floor squares in the order they light up. At home, consider investing in a Wii gaming console. Wii games require players to move around as they compete against one another. It's great fun and it will get everyone in the family moving more as you play together.

● **Create an obstacle course.** Set out hula hoops, pillows and other devices that you can imagine as "rocks." Then tell your children that the hoops are rocks in a turbulent river. You all must jump from rock to rock to avoid falling in and getting swept away, or eaten by a crocodile.

● **Try out the hula hoop and other toys.** You and your children will bond, and you'll be the coolest parent around if you can master the hula hoop.

● **Crawl with your baby.** Too often, once babies start to crawl, we confine them to a bouncy chair. Crawling helps to develop upper-body strength for both you and your baby, and it's a great aerobic activity. So get down on all fours and crawl around the room together. To add to the challenge, take a large, air-filled ball (perhaps your exercise ball) and push it with your nose as you crawl.

● **Play tug-of-war.** You'll develop upper-body and lower-body strength as you tug on the rope. To keep it fair, place two children on one side of the rope and yourself on the other. Bend your knees and bring your legs into a lunge position to get a leg workout as you tug the rope.

● **Learn a sport together.** How about roller skating or golf? Or plan a winter skiing vacation where you can all take lessons together. Or try martial arts. Many local community and fitness centres offer martial arts classes designed for adults and children, and many forms of martial arts provide aerobic, strength and flexibility training. In these classes, your children will also learn self-control and discipline as well as boosting their self-esteem, balance and posture.

● **Play "Pinja."** This is a fun game based on the *Lion King* film, in which Nala plays with Simba and says "pinned ya" every time she manages to get him on his back. Pretend you and your children are all characters from the film and wrestle each other around the living-room floor. The game is over when you are wiped out (the children could probably go on all night).

● **Plan pedometer competitions.** Pick a week in which each member of the family wears a pedometer and you compete to see who can achieve the most steps.

☺ **Set a good example with simple habits.** Use the stairs instead of the escalator, park far from the entrance of a building. Your children will think this is simply the way things are done, and will carry these good health habits into adulthood.

● **Add fun to physically active obligations.** Put on music when sweeping, vacuuming or doing the dishes. Make things a little more fun by creating a game out of chores (who can find the biggest dust bunny?).

● **Look into family fitness programs at your local health club.** Many fitness clubs offer fitness programs for families, ranging from aerobics to swimming to roller skating. Don't just sign everyone up and hope for the best, though. For best results, sit down with your family and go over your options together.

● **Organize a playgroup with other parents and children in your area.** As the toddlers actively play together, the adults can exercise around the periphery.

Healthy INVESTMENT

Water shoes
Get a pair for every member of the family. With aqua or watersport shoes, you're all set for exploring wildlife in a stream and searching the shoreline without any fear of cutting your foot. And they're often great on dry land too – lightweight, snug, comfortable with a strong rubber sole to protect the bottoms of your feet. And no socks needed. They're easy to clean, simple to slip on and off and inexpensive compared with most sandals.

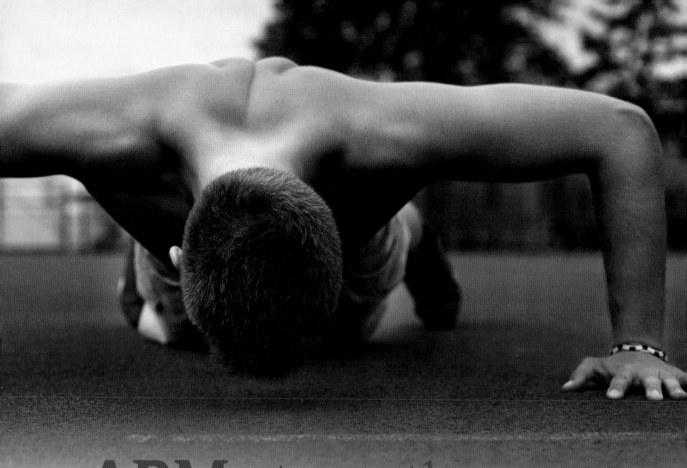

ARM strength

More than 70 years ago, you rarely heard of people lifting weights to keep their arms strong. They didn't have to. Washing clothes by hand, scrubbing pots, chopping wood and scrubbing floors all maintained the muscle mass we needed to stay strong as we aged. Today, of course, things have changed. Modern conveniences mean we rarely call upon our arm muscles to do much of anything. Over a lifetime, this can cause your muscles to wither away. You get weaker and weaker, daily tasks become harder and your body puts on weight and grows more susceptible to disease as you become more and more sedentary. So don't think of strengthening your arms as an act of vanity. The tips in this chapter will help you to fit some arm-strengthening moves into your routines.

17 WAYS TO EXERCISE WITH – OR WITHOUT – WEIGHTS

● **Each autumn, plant bulbs on three consecutive weekends.** Make each planting session last at least an hour. Congratulations – that's your arm workout for the week. Digging in your garden will strengthen your hands, wrists, forearms, upper arms and shoulders. Your hard work will pay off in the spring, when your daffodils and tulips bloom.

● **Stop using weedkiller on your garden.** Yes, this will encourage weeds to grow with wild abandon (even with mulch). That's good, because your job is to get down on your hands and knees once a week to rip weeds out of the ground. Leaning onto your hands as you weed will build arm, shoulder and upper back strength, and yanking the weeds provides an extra dose of arm-building strength. Just remember to alternate hands as you reach and pull so that you work both arms equally.

▶ **Cut your own wood.** If you have a real fire, the chances are you're burning pre-cut logs. If you have the option, though, go out and chop your own wood. Do 30 minutes of log chopping every weekend. Too much at once and it's bad for your back. But in small doses, cutting wood is amazingly good exercise.

● **Scrub the floors on your hands and knees once a week.** Not only will you have cleaner floors than a mop provides, but you'll strengthen your arms at the same time.

● **Bake bread once a week.** You'll strengthen your arms, shoulders and hands as you simultaneously soothe away stress. There's little more calming than the repetitive motion of kneading dough and nothing more pleasing than the smell of bread in the oven. Plus, home-baked

bread – kneaded with your own two hands – tastes better than anything from the store or made in a bread maker.

● **Make your own pizza dough instead of buying it pre-made.** The forward and back action of using a rolling pin is a great arm and shoulder workout. And your family will thank you for your effort later, as no store-bought product compares to homemade.

In PERSPECTIVE

Build strength

When people in their 20s are described as "strong," chances are the subject is muscles. Call someone in his or her 60s "strong," and you're probably talking about character. It's time to change that perception.

The benefits of strong muscles – particularly for people above 50, especially women – are vast. Steve Nance, Performance Director at Pure Sports Medicine in the U.K., says it's also very good for women to do strength training to prevent osteoporosis. Here's why building stronger muscles is one of the best health-boosting pursuits:

● Strong muscles help you to lose weight. Muscle tissue burns as much as 15 times more calories per day than fat tissue does – even when at rest.

● Strong muscles are healthy for your heart. That's because they can perform better with less oxygen, meaning the heart doesn't have to pump too hard when you are active. By extension, strong muscles are good for your blood pressure.

● Strong muscles protect your joints and your back. More muscle power means you put less strain on your joints and connective tissue when lifting or exerting yourself. And that's important both for treating and preventing arthritis.

● Strong muscles improve your looks and give you a mental boost. You feel more energized, and prouder about yourself.

● Strong muscles require active living. You can't get strong muscles from a pill, a meal or a herb. The mere fact that you have strong muscles means you're being active.

● Strong muscles help to fight free radicals (see page 91). Research shows that when people lift weights regularly, they suffer less damage from free radicals than those who are sedentary.

ARM EXERCISES for TV ad-breaks

⭐**Do each of the following exercises at least once a week.** For even better effect, do them twice a week. An easy system: do one exercise each night during a 3 minute commercial break on television (have a rest day on Sunday). Do three slow sets of 10 to 12 repetitions, with 20 seconds of breathing time between sets. This will require keeping a set of dumbbells next to the couch. Beginners should use 2 kg (4 $^1/_2$ lb) dumbbells, and more active adults should try 5 kg or 7 kg (11 or 15$^1/_2$ lb) versions.

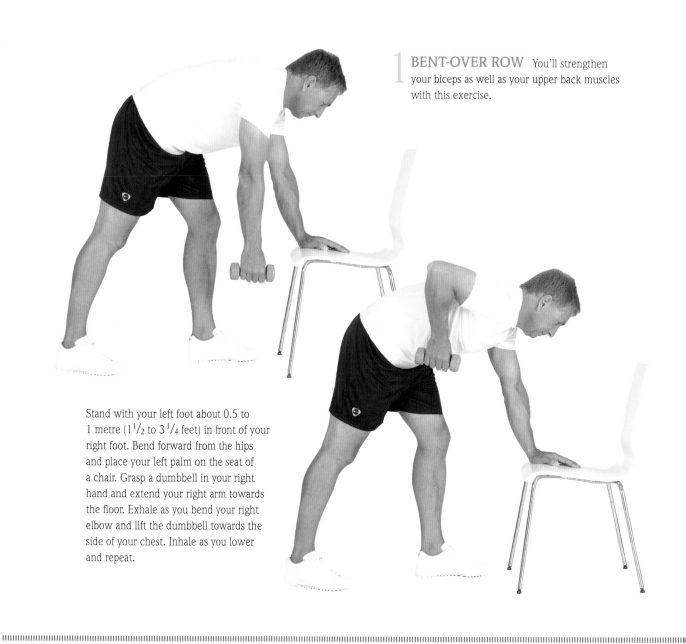

1 **BENT-OVER ROW** You'll strengthen your biceps as well as your upper back muscles with this exercise.

Stand with your left foot about 0.5 to 1 metre (1$^1/_2$ to 3$^1/_4$ feet) in front of your right foot. Bend forward from the hips and place your left palm on the seat of a chair. Grasp a dumbbell in your right hand and extend your right arm towards the floor. Exhale as you bend your right elbow and lift the dumbbell towards the side of your chest. Inhale as you lower and repeat.

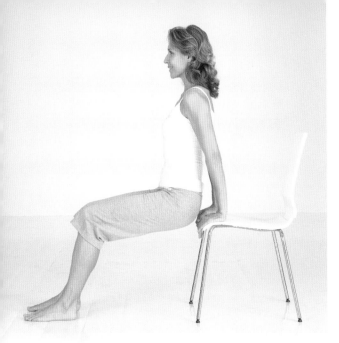

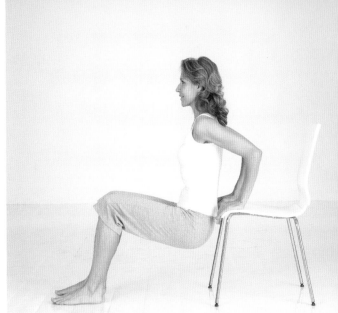

2 **CHAIR DIP** This exercise, above, strengthens your triceps, the muscles along the back of your upper arms (the ones that flap about when you wave goodbye) and your chest muscles.

Sit on the edge of a sturdy chair. Place your palms on the seat of the chair, at either side of your bottom, with your fingers facing forward. Place your feet flat on the floor with your knees bent. Press into your hands and lift your butt about 3 centimetres (1 inch) up and forward, until you can clear the seat of the chair. Inhale as you bend your elbows, lowering your butt towards the floor. Keeping your elbows close to your sides, exhale as you extend your arms and return to the starting position. Be careful you're not cheating by pushing yourself back up with your legs rather than your arms.

   As you gain strength, you can increase the challenge by extending your legs and placing only your heels on the floor.

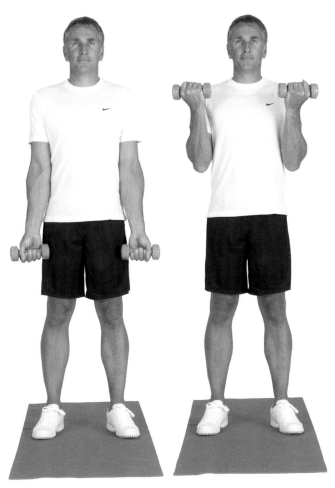

3 **BICEPS CURL** This exercise, right, strengthens your biceps, the muscles along the front of your upper arms.

Grasp a dumbbell in each hand. Extend your arms at your sides with your palms facing forward. Exhale as you curl your hands towards your shoulders, keeping your elbows close to your sides. Inhale as you lower the weights.

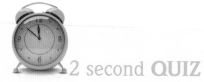

2 second QUIZ

Fast lifting or slow lifting?
ANSWER: **SLOW LIFTING.**

The research is clear: the slower you move the weight, the better. In one American study involving 147 people, participants who lifted slowly – taking a full 14 seconds to complete one repetition – gained more strength than participants who spent just 7 seconds on each repetition. Plus, even though the slow weightlifting group completed fewer repetitions of each exercise (just 4 to 6 compared to the faster group's 8 to 12), they still gained more strength. Slower lifting may help to increase strength because it prevents you from using momentum or cheating with improper technique.

● **Trade in your electric mixer for a whisk and wooden spoon.** You'll build arm strength as you use your own elbow grease to mix batter. Be sure to use both hands to work your arms evenly.

● **Make an omelette rather than fried eggs.** Fill it with at least three different vegetables, such as spinach, mushrooms and onions. You'll not only use your arms to whisk the eggs and chop the veggies, but you'll also improve your health by incorporating veg into your morning meal.

☺ **Use a cast-iron pot for most of your cooking** – and store it in the drawer under the oven. That way, you need to lift the heavy pot onto the stove each time you need it – building more arm strength with every meal.

☺ **Have a large cleaver for everyday chopping and cooking.** Professional chefs love cleavers for their weight and super-sharp, slightly rounded edge. Use one too and you'll give your hand and arm a great workout while you cook.

● **Pour water out of a large jug.** The weight of a large jug may do wonders for your arms (4 litres of water weighs more than 3.5 kg or 8 lb). Bend your elbow and bring your hand to your shoulder five times before pouring.

● **Spend 10 minutes every working day building up resistance in your office.** You have everything you need in the office to keep your arms in great shape. Here are some great office-based arm exercises:
● Desk curl. Place your palms against the underside of your desk with your elbows bent. Push up into the desk with your palms, as if you were trying to lift the desk off the floor. Hold for a count of five, release, then repeat until you feel the burn. This strengthens your biceps.
● Desk push. Place your palms against the top of your desk with your elbows bent. Press into the desktop with all your might. Hold for a count of five, release, then repeat until you feel the burn. This strengthens your triceps.
● Desk push-up. Stand about a half-metre (1½ feet) away from your desk. Keep your feet in place and lean forward from your ankles, placing your palms on top of the desk. Your body should form a straight line from your ankles to your head. Bend your elbows as you lower your chest towards the desk. Straighten your elbows as you push away. Keep your elbows in close to your sides the entire time. This works your triceps.

● **Eat a steak on the nights you work out.** Researchers at the University of Wollongong in New South Wales, Australia, put 28 participants aged 60-plus on one of two diet and exercise programs. Both programs contained weightlifting exercises and a diet that included 20 per cent protein. One diet, however, included 700 g of red meat a week (the amount in three medium steaks), whereas the other included just over 350 g of red meat (the amount in $1\frac{1}{2}$ medium steaks). After 12 weeks, those with the extra red meat increased their muscle strength more than those who ate less red meat. Researchers suspect the extra red meat supplies additional amino acids needed for muscle growth. If you plan to increase your consumption of red meat, choose lean cuts, such as sirloin, rather than rib-eye. That helps to protect your heart as you build up your strength.

● **Hang your laundry outside instead of using the dryer.** As well as saving money on your electricity bill, you'll get in a mild arm workout. As you carry the laundry basket to the clothes line, curl it up and down, bringing your hands to your shoulders. You can also hold it overhead, bending, then extending your elbows.

● **Curl your groceries.** When you get home from the supermarket, carry one bag in each hand. As you walk from the car to the kitchen, curl your groceries by lifting your hands towards your shoulders, keeping your elbows close to your sides. By the time you bring in all of the bags of shopping, you'll have given your biceps a good workout – and you'll have burned some extra calories by making the extra trips to and from the car.

 Try these isometric exercises. These types of exercise are performed against something that doesn't move, like a wall. By pushing against the immovable object, tension builds up in your muscles, increasing their strength. Hold each for 5 to 8 seconds, and repeat five to ten times.
● Press your hands together as hard as you can ten times for 5 seconds at a time. This will really make a difference to your arm strength after a couple of weeks. Try it every time you sit down to watch TV.
● Stand with your legs apart about 30 cm (1 foot) from the wall and push against the wall as if you were trying to move it.
● Stand in the doorway with your legs straight and knees locked. Press your hands upwards against the top of the door frame, holding for several seconds, then relaxing. Repeat at least ten times.
● Extend both arms to the side of the doorway with your palms shoulder high, facing outwards. With both arms, press hard against the sides of the door frame. Hold for several seconds, relax, then repeat up to ten times.
● Extend both arms to the sides of the doorway, arms down, palms facing in. With the back of your hands, press hard against the sides of the frame. Hold for a few seconds, relax, then repeat up to ten times.

Hang your laundry for a swift arm workout.

Reminder

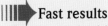 **Fast results**
These are tips that deliver benefits particularly quickly – in some cases, immediately.

 Easy gains
These are health boosters that offer the best value for the least amount of effort.

 Super-effective
This is advice that scientific research or widespread usage by experts has shown to be especially effective.

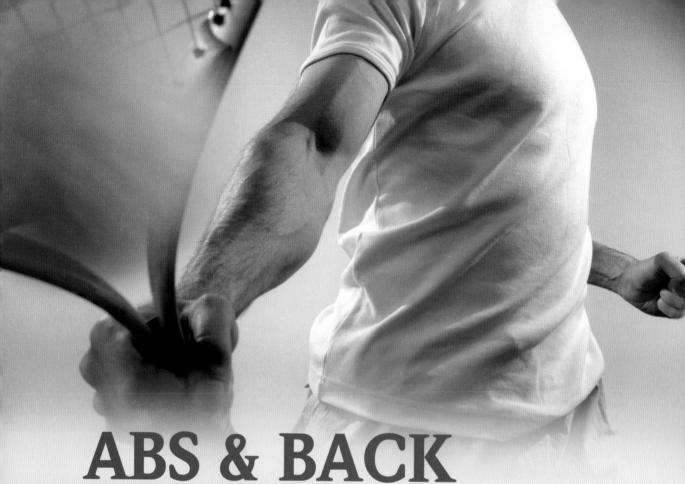

ABS & BACK
strength

Your abs (abdominal muscles) and back are the core of your body, the power centre from which all movement originates. Strengthen them and you'll move with more power and grace. Strong abdominal muscles also help to support and move your spine, protecting your back from injury. Finally, strengthen the lowest part of your core – your pelvic-floor muscles – and you'll prevent incontinence and may even improve your sex life. In this chapter, you'll discover a whole new world of opportunities for abdominal and back strengthening beyond the basic crunch.

17 WAYS TO FEEL LESS CRUNCHED DURING YOUR ROUTINE

● **If you walk for fitness, squeeze your butt.** When you are walking, imagine that you're holding a $50 bill between your butt cheeks As you firm and lift your butt muscles, you'll strengthen your back muscles as well. You can also work your abs as you walk by imagining you have a zipper along the midline of your abdomen. Picture yourself zipping up a tight pair of jeans. As you pull the zip up your abdomen, feel your torso lengthen and your abdomen firm up. Keep your abs zipped up and your bottom tucked under throughout your walks and you'll strengthen your core even as you burn fat.

● **While driving, tighten your stomach and pelvic-floor muscles.** Starting with your pubic area, begin to tighten from the bottom up. Once you squeeze your pelvic floor, suck in your lower belly and then upper belly towards your spine as you exhale. Hold for a count of five, then release and repeat 10 to 20 times.

● **When you're nervous,** tighten and release your abdominal muscles over and over again. You'll strengthen your abs and take your mind off your anxiety. This is a particularly good exercise for when you are nervous about an upcoming speech or presentation.

● **During commercial breaks on TV,** sit on the edge of your chair and lift your feet off the floor, bringing your knees into your chest. Lower and repeat 10 to 15 times.

● **Whenever you find yourself standing in a line,** lift one foot off the floor and try to hold your balance. You'll feel the myriad muscles in your abdomen and back firing up to help to steady your body. Be sure to alternate your feet.

In PERSPECTIVE

Achieving flat abs

So what does it take to have an abdomen that is so strong, so slender, that it reveals beautifully symmetric, perfectly arranged muscles? There are a few surprises in the answers.

Most of all, it takes being very, very lean. For most people, much of their fat lies in the abdomen, and much of that abdominal fat lies between the skin and abdominal muscles. That layer of fat covers up the shapeliness of the muscles. So models and athletes with "six-pack abs" must have very low body fat to reveal that musculature. Sit-ups didn't get them that way – you cannot "spot reduce" fat from your belly using abs exercises. To melt the fat off your body, it requires a low-calorie diet and lots of aerobic exercise such as cycling, walking or running.

Of course, it does take targeted exercise to create big, shapely abdominal muscles. A lot, in fact. While most of us think of the abs as a simple band of muscles across the top of the abdomen, there are many separate abdominal muscles, with names such as "obliques" and "transversus abdominis." People serious about their abs know all these muscles, and target each one for exercise. A thorough abs workout could involve ten different abdominal exercises.

Is all this necessary? Maybe for models, but not for you. What's important is that your ab muscles are conditioned well enough to support your back and allow you to twist, turn and lift without a challenge. If you are at a healthy weight but have a little fat covering your abdominal muscles, consider yourself well ahead of the game.

☺ **Do abdominal exercises as a warm-up for your workout.** The typical workout starts out with 5 or 10 minutes of walking or marching to get your body warmed up and your blood flowing. In truth, that can be boring. Instead, do your abdominal work. Because your abdomen consists of large muscle groups, abdominal work is very warming for the body. Just 5 to 10 minutes of abdominal exercises will warm you up just as well as walking, and give you some good muscle building at the same time.

ABS & BACK ball exercises

● **Use your exercise ball to do abs and back exercises.** Whenever you perform abdominal-strengthening movements on a ball, you use more of your core muscles for every movement. Try the traditional crunch on the ball, shown on page 174, along with these additional ball moves, courtesy of musculoskeletal physiotherapist Claire Small.

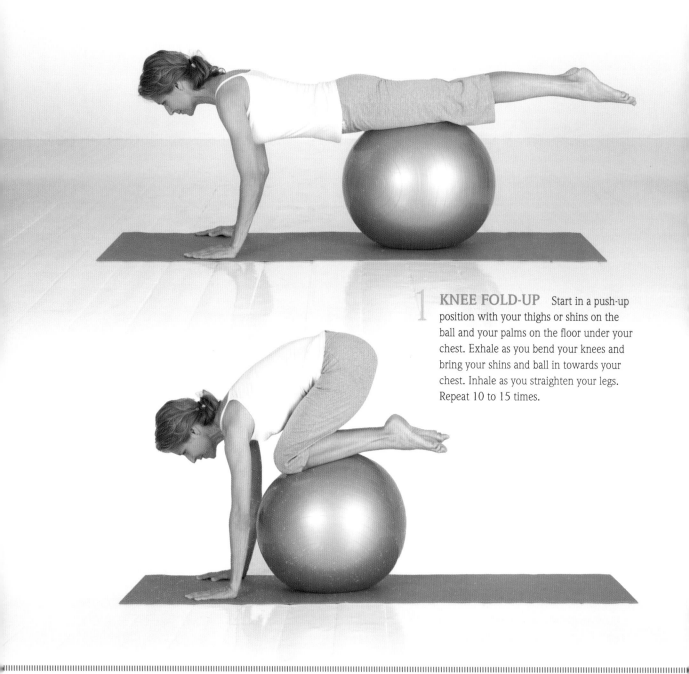

1 **KNEE FOLD-UP**   Start in a push-up position with your thighs or shins on the ball and your palms on the floor under your chest. Exhale as you bend your knees and bring your shins and ball in towards your chest. Inhale as you straighten your legs. Repeat 10 to 15 times.

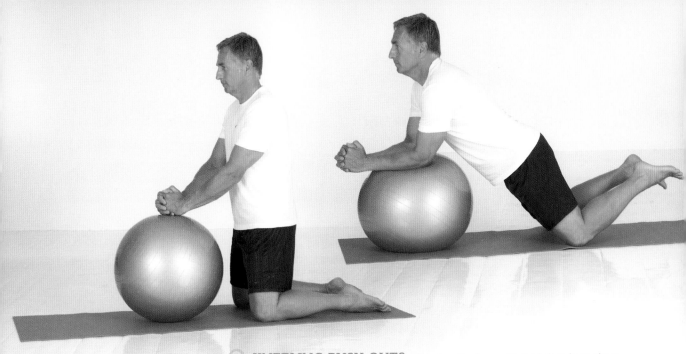

2 **KNEELING PUSH-OUTS** Kneel on the floor with the ball in front of you, keeping your head in a neutral position, with your chin tucked in and your spine stable. Clasp your hands and press the bottoms of your hands into the ball. Lift your feet and shins and balance on your knees. Exhale as you press your hands into the ball and roll the ball forward. Your knees will stay in place, but your feet and shins will rise and your torso will lean forward. Raise yourself back up and repeat 15 times.

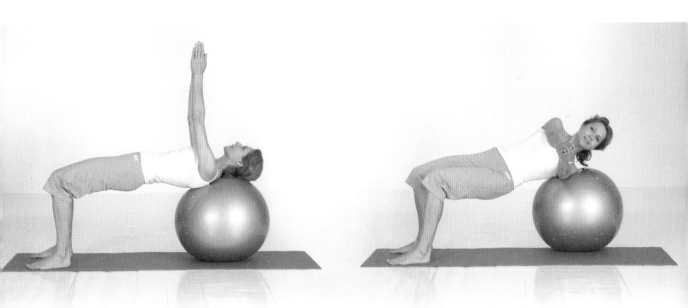

3 **ARM SWING** Lie with your upper back on the ball, your knees bent and your feet on the floor. Clasp your hands together and extend your arms towards the ceiling, so that they are perpendicular with your torso.

Exhale and roll your torso to the left, lifting your right shoulder off the ball. Return to the starting position and repeat to the right, alternating sides. Complete 10 to 15 rolls on each side.

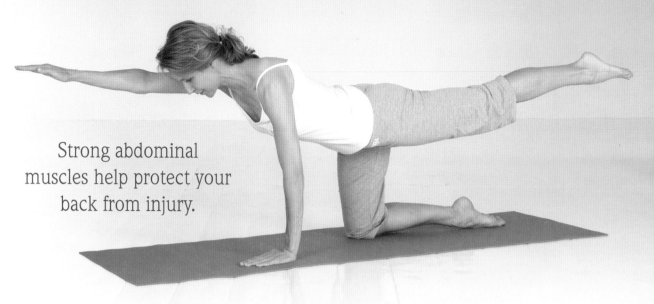

Strong abdominal
muscles help protect your
back from injury.

● **Three times a week, when you get home from work,** try the stretching exercise above. It's called the reciprocal reach (or sometimes the opposite limb extension) and it helps you to strengthen your abdominal muscles and back at the same time. Get on all fours with your hands flat on the floor directly under your shoulders and your knees under your hips. Extend your left leg behind, placing the ball of your left foot against the floor. Tuck in your tail bone and try to keep it tucked in throughout the exercise. Lift your left foot off the floor as you lift your right arm, reaching your right hand and left foot away from each other. Keep your hips level. Do not let your back arch during this exercise. Imagine you have a large glass of water standing on your lower back as you do it. As you move your arms and legs, your back must stay stable so as not to spill the water. Hold for 10 to 20 seconds, release, then repeat on the other side. Work up to two to three sets.

☺ **Set the alarm on your watch or computer to do hourly posture checks.** Your abdominal muscles support your spine; strengthening them will help to improve your posture, and improving your posture will help to strengthen your abdominal muscles. So do a posture check. Set your alarm (but quietly, so as not to annoy colleagues). Every hour, imagine you are zipping up a tight pair of jeans. Extend your spine, bringing the top of your head towards the ceiling. As you do so, your lower abdomen should pull up and in towards your spine and your lower back should flatten slightly as your tail bone reaches towards the floor.

● **Strengthen your waist and back with a medicine ball twist.** Stand back-to-back with a friend. Hold a heavy medicine ball with both hands and rotate to your right to hand the ball off to your friend. Your friend takes the ball, rotates and hands it off to your left. Continue to receive and hand off the ball for 1 minute, then change direction.

● **As you watch television, fly like Superman.** This simple exercise will strengthen your lower back. Lie on your stomach with your legs extended. Extend your arms in front. Inhale as you lift your shoulders and feet, reaching your hands and feet away from each other. Hold for 10 to 20 seconds. Lower and repeat once or twice.

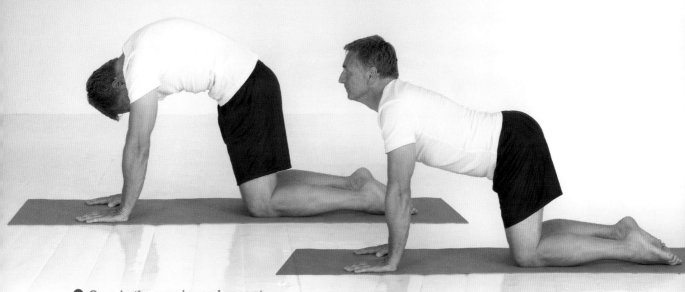

● **Once in the morning and once at night, pretend you're a scared cat.** Get on the floor on your hands and knees (as above). Exhale as you curl your spine towards the ceiling, tucking in your tail bone and bringing your chin to your chest. As you do so, bring your navel up and in towards your spine. Inhale as you gently flatten your back, raise your head and push up your hips, letting your back dip in the other direction to mobilize your spine really effectively. Continue to curl and flatten your spine as you breathe, doing ten repetitions. This stretch will help to work the kinks out of your spine before bed and first thing in the morning.

● **Take a Pilates class once a week.** This method of exercise was developed by Joseph Pilates in the early 1920s. It places a heavy emphasis on the abdominals and core as it simultaneously strengthens the arms and legs. Although many books and DVDs teach Pilates, you'll get the best results by taking a few classes with a certified instructor. Then you can practise at home with a DVD.

● **For a simple, effective back stretch, lie flat on your back.** Lift one knee to your chest, then the other, keeping your lower back on the floor. Wrap your arms behind your knees, using them to support

your legs and, if necessary, pulling them so that your butt rises off the floor. You should feel your back muscles stretching. Hold for 30 seconds, then release.

● **Try a handbag or briefcase side bend.** This is another exercise that's great for your obliques and can be done anywhere, at any time. Stand upright with your briefcase or bag in your right hand, palm facing in, your feet about shoulder-width apart. Slowly bend to your right, allowing the item to drop directly down your right leg until you feel a stretch along your left side. Keep your body facing forward the whole time. Once you've gone as low as possible, slowly return to upright, repeat for a set of 10 to 20 repetitions, then switch hands and repeat on the other side.

● **For upper-back strength, do shrugs – with weights.** Hold a light dumbbell in each hand, allowing your arms to hang down naturally at your sides, palms facing in, with legs about shoulder-width apart. Slowly shrug your shoulders straight up towards your ears. Pause, then lower them back to the starting position. Repeat until your muscles feel fatigued. Don't rotate your shoulders – that will strain them. Concentrate on going up and down.

The most effective
ABDOMINAL EXERCISES

Researchers at San Diego State University have tested numerous abdominal exercises for their effectiveness; surprisingly, the quintessential crunch ranked only 11th out of the 13 exercises tested. Here are five of the best.

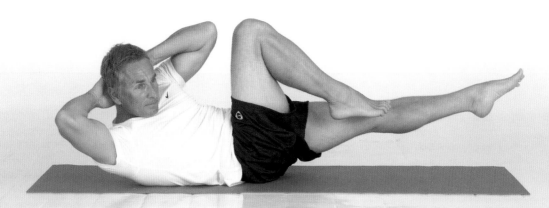

1 BICYCLE Lie on your back. Tuck in your tail bone and press your lower back against the floor. Place your fingertips behind your head and your elbows out to the sides. Bend your knees and lift your feet off the floor, keeping a 45 degree bend in your knees. Begin to pedal your legs, bringing your opposite elbow to the opposite knee as you extend your free leg.

2 BALL CRUNCH A large, air-filled exercise ball will wiggle under your back, causing you to recruit more muscles as you crunch.

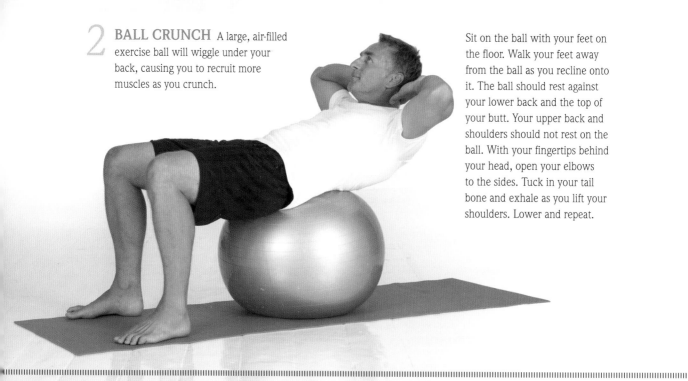

Sit on the ball with your feet on the floor. Walk your feet away from the ball as you recline onto it. The ball should rest against your lower back and the top of your butt. Your upper back and shoulders should not rest on the ball. With your fingertips behind your head, open your elbows to the sides. Tuck in your tail bone and exhale as you lift your shoulders. Lower and repeat.

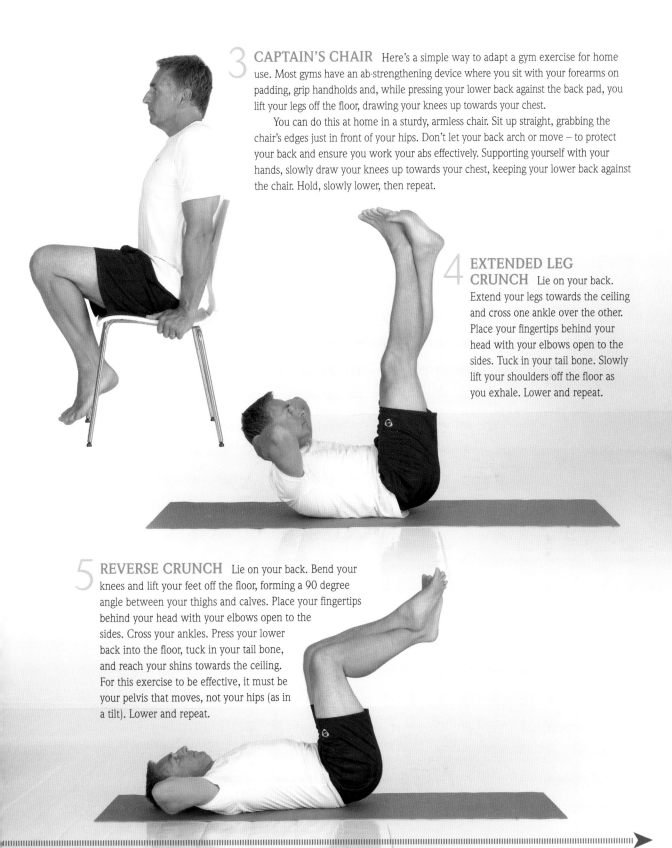

3 CAPTAIN'S CHAIR Here's a simple way to adapt a gym exercise for home use. Most gyms have an ab-strengthening device where you sit with your forearms on padding, grip handholds and, while pressing your lower back against the back pad, you lift your legs off the floor, drawing your knees up towards your chest.

You can do this at home in a sturdy, armless chair. Sit up straight, grabbing the chair's edges just in front of your hips. Don't let your back arch or move – to protect your back and ensure you work your abs effectively. Supporting yourself with your hands, slowly draw your knees up towards your chest, keeping your lower back against the chair. Hold, slowly lower, then repeat.

4 EXTENDED LEG CRUNCH Lie on your back. Extend your legs towards the ceiling and cross one ankle over the other. Place your fingertips behind your head with your elbows open to the sides. Tuck in your tail bone. Slowly lift your shoulders off the floor as you exhale. Lower and repeat.

5 REVERSE CRUNCH Lie on your back. Bend your knees and lift your feet off the floor, forming a 90 degree angle between your thighs and calves. Place your fingertips behind your head with your elbows open to the sides. Cross your ankles. Press your lower back into the floor, tuck in your tail bone, and reach your shins towards the ceiling. For this exercise to be effective, it must be your pelvis that moves, not your hips (as in a tilt). Lower and repeat.

AB-STRENGTHENING ball routine

● **Use a children's ball as an abdominal strengthening aid.** Children's play balls or small (about 20 cm/8 in.), fitness balls make great workout aids. To start, use one in the kitchen while cooking. Place the ball between your thighs, just above your knees. As you work, squeeze your inner thighs to hold the ball in place. This action fires up your pelvic floor and lower abdominal muscles. You can also use a small ball to increase the effectiveness of traditional abdominal exercises. Here are a few to try:

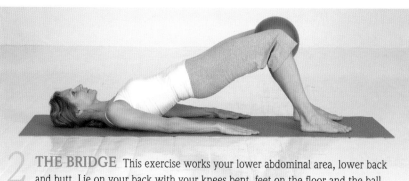

2 **THE BRIDGE** This exercise works your lower abdominal area, lower back and butt. Lie on your back with your knees bent, feet on the floor and the ball between your thighs. Rest your arms at your sides with your palms down. Tuck in your tail bone and lift your hips and lower back off the floor. Lift only as high as you can while still keeping your tail bone tucked in. Hold for 10 to 20 seconds. Lower and repeat once or twice.

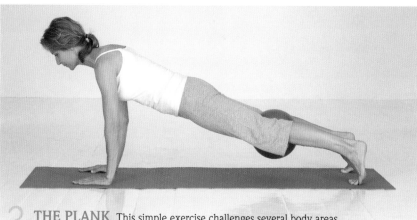

1 **THE MOUNTAIN** This exercise stretches your calves, helps your posture and, by adding in the small exercise ball, it works your lower abdominals as well.

Stand tall with the ball between your thighs. Lift your arches and squeeze the ball. Hold for 10 to 20 seconds. Release the ball, walk around a bit, then repeat the exercise once or twice.

3 **THE PLANK** This simple exercise challenges several body areas, including the shoulders, backs and abs. The small exercise ball brings even more pelvic muscles into the mix.

With the ball between your knees or thighs, come into a push-up position with your hands under your chest. Reach back through your heels and forward through the top of your head. Tuck in your tail bone. Hold for 10 to 20 seconds. Repeat once or twice.

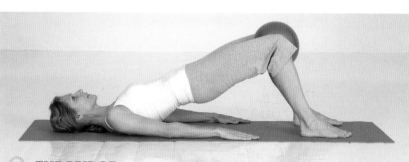

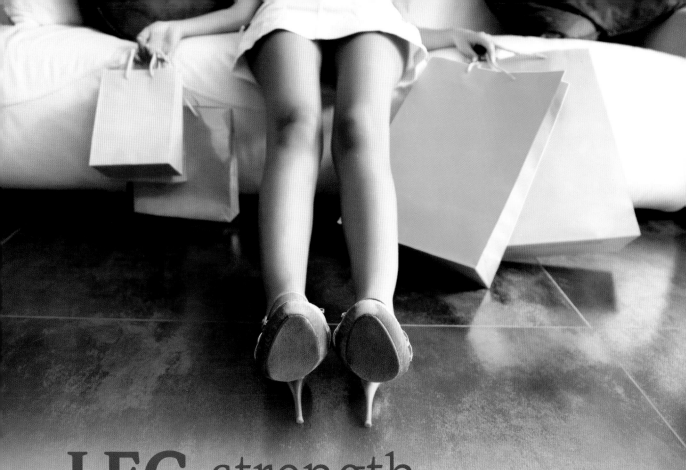

LEG strength

Your legs contain perhaps the easiest muscles in your body to keep in shape. After all, they support the weight of your body and you use them every time you walk. Just being on the go can help you to tone and fine-tune them, and they, in turn, will help you to burn calories and keep the rest of your body fit. Add some leg-strengthening exercises, and you'll gain even more benefits without a lot of effort. A stronger pair of legs will help you to accomplish more every day. You'll climb stairs more easily and be able to bend your knees and squat down to pick up heavy objects, protecting your lower back from strain. To strengthen your legs and avoid injury, you must work all of the muscles in your legs equally. The following tips will incorporate thorough leg work seamlessly into your day.

19 WAYS TO FIRM UP YOUR HIPS, THIGHS AND BUTTOCKS

● **Whenever you stop at traffic lights,** tighten your thighs and buttocks, over and over again. You will firm your leg muscles, boost blood flow (thus preventing the pins-and-needles sensation that tends to attack your butt when you've been sitting in a car seat for too long) and give yourself something to focus on.

● **Before you get out of bed in the morning, do the clam.** Lie on your back, bring your feet together, and open your knees out to the sides. Then, as you exhale, lift your knees, bringing them together. Lower and repeat this exercise 10 to 15 times and you'll strengthen your inner thighs.

● **Do leg lifts as you cook dinner.** Flex your foot and lift your leg out to the side, lower it, then repeat 10 to 15 times. Make sure you move only at the hip – don't let your waist move. Then swap legs. You'll finish your leg workout before dinner time.

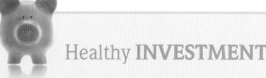

Healthy **INVESTMENT**

Ankle weights
One set of ankle weights allows you to do just about any leg exercise at home and you'll never have to set foot in the gym again to maintain shapely legs. In addition to the traditional leg lifts, you can use ankle weights to do other popular leg exercises such as hamstring curls and leg extensions, often performed on a machine at the gym. Look for ankle weights that allow you to add weight as you get stronger, and with Velcro straps rather than shoelaces for easy access and removal. Many of these weights contain small pockets into which you can insert or remove weighted bags. Try on the weights in the store to make sure they feel comfortable.

● **If you walk for fitness, switch to a softer surface.** Your legs get a better workout when you walk on trails or sand rather than pavement. And softer surfaces transfer less impact to your joints, preventing strain to your knees and back.

☺ **Get up, place your palms against your desk** and do a series of donkey kicks when you find yourself falling asleep at your keyboard. Bend one knee, flex that foot and kick your leg back, as if you were a donkey kicking someone behind you. Alternate legs for 15 kicks in total. Then return to work refreshed and with a stronger butt.

● **Instead of straining and reaching to get something** off a high shelf, step up on a stool. You'll strengthen your legs and protect your back.

● **Next time you find yourself at a wedding or other function** with a dance floor, do the twist. Or, do it in your living room tonight. Bend your knees and squat down as far as you comfortably can as you shimmy from side to side. You'll burn calories, have a few laughs and strengthen your legs – all at the same time.

● **Do the "lunge walk" in the backyard.** Your neighbours might laugh if they see you, but you'll have the last laugh when, in just minutes each day, you sculpt a toned pair of legs. During each step forward, bend your knees and sink down until both legs form 90 degree angles. Then press into your front heel to rise. Lift your back leg and knee all the way into your chest before planting it in front of you for the next lunge. This takes a little practice (see also page 182), but if you "lunge walk" for 20 or 30 steps a day, your legs will be far stronger and shapelier.

THE SQUAT: king of the leg exercises

Can you do only one leg exercise and still see results? Yes, if that exercise is a squat. You can strengthen all of the muscles in your legs and butt with either full squats or quarter-squats, says Jose Antonio, president of the International Society of Sports Nutrition.

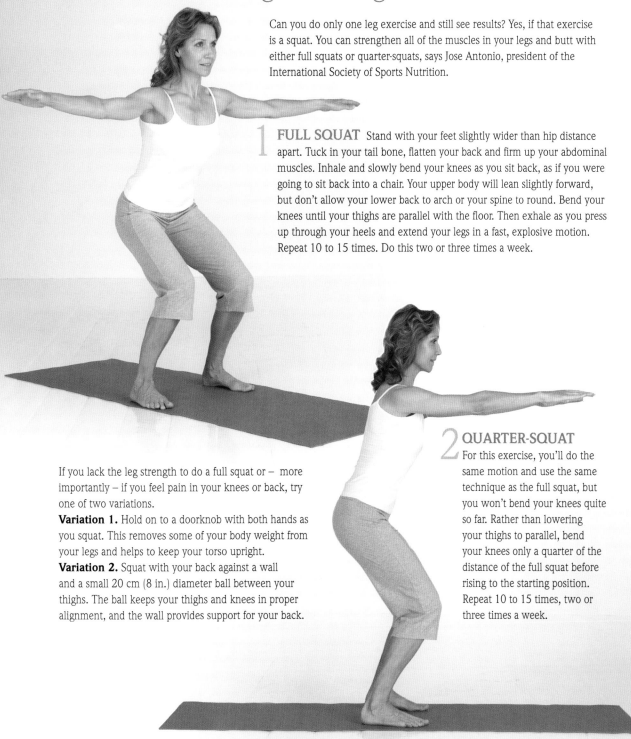

1 FULL SQUAT Stand with your feet slightly wider than hip distance apart. Tuck in your tail bone, flatten your back and firm up your abdominal muscles. Inhale and slowly bend your knees as you sit back, as if you were going to sit back into a chair. Your upper body will lean slightly forward, but don't allow your lower back to arch or your spine to round. Bend your knees until your thighs are parallel with the floor. Then exhale as you press up through your heels and extend your legs in a fast, explosive motion. Repeat 10 to 15 times. Do this two or three times a week.

If you lack the leg strength to do a full squat or – more importantly – if you feel pain in your knees or back, try one of two variations.

Variation 1. Hold on to a doorknob with both hands as you squat. This removes some of your body weight from your legs and helps to keep your torso upright.

Variation 2. Squat with your back against a wall and a small 20 cm (8 in.) diameter ball between your thighs. The ball keeps your thighs and knees in proper alignment, and the wall provides support for your back.

2 QUARTER-SQUAT For this exercise, you'll do the same motion and use the same technique as the full squat, but you won't bend your knees quite so far. Rather than lowering your thighs to parallel, bend your knees only a quarter of the distance of the full squat before rising to the starting position. Repeat 10 to 15 times, two or three times a week.

KICKBOXING

● **Practise kickboxing moves** for 5 minutes every morning before putting on your pants or skirt. There's nothing like seeing your bare thighs in the mirror to motivate you to do your kicks. Kick in all directions, mixing in front kicks, roundhouse kicks, side kicks and back kicks. No matter what kick you do, never fully extend your knee. This protects your knee joint.

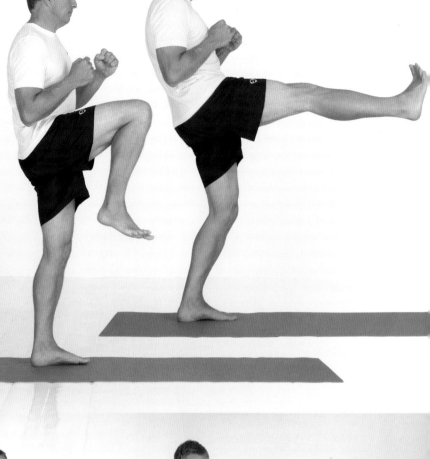

1 FRONT KICK Pretend an opponent is standing in front of you and you wish to kick him or her in the groin (or in the stomach). Lift one knee into your chest, then forcefully extend your leg, smacking the top of your foot into your imaginary target. Recoil your leg quickly and follow up with the other leg in quick succession.

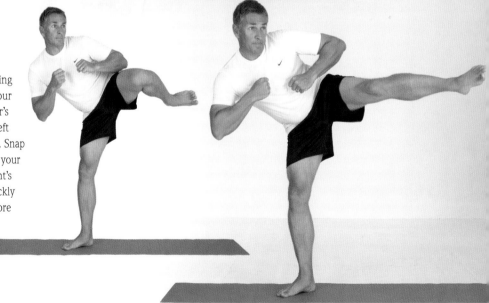

2 ROUNDHOUSE KICK Pretend your opponent is standing in front of you and slightly to your left. Place your hands in a boxer's stance for balance. Bring your left knee diagonally into your chest. Snap your leg forward as you extend your foot and shin into your opponent's imaginary abdomen. Recoil quickly and follow up with 10 to 20 more kicks before switching sides.

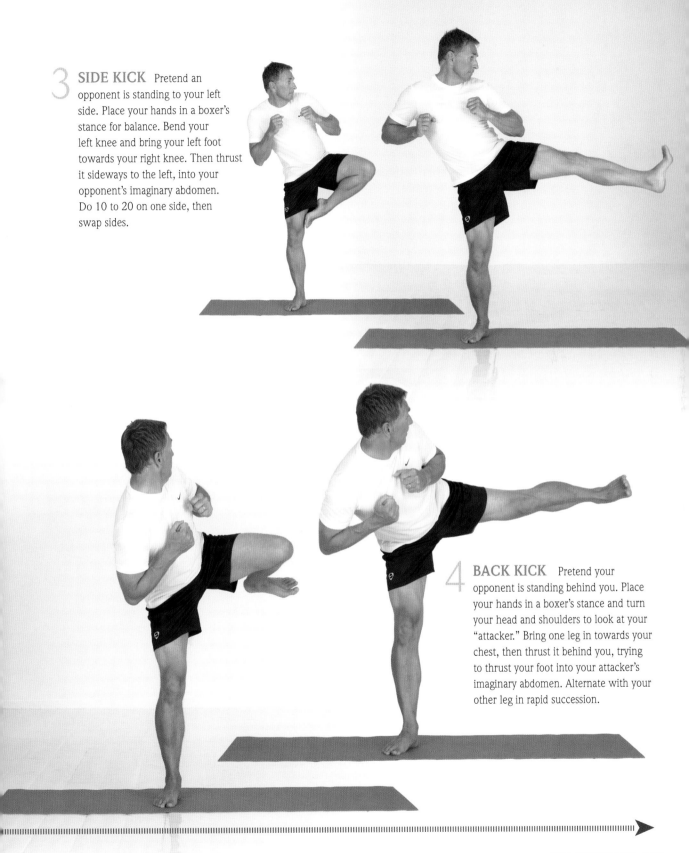

3 SIDE KICK Pretend an opponent is standing to your left side. Place your hands in a boxer's stance for balance. Bend your left knee and bring your left foot towards your right knee. Then thrust it sideways to the left, into your opponent's imaginary abdomen. Do 10 to 20 on one side, then swap sides.

4 BACK KICK Pretend your opponent is standing behind you. Place your hands in a boxer's stance and turn your head and shoulders to look at your "attacker." Bring one leg in towards your chest, then thrust it behind you, trying to thrust your foot into your attacker's imaginary abdomen. Alternate with your other leg in rapid succession.

☆ **Jump into the pool once or twice a week.** Literally. Sports coaches often tell their runners, hockey players and other athletes to increase their leg strength through plyometrics, which is a series of skipping, jumping and bounding exercises usually done on land. Because of the force of gravity and the impact of the body as it hits the ground, these exercises result in quite a bit of post-exercise muscle soreness, which is why you're not advised to do them.

That said, U.S. researchers have developed a way to get the leg-strength benefits from plyometrics without the post-exercise soreness: complete the exercises in a swimming pool. Researchers split 32 women into two groups. One group performed plyometrics on land for eight weeks; the others did the same routine in the water. After eight weeks, both groups increased their leg strength, but the group that did their exercises on land experienced much more muscle soreness than the others.

So the next time you find yourself entertaining your children or grandchildren at the local pool, try the following routine in the shallow end and see if they can keep up with you:

● Hop. With your legs together, hop the width of the pool from one side to the other and back. Rest for up to a minute, then repeat twice.

● Exaggerated running. Run the width of the pool slowly with an exaggerated motion, lifting your knees into your chest and pushing off with your rear foot just enough to lift your entire body off the bottom of the pool. When you reach the other side, turn around and run back. Rest for up to a minute, then repeat twice.

● Hop on one foot. Hop on the spot on one foot for 30 seconds, trying to get as high as possible. Then switch legs. Rest for up to a minute, then repeat twice.

Four other great
LEG EXERCISES

While squats strengthen all of the muscles in your legs, you should do other leg exercises to balance your muscles. So include the following leg-strengthening movements with your squats, completing the entire routine two to three times a week.

1 **LUNGE** Stand with your feet under your hips. Take a large step forward with your right foot. Bend both knees up to 90 degrees until your right thigh is parallel with the floor. Exhale as you straighten your legs and step back to the starting position. Repeat with the left leg. Continue alternating stepping forward with your right and left leg for a total of 10 to 15 repetitions on each leg.

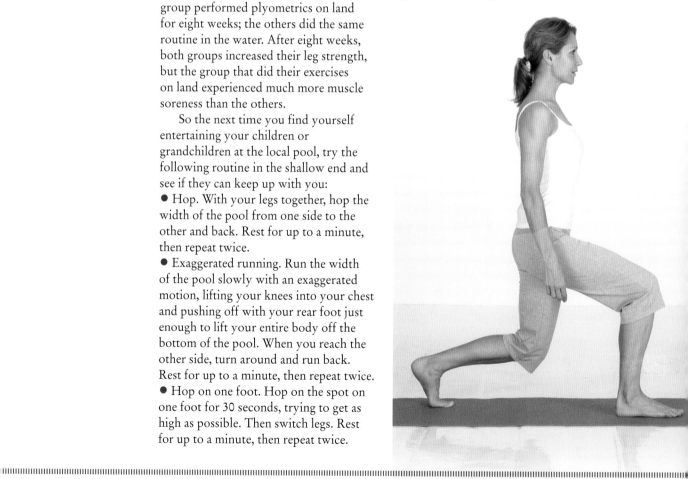

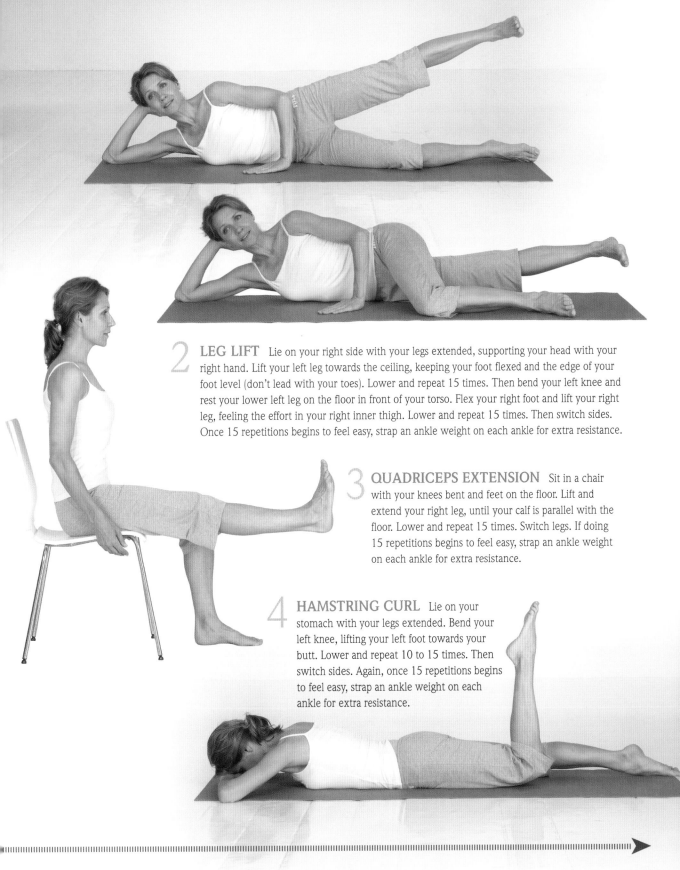

2 **LEG LIFT** Lie on your right side with your legs extended, supporting your head with your right hand. Lift your left leg towards the ceiling, keeping your foot flexed and the edge of your foot level (don't lead with your toes). Lower and repeat 15 times. Then bend your left knee and rest your lower left leg on the floor in front of your torso. Flex your right foot and lift your right leg, feeling the effort in your right inner thigh. Lower and repeat 15 times. Then switch sides. Once 15 repetitions begins to feel easy, strap an ankle weight on each ankle for extra resistance.

3 **QUADRICEPS EXTENSION** Sit in a chair with your knees bent and feet on the floor. Lift and extend your right leg, until your calf is parallel with the floor. Lower and repeat 15 times. Switch legs. If doing 15 repetitions begins to feel easy, strap an ankle weight on each ankle for extra resistance.

4 **HAMSTRING CURL** Lie on your stomach with your legs extended. Bend your left knee, lifting your left foot towards your butt. Lower and repeat 10 to 15 times. Then switch sides. Again, once 15 repetitions begins to feel easy, strap an ankle weight on each ankle for extra resistance.

● **Climb the stairs two or three at a time.** This strengthens the gluteal muscles in your buttocks and revs up your heart rate, boosting your cardiovascular fitness.

● **Play leapfrog.** You'll get a good leg and cardiovascular workout – and lots of fun. Everyone squats down low, imitating a frog on a lily pad. To leap over the person in front of you, place your hands on his or her back, then spring forward and up. Keep your legs and feet wide, in case you need to take two hops to clear your obstacle. Land with your knees soft and slightly bent to protect whoever's in front.

Play leapfrog with your children.

● **Challenge your children, grandchildren, partner or colleagues to a toe-walking contest every other day.** Rise onto the balls of your feet and walk across the room. Whoever lowers his or her heels to the floor first loses. You'll have plenty of laughs and strengthen your arches, ankles and calves.

● **Add a hill to your walking route.** As you trudge up, you'll feel the muscles in the backs of your legs working hard to push off with every step.

● **Practise "hot seats" as you watch TV.** Television time doesn't have to be couch potato time. Pledge that you won't sit down on your favourite recliner until you've done 15 to 20 hot seats during the commercials. To do a hot seat, stand with your feet slightly wider than your hips. Sit back into a squat, just until your butt touches the seat of the chair. As soon as you feel the seat of the chair under your bottom, spring up to a standing position, as if the seat were "hot."

☺ **Whenever you stand in a line, balance on one foot.** As soon as you lift one foot off the ground, the muscles in the foot, ankle, calf, thigh and buttock of the opposite leg firm up as they work harder to keep you upright. If you're worried about what other people might think, relax – no one will notice.

☆ **Do a squat every time you pick something up off the floor.** Bending over to pick something up from the waist puts stress on the lower back, especially if you're lifting something heavy. But a squat forces you to use your legs, building up your leg strength. The best way to squat: with your feet hip-distance apart or wider, knees bent and your butt stuck out as you squat down. Then bend forward and pick up your object. Bring your torso upright, then rise by pressing up through your heels. Even if you just squat to pick up a pencil, it will help you to build more leg strength.

● **Exercise your calf muscles while you brush your teeth.** Place your feet flat on the floor, then rise up onto the balls of your feet, hold for 2 seconds, and sink down. Repeat 20, 30, 50 or more times. You can do this not only while brushing your teeth, but any time you are waiting.

☆ **Push against immovable objects.** Isometric exercises are the best way to exercise without moving. Your goal: to put your foot or upper thigh against a surface that won't move or break, and to press against it hard (but not so hard as to strain your muscles or joints). Hold each position for 6 to 8 seconds, relax for a few seconds, then repeat five to ten times on each side.

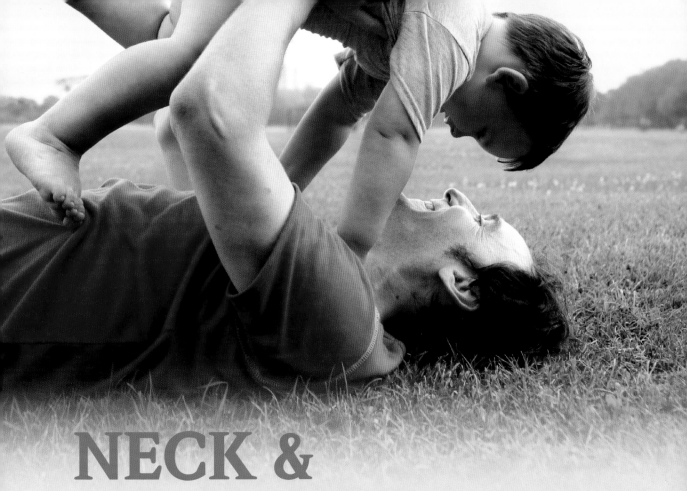

NECK &
SHOULDER strength

You might wonder why neck and shoulder strength matters. You're not training for a football team or pulling a plow. Yet strength in these areas is vital to your overall well-being. Neck pain, be it caused by bad sleep, bad posture or too much stress, is among the most common everyday complaints. Research shows that neck-strengthening exercises may be more important than stretching when it comes to preventing neck pain. The same goes for shoulder strength. Weak shoulders increase the stress on your elbows and wrists. Here are some simple ways to build neck and shoulder strength.

12 SIMPLE STRATEGIES THAT DECREASE PAIN AND STIFFNESS

● **Whenever you feel exasperated at work,** press your forehead into your palms. Many of us tense up our neck muscles when under stress, which can lead to pain and stiffness over time. You can reduce tension and strengthen your neck at the same time with this simple exercise.

● Sitting at your desk, lean forward and place your elbows on your desk. With your head centred over your shoulders, press your forehead into your palms, using your palms to resist the pressure of your head. Hold this position for 3 to 5 seconds, release and repeat three to five times. Now sit up straight and place your palms on the back of your head with your elbows out to the sides. Press your head back into your palms as you use your palms to resist the pressure of your head. Hold for 3 to 5 seconds, release, then repeat three to five times.

● **Boost yourself up twice a day.** Here's another great exercise for the office. Place your palms on the edge of your chair and press down into your hands, lifting your hips and butt a few centimetres (1 or 2 inches) into the air. Hold for 5 seconds, lower and repeat five times for a great shoulder muscle strengthener.

☆ **Rent a rowboat** and take your partner for a romantic jaunt on a lake or pond. As you row out onto the water, you'll strengthen the weakest section of your shoulders, behind your shoulder blades. When these muscles are weak, your shoulders slump forward. If rowing's impractical, simulate the motion for a few minutes, moving slowly and carefully, with a piece of rubber tubing attached to a door handle. Or use a rowing machine at home or at the gym.

● **Practise shrugging your shoulders.** The action of lifting your shoulders up to your ears will strengthen your neck and shoulder muscles. For a fuller workout, do three sets of ten shrugs.

▐▐▐➡ **Make sure you're sleeping on the right pillow.** The best pillow for you depends on your own preferences, but generally stomach sleepers should go for soft, side sleepers for medium, and back sleepers for firm.

Do **THREE** things...

The repetitive movements involved in working at a computer all day – making micro-movement after micro-movement and staring at your screen for hours on end – can, over time, stiffen the muscles in your arms, shoulders and neck, causing pain. A number of treatments can be used to prevent and reverse "computer neck," ranging from chiropractic manipulation to massage. Here are three tactics that have been proven by research to reduce neck pain.

1 Exercise aerobically for at least 30 minutes three to four times a week. Regular aerobic exercise increases blood flow to your muscles, helping them to heal faster. A brisk walk works just fine.

2 Lose weight. Excess pounds not only encourage you to sit with poor posture, they also impede blood circulation, slowing the healing process. You can lose 500 g (1 lb) a week by eliminating 250 calories a day from your diet and walking for 20 additional minutes a day.

3 Quit smoking. Research shows that smoking can cause all types of pain, including neck and back pain. The nicotine in tobacco is toxic to all body tissues and may damage the blood vessels in your neck and shoulders, preventing blood from getting to your spine.

Exercise your **ROTATOR CUFF**

● **Exercise your rotator cuff once a week.** Your rotator cuff is actually a group of muscles and tendons that holds your shoulder joint in place. Most people neglect to strengthen this area of the body because these deep muscles don't play much of a role in shaping sexy shoulder contours and, quite frankly, no one tells you about these muscles until after you've already injured them. Yet strengthening them will go a long way towards preventing shoulder problems later in life. You can do the following exercises at home.

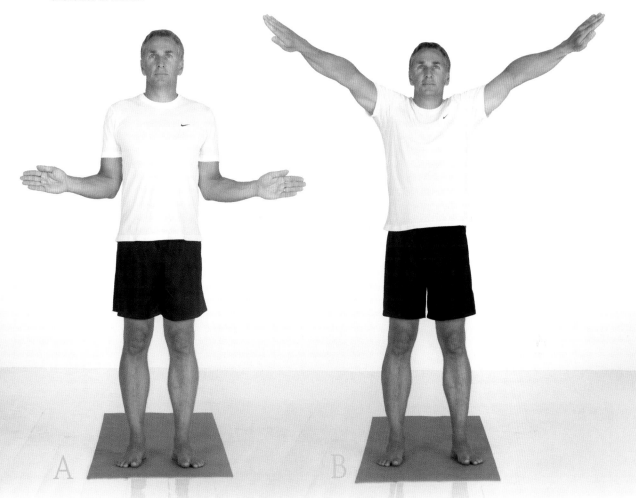

A

Stand with your elbows pressed into your waist, your upper arms snuggled next to your ribs, your elbows bent at 90 degrees, and your palms facing each other. Open your shoulders by pulling your shoulder blades together behind your back. Keeping your upper arms and elbows touching your sides, open your hands slowly out to your sides. You should feel tension between your shoulder blades. Hold for five, bring your palms together, and repeat ten times.

B

Stand with your feet under your hips and your arms at your sides. Raise your arms out to the sides and forward at an angle of 45 degrees to your torso as high as you can with your little fingers facing up. Keep your shoulders relaxed away from your ears as you raise your arms. Lower and repeat 10 to 20 times. As the exercise becomes easier, attach ankle weights to your wrists to increase the challenge.

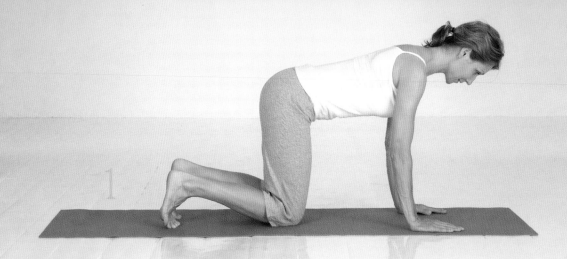

Morning STRETCH

● **Every morning before you get dressed, stretch into a yoga down dog.** This quintessential yoga posture stretches your calves, hamstrings, chest and spine, while it strengthens and stretches your shoulders. Kneel with your palms on the floor under your shoulders and knees under your hips. Spread your fingers as wide as you can, with your middle fingers pointing forward. Tuck your toes under, coming onto the balls of your feet. Roll your shoulder blades away from each other, bringing the creases of your elbows towards each other. Lift your tail bone. Then exhale as you extend your legs and lift your hips towards the ceiling, forming an upside-down V shape with your body. Relax your head between your arms. Press into your palms to bring more body weight back into your legs. Continue to roll your shoulder blades away from each other and the inner creases of your elbows towards each other. Hold for five to ten breaths. Lower and repeat.

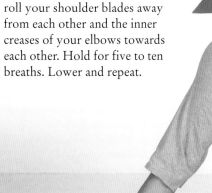

☺ **As you watch television at night, retract your shoulder blades.** Sit on the edge of your chair and lengthen your spine, as if you were trying to grow taller. Place your hands in your lap. Bring your shoulders as far back as you can, pinching your shoulder blades together. Hold for the length of an entire commercial. Relax, then repeat one more time during the course of the evening.

▌▶ **When you get home from work,** stuff a tube sock three-quarters full with white rice, 2 cinnamon sticks and 1 tablespoon of cloves. Seal the end tightly with a rubber band. Heat for 2 minutes in the microwave, then drape the sock around your neck for a surprisingly pleasing aromatherapeutic remedy for sore shoulders and neck. There's no need to empty the sock when you're finished – you can use it over and over, until the spices lose their fragrance.

● **Whenever you spend more than 45 minutes in the driver's seat or in front of the computer, practise the "turtle" exercise.** Often during driving and when staring at a computer screen, we tend to jut our heads forward, as if sticking our nose out is going to get us to our destination faster or help us to finish that project quicker. Because the head weighs about 4.5 kg (10 lb), this puts quite a bit of stress on the back of the neck. Before you know it, you've got a headache. You can both strengthen the muscles in the back of your neck and train yourself to sit with proper posture with the following exercise. As you drive or type, pretend you're a turtle retracting your head into your shell. Keeping your chin level, bring your head back, flattening the curve in the back of your neck. Hold for a count of five, release, and repeat ten times.

● **Every hour, drop your chin to your chest,** then roll your neck to the left, back, to the right and down again in a circular motion. Repeat five times, then switch direction, starting with a roll to the right.

● **Start each working day with a chair exercise.** Sit on the edge of a chair with your knees bent and feet on the floor. Extend one arm overhead and the other towards the floor, with your palms facing in. Keeping your shoulders low on your back and away from your ears, reach back through both arms, feeling a stretch through your top armpit and front of your lower shoulder. You'll also feel muscles in the backs of your shoulders and upper back firming up as they work to keep your arms in place. Hold for 2 seconds, then switch positions, so the top arm is now facing towards the floor and the bottom arm is facing the ceiling, and repeat. Continue to hold for 2 seconds, then switch positions 20 times. Then do the same movement 20 times, but turn your hands so that your palms face behind your torso. Finally, repeat the exercise again, but turn your hands so that your palms face forward. Each new palm position strengthens and stretches a slightly different area of your shoulders.

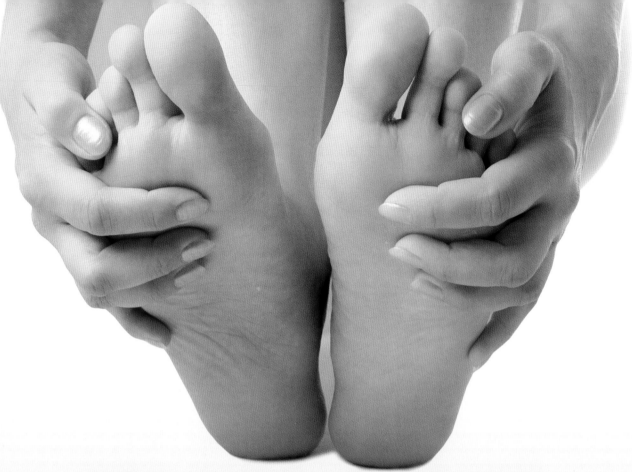

SELF-MASSAGE

Have you ever had a professional massage? If you have, you know what a terrific experience it is. A massage helps to reduce muscle tension in many ways, including increasing blood flow to your muscles. Some research shows that having a regular massage may also boost your immunity by stimulating the production of white blood cells. Not only that, a massage may also make you more productive at work. Researchers have found that a brief self-massage at work reduced stress and boosted job performance. Fortunately, you have your very own massage therapist with you at all times – your hands! The tips that follow give you advice on how to reduce tension from head to foot.

16 WAYS TO REDUCE TENSION IN SECONDS

☆ **Every morning and evening, hammer out the kinks.** Using your fists, gently thump the outside of your body, starting with your legs and arms, working from top to bottom. Then move inwards to your torso and thump from bottom to top. Pummelling your muscles and bones will help to strengthen your body, stimulate blood circulation and relax nerve endings. If you do it in the morning, this self-massage technique will waken and prepare your body – and mind – for the day ahead. When done before bed, it calms down the mind and beats out the stress and tension of the day. One warning: don't do this if you're taking any kind of blood thinner, such as warfarin; you could end up with bruising.

● **Rub your stomach after every meal.** Most of us do this instinctively, especially after overeating. Place one or both palms on your abdomen and rub it in clockwise circles. This is the same direction that food naturally moves through your intestine, so your circular massage will help to stimulate digestion.

☺ **Rub yourself down before and after exercise.** Massaging your body before your stretching, cardio or strength training increases blood flow to the muscles. Massaging your muscles after exercise may help to encourage waste removal and speed muscle recovery. Before exercise, use a pummelling motion with your fists to bring blood flow to your leg and arm muscles. After exercise, rub along your muscles with your palm or fist, moving in the direction of your heart.

● **Give your hands a massage every day** – whenever you put on lotion. Start with the bottom of your palms by clasping your fingers and rubbing the heels of your palms together in a circular motion.

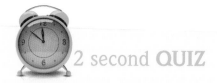

2 second **QUIZ**

Hard or soft massage?
ANSWER: **HARD.**

The point of massage isn't to stimulate the skin; it's to relieve the muscles lying deep below the skin. While you're not advised to massage to the point of pain, you need to use enough effort to work the muscles thoroughly. And that takes more force than many home massagers assert. If your hands and arms aren't getting strained or tired giving a massage, you're probably not pressing hard enough.

Then, with your hands still clasped, take one thumb and massage the area just below your other thumb in circular motions, moving outwards to the centre of the palm. Repeat with the other hand. Then release your fingers and use your thumbs and index fingers to knead your palms, wrists and the webbing between your fingers. With one hand, gently pull each finger of the other hand. Finish by using your thumb and index finger to pinch the webbing between your other thumb and index finger.

● **Roll on a tennis ball to release tension.** If your foot feels tense, stand with one hand on a wall for support and place the arch of the foot on top of the ball. Gradually add more body weight over the foot, allowing the ball to press into your arch. Begin to move your foot slowly, allowing the ball to massage your heel, forefoot and toes. If the tennis ball seems too big for your foot, try a golf ball instead.

You can also lie on the ball to get at that hard-to-reach spot between the shoulder blades or to soothe tension in your lower back. For tight hips, sit on the ball, wiggling your butt around and holding it in any spot that feels good.

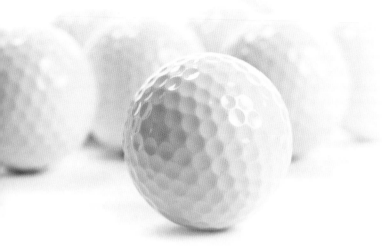

The secret of happy feet is a hidden box of golf balls.

● **Fill the bottom of a shoebox** with golf balls and stick it under your desk at work. When you need to soothe your feet, take off a shoe and rub your feet over the balls.

● **Whenever you take off a pair of high heels,** give your calves some attention. Elevating your heels all day long can eventually shorten your calf muscles. To release them, sit with your knees bent and feet on the floor. Grasp one ankle, placing your thumb just above your Achilles tendon. Press your thumb into the bottom of your calf muscle, hold for 5 seconds, then release. Move 2 centimetres (1 inch) up your calf and repeat the pressure. Continue pressing and releasing until you get to your knee.

▶ **Use your hands to _heel_ your neck.** Once an hour, take a break and clasp your fingers behind your neck, pressing the heels of your palms into your neck on either side of your spine. Massage the heels of your hands up and down in slow, deliberate motions. Then place the fingers of your right hand on your trapezius muscle along the left side of your neck just below the base of your skull. Press into that muscle, tilt your head to the left and rub downwards until you reach your shoulder. Repeat three times, then switch

sides. Finish by stretching your head back so that the top of your office chair presses into your neck just below your skull. This also stretches out the front of your neck, which tends to get tight during desk work. Hold for 20 seconds.

● **Make congested sinuses more comfortable with some finger pressure.** If you have clogged sinuses due to a cold or allergies, rub them with your index fingers. Start just above your brow line. Place your finger pads just above your nose, press down and rub outwards, tracing your brow line as you go. Repeat two or three times. Then place the pads of your fingers below your eyes and to the sides of the bridge of your nose, rubbing outwards and moving downwards with each stroke. Now use your thumbs to massage your cheekbones, making small circles starting at the centre of your face and moving out towards your ears. Finally, place your thumbs on your temples and massage them in small circles.

● **When your eyes feel tired** from staring at your computer screen all day long, give them some heat. Rub your hands together vigorously until you feel the skin on your palms begin to warm up. Then cup one hand over each eye, feeling the heat from your hands relax your eyes.

☺ **If your feet are sore after a long day** of standing, take off your shoes and socks, wash your feet and give them a rub-down. Sitting on a comfortable couch or chair, thread the fingers of one hand through the toes of one foot, spreading out your toes and placing the palm of your hand against the bottom of your foot. Use your palm to rotate the joints of your forefoot forward and back gently for 1 minute. Then remove your fingers from your toes, hold your ankle with one hand, and gently rotate the entire foot with the other hand, starting with small circles and progressing to larger circles as your ankle warms up. Switch directions, then repeat with the other foot.

● **Give yourself a bear-hug to relax away shoulder tension.** Cross your arms over your chest and grab a shoulder with either hand. Squeeze each shoulder and release three times. Then move your hands down your arms, squeezing and releasing until you get to your wrists.

☆ **Rub lavender oil onto your feet before you go to bed.** Lavender-scented oils are available at most health-food stores. The smell of lavender and the gentle massaging motions you make as you work the oil into your feet will help you to unwind. An added bonus: the nightly oil treatment softens and hydrates any rough, dry spots on your feet. Once you've finished your massage, put on a pair of socks to prevent the oil from rubbing off onto your sheets.

● **After tennis, cycling, rock climbing,** and other arm-tiring sports, give your arms a pinch. Place your right arm across your chest with your elbow bent. Reach across your chest with your left arm and pinch your right arm's triceps, near the shoulder, with the thumb and index finger

of your left hand. Hold for a few seconds, release, then pinch again 2 centimetres (1 inch) lower on the arm. Continue pinching and releasing until you've made your way to your elbow. Then pinch your right arm's biceps near your armpit and work your way in the same way down to the elbow. This will release the tension in your muscles and help to improve blood circulation.

● **When you have a headache,** stand up, bend forward from the hips and place your forehead on a padded chair. The chair will gently place pressure on your head as you relax in the forward bend. Hold for about 30 seconds. When you rise, sit down and spread your fingers through your hair, making a fist. Gently pull the hair away from your head. Hold for 2 or 3 seconds, then release. This stretches the fascia, the fibrous tissue, along your scalp, releasing tension. Continue to grab different clumps of hair all over your head, working from the top front of your head, progressing to the sides, and then to the back. Once you have grabbed and released your entire scalp, return to work refreshed.

● **Keep a tennis ball on your desk and squeeze it regularly.** The squeezing motion helps to rejuvenate tired fingers and hands, and strengthens your hands for other self-massage techniques.

Reminder

 Fast results
These are tips that deliver benefits particularly quickly – in some cases, immediately.

 Easy gains
These are health boosters that offer the best value for the least amount of effort.

 Super-effective
This is advice that scientific research or widespread usage by experts has shown to be especially effective.

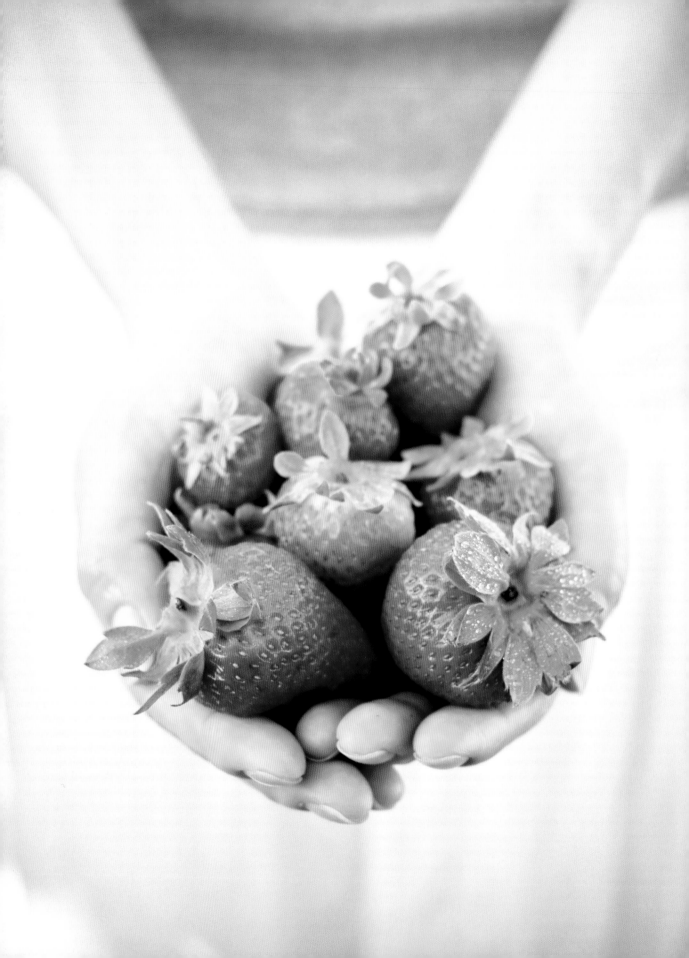

part 5

TARGETED HEALTH GOALS

As we travel through life, each of us encounters unique health challenges and concerns. To help you make your journey as disease – and worry – free as possible, we've put together proven health tips for 18 common health goals, from losing weight to helping prevent cancer.

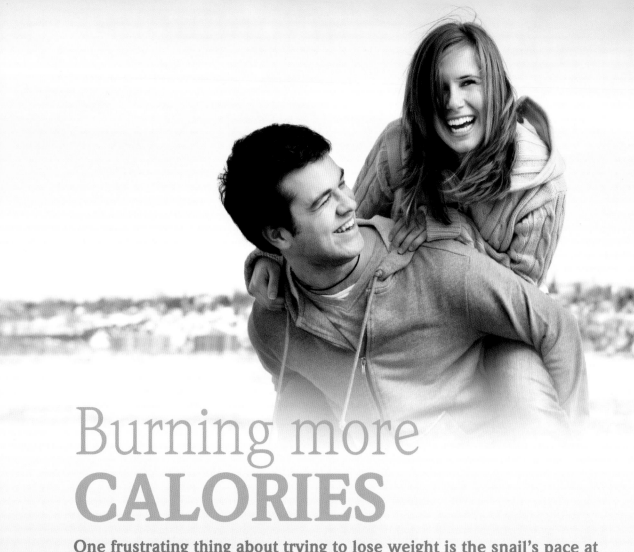

Burning more
CALORIES

One frustrating thing about trying to lose weight is the snail's pace at which it seems to drop off. The more weight you lose, the harder your body fights to hold on to the calories it gets and the fewer calories it burns. That's usually when you hit the infamous weight-loss plateau. But what if you could turbo-charge your weight-loss efforts? That's where this chapter comes in. It lists easy ways to boost your metabolism – the rate at which you burn calories – as well as tips on cranking up the calorie burn of your workout. Still, it's important to maintain a realistic expectation of what's considered "healthy" weight loss; about 0.5 to 1 kg (1 to 2 lb) a week is ideal.

12 WAYS TO BOOST YOUR METABOLISM AND KICK-START YOUR WEIGHT LOSS

A good dose of chili may increase your metabolism.

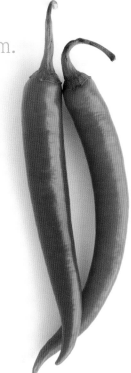

● **Use interval training to rev up your workout.** Walk for the same amount of time at the same intensity day in and day out and your body will get as bored with your workout as you do. Throw in some variety with interval training, which involves changing the intensity of your workout throughout your exercise session. Every 5 minutes of your walk, jog for 1 minute. Every 5 minutes of your bike ride, shift into a higher gear and pedal hard for a minute. If you swim, speed up every other length. You'll burn more calories in the same amount of time.

▶ **Fidget.** People who drum their fingers or bounce their knees burn at least 500 calories a day. That adds up to losing 500 g (1 lb) a week.

● **Keep a small squeeze ball with you** and grip and squeeze it frequently during the day. It's one of the few exercises you can do at any time. You'll build up the muscles in your hands – and muscle, wherever it is, burns a lot of calories.

● **Don't starve yourself.** Cutting out too many calories can backfire in more ways than one. Try to subsist on morsels and your metabolism will slow down so much that you'll not only stop losing weight, but you'll be lucky if you can peel yourself off the couch.

✡ **Put five rubber bands around your wrist every morning.** That's how many 500 ml bottles of water you should drink during the day to rev up your metabolism, helping to burn more calories. At least, that's what German researchers found when they got 14 participants to drink about 500 ml of water. The volunteers' metabolic rate – or how quickly they burned calories – jumped a third within 10 minutes of

drinking the water and remained high for another 30 or 40 minutes. The researchers estimated that, over a year, increasing your water consumption by 1.5 litres a day would burn an extra 17,400 calories, or about 2.25 kg (5 lb) worth. Since much of the increased metabolic rate is due to the body's efforts to heat the liquid, make sure the water you're drinking is icy cold.

● **Turn up the heat with hot peppers.** Some studies show that very spicy foods can temporarily increase your metabolism. Specialist grocers often stock many different kinds of peppers. Buy one type a week and add some to various meals. Spice up your scrambled eggs with minced jalapeño, add a little fire to beef stew with half a Scotch bonnet pepper.

In **PERSPEC**Tive

The weight-loss plateau

There's nothing more frustrating than hitting a weight-loss plateau, particularly if you're doing everything right – eating well and exercising. So what happens?

First, it's not your fault. Weight-loss plateaus are perfectly normal and easily explained. Your basal metabolism, or the energy your body consumes just to survive, accounts for about 70 per cent of all the calories you burn – and it depends on how much you weigh. The less you weigh, the lower your basal metabolic rate (BMR). Lose enough weight, and boom! Your metabolism slows down and you hit the weight-loss plateau. The only way to lose more weight is to decrease the calories you take in, increase the calories you burn, or both.

You can boost your BMR by building up muscle. Muscle tissue requires more energy than fat does, even at rest. In fact, every kilogram of muscle burns another 65 to 110 calories (1 lb/30 to 50 calories) a day. Walking helps a bit, but resistance training helps even more.

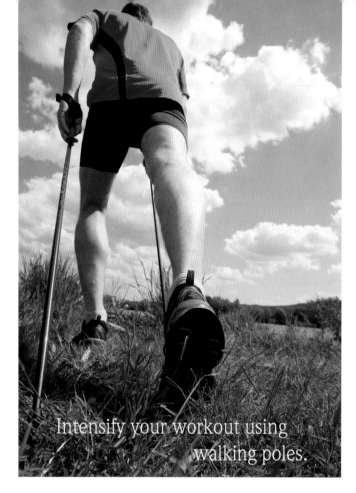
Intensify your workout using walking poles.

● Exercise outside. Maybe it's the fresh air, maybe it's the sunshine, but something about exercising out in the open makes you walk or run faster than doing the same exercise in the gym.

☺ Eat five small meals throughout the day instead of three large meals. You might think you should eat less often if you want to lose weight, but that's just not the case. By eating every few hours, you keep your metabolism fired up and ensure it doesn't slow down between meals in order to hang on to calories. A "meal" can be as small as a cup of soup.

● Sip a couple of cups of coffee throughout the day. Studies find that the caffeine in coffee increases the rate at which your body burns calories. This does not mean, however, that you should

order a fancy calorie-packed frappuccino. And skip the espresso if it makes you toss and turn at night.

● Don't worry if you've been yo-yo dieting. There's a myth that if you've spent your life losing and gaining the same 4.5 to 9 kg (10 to 20 lb), your metabolism gets out of kilter and ends up slowing right down. Don't believe it. When researchers reviewed 43 studies on the topic, they found no difference in the metabolic rates of yo-yo dieters compared to those of everyone else.

● Walk with intent – and intensity. Burn more calories in the same amount of time with these strategies:
● Swing your arms when you walk. You'll burn 5 to 10 per cent more calories.
● Wear a weighted vest – another great way to burn calories. But leave the hand and ankle weights at home. They throw you off balance and could result in injury.
● Walk on grass, sand or a gravel path instead of the road. It takes more muscle power to glide smoothly over these uneven surfaces (especially sand) than over asphalt.
● Use walking poles. A U.S. study found that you get a much more intense workout than you would without the poles.
● Walk along the shore of a river or lake with your ankles in the water. The resistance burns more calories and gives your muscles an added workout.

● Increase the protein in your diet. There is some evidence that if you increase your protein intake to the upper end of the recommended range (roughly 20 per cent of overall calories), the amount of energy you expend at rest will remain the same even while you're losing weight. Normally, as you lose weight, your body adjusts and you burn fewer calories at rest.

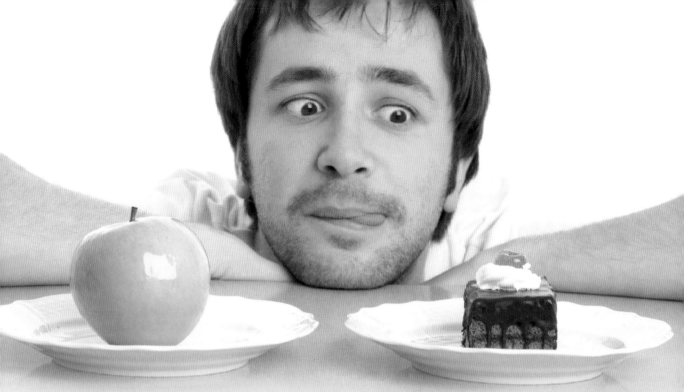

LOSING weight

If you're overweight, one of the best things you can do for your overall health is lose a few kilos. Or maybe more than a few kilos. Carrying too much weight significantly increases your risk of heart disease, diabetes, stroke, high blood pressure, cancer … the list seems almost endless. Plus, if you do get sick or need surgery, being overweight can make any treatments riskier.

You know the drill by now when it comes to losing weight – take in fewer calories than you burn off. But you probably also know that most diets and quick weight-loss plans are not really sustainable. You're better off finding several simple things you can do on a daily basis – and following the cardinal rules of eating more fruit and vegetables and less fat while making sure you get more physical activity.

Together with our tips, these actions should send the numbers on your scales in the right direction: down.

47 OF THE BEST TIPS FOR EASY SLIMMING

Once a week, indulge in a treat that tastes as if it's high in calories but isn't. This should stop you feeling deprived and therefore bingeing on higher-calorie foods. For instance:

- **Olives.** Just 25 calories in 5 olives.
- **Shrimps.** A mere 58 calories in 75 g.
- **Smoked salmon.** Only 58 calories in 50 g. Sprinkle with capers for an even more elegant treat.

Serve high-calorie foods as the jewels in the crown. Make a spoonful of ice cream the jewel and a bowl of fruit the crown. Cut down on the tortilla chips by pairing each bite with lots of chunky, filling fresh salsa. Balance a little cheese with a lot of salad.

After breakfast, drink water. At breakfast, go ahead and drink orange juice. But throughout the day, focus on water instead of juice or soft drinks. A 355 ml can of cola contains around 160 calories. Research shows that despite the calories, sugary drinks don't trigger a sense of fullness in the way that food does.

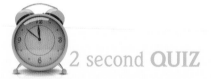

2 second QUIZ

Organized weight-loss plan or solo weight loss?
ANSWER: **ORGANIZED WEIGHT-LOSS PLAN.**

Join the group. When researchers assigned 413 overweight and obese men and women to either a self-help program, in which they met twice with a nutritionist then followed a program on their own, or to Weight Watchers, they found that after two years, those in the organized Weight Watchers group lost more weight than those going it alone.

Carry a palm-sized notebook everywhere you go for one week. Write down every single morsel that passes your lips – even water. Studies have found that people who maintain food diaries end up eating about 15 per cent less food than those who don't.

Buy a pedometer, clip it to your belt and aim first for an extra 1,000 steps a day. On average, very sedentary people might take only 2,000 to 3,000 steps a day. Upping the ante to add 2,000 steps will help you to maintain your current weight and stop you gaining weight; adding more than that will help you to lose weight.

Add 10 per cent to the amount of daily calories you think you're eating, then adjust your eating habits accordingly. If you think you're consuming 1,700 calories a day and don't understand why you're not losing weight, add another 170 calories to your guesstimate. Chances are, the new number is more accurate.

Eat five or six small meals or snacks a day instead of three large meals. A 1999 South African study found that when men ate parts of their morning meal at intervals over 5 hours, they consumed almost 30 per cent fewer calories at lunch than when they ate a single breakfast. Other studies show that even if you eat the same number of calories distributed this way, your body releases less insulin, which keeps blood sugar steady and helps to control hunger.

Walk for 45 minutes a day. Why 45 minutes rather than the typical 30? One American study found that while 30 minutes of daily walking is enough to prevent weight gain in most relatively sedentary people, exercise beyond 30 minutes results in weight and fat loss.

Surround yourself with blue. It's an appetite-suppressing colour that will help you to stick to your weight-loss goals.

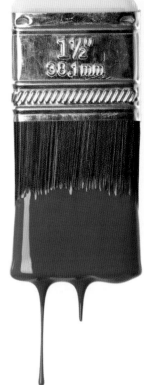

Burning an additional 300 calories a day with 5 kilometres of brisk walking (45 minutes should do it) could help you to lose 14 kg (30 lb) in a year without you even having to change how much you're eating. See "Walking," on page 140, for ways to make doing this more fun.

Bring the colour blue into your life more often. There's a good reason why you won't see many fast-food restaurants painted blue: believe it or not, the colour blue functions as an appetite suppressant. So serve up dinner on blue plates, dress in blue when you eat and have a blue tablecloth. Conversely, avoid red, yellow and orange in your dining areas. Studies find they encourage eating.

Clear your wardrobe of the "fat" clothes. Once you've reached your target weight, throw out or give away every item of clothing that doesn't fit. The idea of having to buy a whole new wardrobe if you regain the weight will be a strong incentive to maintain your new figure.

Hang a mirror opposite your seat at the table. One study found that eating in front of mirrors reduced the amount people ate by nearly a third. It seems that having to look yourself in the eye reflects back some of your own inner standards and goals, and reminds you of why you're trying to lose weight in the first place.

Downsize your dinner plates. Studies find that the less food put in front of you, the less food you'll eat. Conversely, the more food in front of you, the more you'll eat – regardless of how hungry you are. So instead of using standard dinner plates, which range these days from 25 to 35 cm (making them look empty if they're not piled with food), serve your main course on salad plates (about 15 to 20 cm wide). The same goes for liquids. Instead of large glasses and coffee mugs, return to the old days of tumblers and even smaller coffee cups.

Serve your dinner restaurant-style (with food already on the plates) rather than family-style (where the food is served in bowls and on platters on the table). When your plate is empty, you're finished; there's no reaching for seconds.

Put out a vegetable platter. A body of U.S. research found that eating water-rich foods such as zucchini, tomatoes and cucumbers during meals reduces overall calorie consumption. Other water-rich foods include soups and salads. You won't get the same benefits by just drinking water, though. Because the body processes hunger and thirst through different mechanisms, it simply doesn't register a sense of fullness with water (or soft drinks, tea, coffee or juice).

Use vegetables to bulk up meals. For the same calories, you can eat twice as much pasta salad packed with veg such as broccoli, carrots and tomatoes as you can pasta salad dressed only with mayonnaise. And add veggies to make a fluffier, more satisfying omelette without increasing the number of eggs.

Avoid any prepared food that lists sugar, fructose or corn syrup among the first four ingredients on the label. You should be able to find a lower-sugar version of the same type of food. If you can't, have a piece of fruit instead. Look for sugar-free varieties of foods such as ketchup.

Eat one less cookie a day. Or have one can less of soft drink, one glass less of orange juice, or three bites fewer of a burger. Doing any of these saves you about 100 calories a day. That's enough to prevent you from gaining the 1 kg (2 lb) or so that most of us put on each year.

Avoid white foods. There is some scientific legitimacy to today's lower-carb diets: large amounts of simple carbohydrates from white flour and added sugar can wreak havoc on your blood sugar and lead to weight gain. But you shouldn't throw out the baby with the bathwater. While avoiding sugar, white rice and white flour, you should eat plenty of whole-grain breads and brown rice. One Harvard study of 74,000 women found that those who ate more than two daily servings of whole grains were 49 per cent less likely to be overweight than those who ate the white stuff.

Eat cereal for breakfast five days a week. Studies find that people who eat cereal for breakfast every day are significantly less likely to be obese and

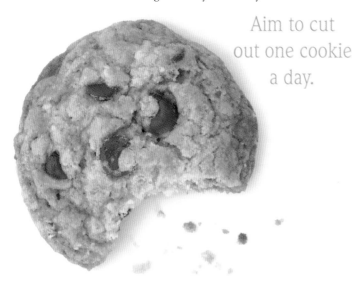

Aim to cut out one cookie a day.

have diabetes than those who don't. They also consume more fibre and calcium – and less fat – than those who eat other breakfast foods. But be sure to choose a high-fibre, low-sugar variety.

Pare your portions. Whether you eat at home or in a restaurant, immediately remove a third of the food on your plate. Arguably the worst food trend of the past few decades has been the explosion in portion size. We eat far, far more today than our bodies need. Studies find that if you serve people more food, they'll eat more, regardless of their hunger level. The converse is also true: serve yourself less and you'll eat less.

Eat 90 per cent of your meals at home. You're more likely to eat more – and eat more high-fat, high-calorie foods – when you eat out than when you eat at home.

Eat slowly and calmly. Put your fork or spoon down between every bite. Sip water frequently. Intersperse your eating with stories of the interesting things that happened during your day. Your brain lags behind your stomach by about 20 minutes when it comes to satiety (fullness) signals. If you eat slowly enough, your brain will catch up and tell you that you no longer need food.

Dine only when you hear your stomach rumbling. It's surprising how often we eat out of boredom, nervousness, habit or frustration – so often, in fact, that many of us have actually forgotten what physical hunger feels like. Next time, wait until your stomach is rumbling before you eat. If you're hankering for a specific food, it's probably a craving, not hunger. If you'd eat anything you could get your hands on, chances are you're truly hungry.

☆ **Find ways other than eating to express love, combat stress and relieve boredom.** For instance, you might make your family a photo album of special events instead of a rich dessert, sign up for a stress-management course (or read the chapter on stress management that begins on page 270) or take up an active hobby, such as bowling.

● **State the positive.** You've heard of a self-fulfilling prophecy? Well, if you keep focusing on things you can't do, such as resisting junk food, chances are you won't do them. Instead (whether you believe it or not) repeat positive thoughts to yourself. "I can lose weight." "I will get out for my walk today." "I can resist the dessert menu." Repeat these phrases like a mantra all day long. Soon, they will become their own self-fulfilling prophecy.

● **Discover your dietary balance point.** If you work hard to control your weight, you may get pleasure from your appearance, but you may also feel sorry for yourself when you forgo a favourite food. There is a balance to be struck between the immediate gratification of indulgent foods and the long-term goal of maintaining a desirable weight and good health. So identify your own personal dietary balance point and stay there.

▷ **Use flavourings such as hot sauce,** salsa and Cajun seasonings instead of buttery, creamy or sugary sauces. As well as providing lots of flavour with no fat and few calories, many spicy seasonings fire up your digestive system, causing you to burn more calories temporarily.

● **Spend 10 minutes a day walking up and down stairs.** That's all it takes to help you to shed as much as 4.5 kg (10 lb), assuming you don't start eating more.

Do **THREE** things...

If you do only three things to lose weight, make them these three, say weight-loss experts:

1 Eat more vegetables. Gram for gram, vegetables have a fraction of the calories that fats, meats and starches contain. Fill up on greens and other colourful vegetables and you'll have less room for the higher-calorie foods.

2 Get more exercise. You'll not only burn calories, but you'll build muscle that will boost your metabolism.

3 Decrease your portions. Most of us simply eat more than we need to. Gradually cut back on how much you serve yourself at mealtimes.

● **Eat equal portions of vegetables and grains at dinner.** A medium-sized portion of boiled rice (150 g) and cooked pasta (230 g) both contain about 200 calories, whereas a portion (80 g) of cooked vegetables contains around 30 calories. To avoid a calorie overload, eat a 1:1 ratio of grains to veggies. The high-fibre veggies will help to satisfy your hunger before you overeat the grains.

● **Wash something thoroughly once a week** – a floor, a couple of windows, the shower cubicle or your car. A 68 kg (150 lb) person who exerts some elbow grease will burn about 4 calories for every minute spent cleaning. If you scrub for 30 minutes, you could work off 120 calories – the calories in two digestive cookies.

● **Take a walk before dinner.** You'll do more than burn calories – you'll cut your appetite. In a study of ten obese women conducted at the University of Glasgow, 20 minutes of walking reduced the appetite and increased sensations of fullness as effectively as a light meal.

☆ **Nibble some almonds instead of a sugary snack.** An American study found that overweight people who ate a moderate-fat diet containing almonds lost more weight than a control group that didn't eat nuts. In fact, any nut will do.

● **Don't eat with a large group.** A study published in the *Journal of Physiological Behavior* found that we tend to eat more when we eat with other people, probably because we spend more time at the table. But eating with your partner or your family, and using table time for talking in between chewing, can help you to cut down on calories – and facilitate bonding.

● **Watch an hour less of TV.** A study of 76 undergraduate students found that the more they watched television, the more often they ate and the more they ate overall. So sacrifice one program and go for a walk instead.

● **Get most of your calories before noon.** Studies find that the more you eat in the morning, the less you'll eat in the evening. And you have more opportunities to burn off those early-day calories than you do the dinner calories.

Healthy INVESTMENT

A kitchen timer
Set it for 30 minutes when you sit down to eat dinner, then eat slowly so that your last bite coincides with the ding, allowing time for fullness signals to make it from your stomach to your brain. Once you've finished eating, set the timer for 2 hours. If you're really hungry when it dings, you can have dessert. Otherwise, pat yourself on the back.

☆ **Close down the kitchen after dinner.** Wash all the dishes, wipe down the counters, turn off the light and, if necessary, tape closed the cupboards and the fridge. Late-evening eating significantly increases the overall number of calories you consume. Stopping late-night snacking can save 300 calories or more a day, or 14 kg (31 lb) a year.

☺ **Sniff a banana, an apple or a peppermint when you feel hungry.** You might feel silly, but it works. When Dr. Alan R. Hirsch of the Smell & Taste Treatment and Research Foundation in Chicago tried this with 3,000 volunteers, he found that the more frequently people sniffed, the less hungry they were and the more weight they lost – an average of 13.5 kg (30 lb) each. One theory is that sniffing the food tricks the brain into thinking you're actually eating it.

☺ **Order wine by the glass, not the bottle.** That way you'll be more aware of how much alcohol you're drinking. Moderate drinking can be good for your health, but alcohol is high in calories. And because drinking turns off our inhibitions, it can drown your best intentions to keep eating and snacking in check.

● **Watch every morsel you put in your mouth on the weekend.** A U.S. study found that people tend to consume an extra 115 calories a day on the weekend, primarily from alcohol and fat.

● **Stock your fridge with low-fat yogourt.** One American study found that people who cut out 500 calories daily and ate yogourt three times a day for 12 weeks lost more weight and body fat than a group that cut out only the calories. The researchers concluded that the calcium in low-fat dairy foods triggers a hormonal response that inhibits the body's production of fat cells and boosts the breakdown of fat.

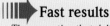 **Brush your teeth after every meal, especially after dinner.** That clean, minty freshness will serve as a cue to your body and brain that mealtime is over.

Serve individual courses rather than piling everything on one plate. Make the first two courses soup or vegetables (such as a green salad). By the time you get to the more calorie-dense foods, the meat and dessert, you'll be eating less or may already be full (leftovers are a good thing).

Passionately kiss your partner ten times a day. According to the 1991 *Kinsey Institute New Report on Sex*, a passionate kiss burns 6.4 calories per minute. Ten minutes a day of kissing equates to about 23,000 calories – or 3.5 kg (8 lb) – a year!

Pack nutritious snacks. Snacking once or twice a day helps to stave off hunger, but healthy snacks can be hard to come by when you're on the go. Pack up baby carrots or your own special mix made with nuts, raisins, seeds and dried fruit.

Weed out hidden calories. It's easy to overlook the extra calories in spreads, dressings, sauces, condiments, drinks and snacks. These all add up, whether or not you've been counting them, and could make the difference between weight gain and weight loss.

When you shop, choose nutritious foods based on these four simple rules:
- Avoid partially hydrogenated oil.
- Reject high-fructose corn syrup.
- Choose a short ingredient list rather than a long one; there will be fewer flavour enhancers and empty calories.
- Look for 2 g or more of fibre per 100 calories in all grain products (cereal, bread, cookies and chips).

When you're eating out with friends or family, dress in your most flattering outfit. You'll get loads of compliments, which will be a great reminder to watch what you eat.

Sniff a banana when you're hungry. You might feel silly, but it works.

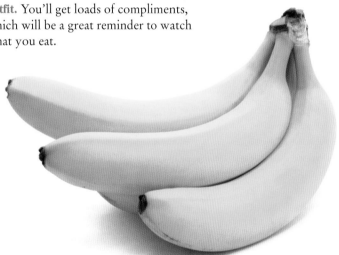

Reminder

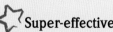

||▶ Fast results
These are tips that deliver benefits particularly quickly – in some cases, immediately.

☺ Easy gains
These are health boosters that offer the best value for the least amount of effort.

☆ Super-effective
This is advice that scientific research or widespread usage by experts has shown to be particularly effective.

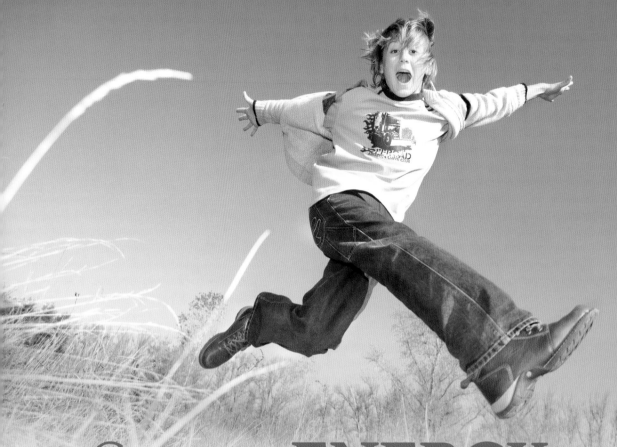

Greater ENERGY

Do you find yourself collapsing on the couch by midafternoon? Are you feeling more sluggish than a hungover sloth? Do you envy the boundless energy of your children or grandchildren – or even your on-the-go next-door neighbour? Don't blame your age; blame your lifestyle. A low-energy lifestyle leaves you with little energy. A high-energy lifestyle gives you lots of energy. For most people, it's that simple.

Indeed, with just a few easy changes to your daily routine, it's guaranteed that the seemingly permanent imprint of your bottom on the sofa will rise up and vanish, along with your inertia.

Your friends and family may start asking what you're taking. Tell them nothing, except some good health-boosting advice.

23 WAYS TO FIND YOUR GET UP AND GO AFTER IT HAS GOT UP AND GONE

☺ **Nurse a coffee throughout the day.** If you need a quadruple shot of espresso just to bring your eyelids to half mast in the morning, you may be driving yourself deeper and deeper into a low-energy rut. Compelling research from various institutions, including Harvard Medical School, finds that frequent low doses of caffeine – the amount in a quarter-cup of coffee – are more effective than a few larger doses of caffeine in keeping people alert.

☺ **Lighten your glycemic load.** Foods with a low glycemic load (see page 100) – such as beans, bran cereal, brown rice, whole-wheat bread and nuts – have less impact on your blood sugar than foods with a high glycemic load – including white rice, spaghetti, potatoes and sugary juices and drinks. Eating more low glycemic-load foods will help you to keep your blood sugar steady and avoid the lightheadedness and "shakes" associated with blood sugar drops, which usually follow rises.

☺ **If you have dried rosemary in your kitchen, crush a small handful and take a whiff or three.** The herb's intense woody fragrance is known to herbalists as an invigorating stimulant.

☆ Once a day, try to go for a 10 minute "thank you" walk. As you walk, focus your thoughts on the things for which you feel most thankful. After the walk, make a mental note of how you feel. This simple technique gives you both a sense of well-being and the positive benefits of walking and exercise, flooding your brain with happy neurotransmitters and endorphins. It's simple, yet it's a powerful exercise that energizes the mind and body, and builds mental and physical muscle.

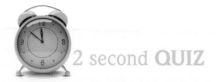

2 second QUIZ

Cup of coffee or 20 minute nap?
ANSWER: **A NAP.**

This is according to a French review of research on techniques that helped night-shift workers to remain alert. Set an alarm to wake you in 20 minutes. A longer nap could interfere with your sleep later that night.

☺ **When you find yourself thinking a negative thought, picture a stop sign.** Then either push the thought out of your mind or replace it with a positive one. Negative feelings take a lot of mental energy. Whenever possible, avoid unnecessary self-criticism. Stop blaming yourself for past events that you cannot change. You deserve the same level of respect and kindness as others.

▐▌▶ **Drink two glasses of icy water.** Fatigue is often one of the first symptoms of dehydration, and if all you've sipped throughout the day is coffee and soft drinks, it's quite likely that you're dehydrated. Plus, the refreshing coldness will serve as a virtual slap in the face.

☺ **Soak a washcloth in icy water and place it over your face.** The icy coolness of the cloth will quickly rejuvenate your facial muscles and eyes. It will probably lift your spirits as well.

☺ **Get enough iron.** Constantly dragging yourself around? You could have iron-deficiency anemia, a common cause of fatigue. Iron is essential for producing hemoglobin, which carries oxygen to your body's cells, where it's used to produce energy. Good food sources of iron are red meat, iron-fortified

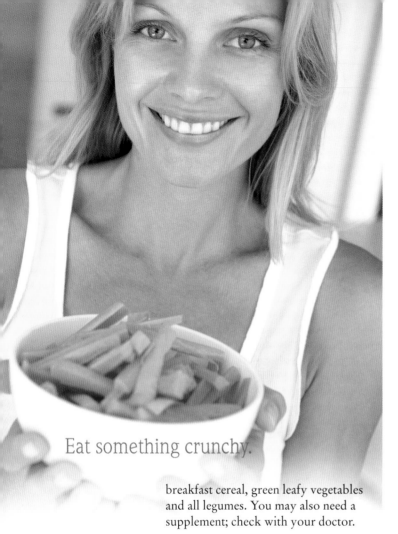

Eat something crunchy.

⚽ **Turn off the news for one week.**
Depressing television news of murders, fires and terrorism can quickly drain your mental reserves. If you're a news junkie, try this experiment for one week: stop reading your newspaper and watch only one television news program a day (or none if you can stand it). Notice how you feel at the end of the week. If you feel more energetic and peaceful, stick to your new habit.

⚽ **List all the people you're angry with and write a friendly letter to each one.** Brooding over past events only drains your energy. Try to accept others for who they are and don't expend a lot of effort on changing them. You don't have to send the letter. Simply writing it is enough.

⚽ **Soak up a little sun in winter.** Do you have all the energy of a hibernating bear in winter months? Make a point of getting outside for 30 minutes to an hour during the day. The natural light can improve your energy levels and help to fight seasonal affective disorder (SAD).

☺ **In the hour before bedtime, turn off the TV,** put away your work and relax with a good book, some embroidery or a crossword puzzle. Take a warm bath and listen to soothing music. This ritual will help you to fall asleep more quickly and experience a more restful slumber, resulting in a more energetic you the following day.

⚽ **Create an area for sorting out the mail.** Clutter is not only distracting, it's frustrating and energy-wasting. (How many times have you scoured the house for lost keys or bills that were right in front of you?) To keep track of your bills and other mail, buy an open box file or some hanging files from an office supply

breakfast cereal, green leafy vegetables and all legumes. You may also need a supplement; check with your doctor.

⚽ **When someone asks you to do something, say,** "Let me check my agenda and I'll get back to you." This gives you time to think about the request and decide if it's something you really want to do, or simply an energy-sucking waste of your time. Don't overextend yourself, especially doing tasks you don't really enjoy. If you don't want to bake for another school sale, say so.

⚽ **Have your thyroid checked.** If it's not producing enough thyroid hormone, it could be making you feel tired and rundown. A simple blood test will show if that's the case. Other symptoms of low thyroid are dry skin, weight gain, constipation and feeling cold.

store. Place it in your kitchen and use it to sort your mail into categories such as bills, receipts and letters.

⚙ **Breathe in new energy.** Sit in a chair with a straight back. Place your hands over your stomach and breathe into your tummy so that your hands rise and fall with your breath. Imagine you're inhaling a white light that fills your body with vital energy. Do this for five full breaths. Then, as you inhale, tighten the muscles that connect your shoulders and neck, pulling your shoulders up towards your ears. When you've inhaled all you can and your shoulders are snug around your ears, hold your breath for just a second. Then exhale as you release the tension and your breath in one big whoosh – as if you were releasing the weight of the world from your shoulders. Repeat until you feel clear, refreshed and revitalized.

⚙ **Make a list of everything you're looking forward to in the next month.** Do this every month when you pay your rent or mortgage. Simply building more anticipation into your life helps to stoke up your energy.

▐▐▐▶ **Eat something crunchy.** Pretzels, carrots and other crunchy foods make your jaw work hard, which can wake up your facial muscles, helping you to feel more alert.

⚙ **Chew a piece of peppermint or spearmint chewing gum.** You'll get a burst of energy from the invigorating flavour and scent, not to mention the physical act of chewing.

⚙ **Eat every 4 hours.** It's much better to refuel your body continually before it hits empty than to wait until you're in the danger zone, then overdo it. So every

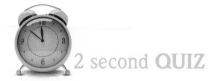
4 hours (except, of course, when you're sleeping), have a mini-meal or snack. A mini-meal might be a handful of roasted peanuts, a hard-boiled egg or a slice of lean cold meat and a sliced apple. Fat-free yogourt sprinkled with flaxseeds makes a good, nutritious snack.

⚙ **Stay still.** You wouldn't think stillness would lead to energy, but often that's just what you need to create your second wind. Simply sit for 10 minutes in a comfortable chair and stare out of the window. Let your mind drift wherever it wants to go. Allow yourself just to "be," something we're often too frenzied to do.

⚙ **Or stretch.** Stand up, get on your toes and lift your fingertips as close as you can to the ceiling. Keep the stretch expanding for several seconds, feeling it in your calves, your abdomen, your shoulders, your arms, your fingers. After a few seconds, relax, take a few deep breaths and do it again. By doing this, you activate almost every muscle you have, sending oxygen-rich blood throughout your body.

⚙ **Make a list of every relationship in your life** and rank how those relationships make you feel, from 1 (terrible) to 5 (fabulous). Bad relationships are known energy sappers. Take note of the relationships that don't add any positive energy, and develop plans to remove yourself from them.

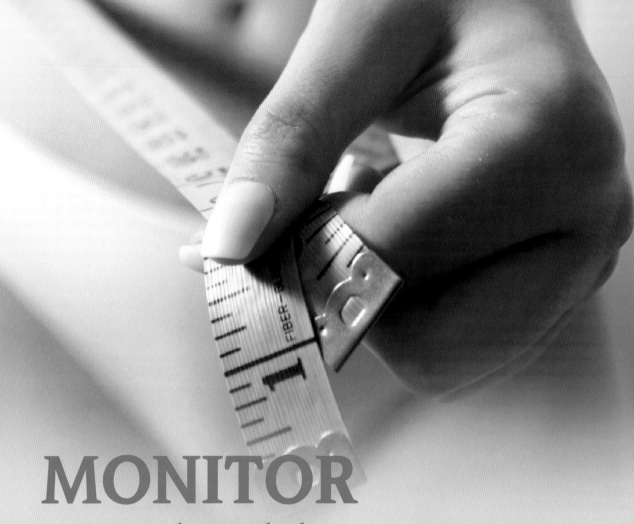

MONITOR
your health

Many of us go for regular check-ups and blood tests. But that's not to say that in between visits you should close your eyes and cross your fingers that all's still well. The fact is that while your doctor may see you once or twice a year, you live in your body every single day, and that makes you the best judge of your own health – if you know what clues to look for. Here are 15 ways to play doctor detective.

15 WAYS TO DO IT WITHOUT A DOCTOR

☆ **Have a PERF-ect day.** Essentially, there are four things you should monitor every day to make sure you are living healthily: the amount of fruit and vegetables you ate that day (fresh Produce); whether you walked and were active (Exercise); whether you got at least 15 minutes of laughter and fun time for yourself (Relaxation); and whether you got enough legumes, grains and other high-fibre foods (Fibre). If you can say you did well on all four, your day has been extremely healthy.

☆ **Monitor your sleepiness.** There are three good ways to tell if you're getting enough sleep. First, do you require an alarm clock to wake up most mornings? Second, do you become drowsy in the afternoon to the point that it affects what you're doing? Third, do you doze off shortly after eating dinner? If the answer to any of these is yes, you need more sleep. And if you're getting enough sleep (about 8 hours) and still have these troubles, talk to your doctor about your low energy.

● **Check your hairbrush.** If your hair's falling out, ask your doctor to check your levels of blood ferritin, an indication of how much iron your body is storing. Some studies suggest low levels may be related to unexplained hair loss. Thyroid disease is another fairly common cause.

● **Measure your height every year after you turn 50.** This is especially important for women as a way of assessing posture and skeletal health. A change in stature can be as informative as a change on a bone density test in terms of assessing your overall bone health. If you're concerned, ask your GP about having a bone density test: it picks up bone loss even before your height changes.

Healthy INVESTMENT

A home blood pressure-monitoring test
A study published in the *Journal of the American Medical Association* found that monitoring your blood pressure at home can save money and give your doctor a valuable insight into your risk of high blood pressure (hypertension). See page 230 for advice on choosing a monitor.

● **Keep a mental colour chart of how dark your urine is.** It may sound weird, but it's a useful health indicator. Your urine should be a clear, straw colour; if it's dark or smells strong, you may not be getting enough fluids. If it stays dark-coloured even after you increase your liquid intake, make an appointment to see your doctor. If it's bright yellow, it may be the B vitamins in your multivitamin.

● **Check your heartbeat after you exercise.** A study published in the *Journal of the American Medical Association* found that women with poor heart rate recovery (HRR) after exercise had twice the risk of having a heart attack within ten years as those who had normal HRR. To test your HRR after regular strenuous activity, count your heartbeats for 15 seconds, then multiply by four to get your heart rate. Sit down and wait 2 minutes before checking again. Subtract the second number from the first. If it's under 55, your HRR is higher than normal and you should talk it through with your doctor.

Your hairbrush may provide valuable health clues.

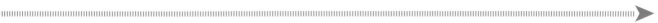

● **If you have diabetes, check your feet every day.** You will be susceptible to foot damage so examine your feet carefully for any blisters, fungus, peeling skin, cuts or bruises. Because people with diabetes often have some nerve damage in extremities such as the feet, these daily self-examinations give critical clues as to how well you're monitoring your blood sugar and if you might have nerve damage.

● **Men only: check down below.** Believe it or not, it's even more important for men to conduct a testicular self-exam than it is for women to conduct a breast check. Catching testicular cancer early is the best way to beat it. Follow these steps every month to become familiar with what's normal so you can recognize if anything feels wrong:
● **The best time to check is after a bath or shower,** when your skin is relaxed. Stand in front of a mirror. Check for any swelling on the scrotal skin.
● **Examine each testicle with both hands.** Place the index and middle fingers under the testicle with the thumbs placed on top. Roll the testicle gently between thumbs and fingers – you shouldn't feel any pain as you do it. Don't be alarmed if one testicle seems slightly larger than the other.
● **If you find a lump on your testicle,** see a doctor right away. It may be only an infection, but if it's testicular cancer, it will spread without treatment. Any free-floating lumps in the scrotum that aren't attached to a testicle are not testicular cancer. But it's still sensible to have a check.

● **Take the fall test.** If you have osteoporosis, you are at great risk if you fall.

So take this simple self-test developed by Dr. Joseph Lane and his colleagues at the Hospital for Special Surgery in New York. Time yourself standing on one leg. Do it in shoes or barefoot, but don't hold onto anything. Try it on both legs (one at a time) three times. A normal 80 year old should be able to stand without difficulty for at least 12 seconds. If your best leg time is less than 12 seconds, or you wobble back and forth, you have poor balance. Talk to your doctor or physiotherapist about different exercises that will help to improve it.

● **Check your blood pressure every six months,** at home with a home blood monitor (see page 228), the pharmacy or at a local health clinic. You'll find plenty of information at www.hypertension.ca – the website of the Canadian Hypertension Society. If the top number is more than 140 (130 if you have diabetes) and the bottom number is higher than 90 (80 for diabetics), wait a day, then check it again. If it's still high, make an appointment with your doctor.

● **Have a cardiovascular check.** If you're over 40 and not on treatment for heart disease or high blood pressure, talk to your doctor about getting a cardiovascular risk assessment. You can also request one if you're under 40 with a strong family history of heart attack or stroke. Blood cholesterol levels are just one of several factors that need to be measured and assessed, including smoking status, fasting blood glucose level, ECG results and blood pressure. Measuring cholesterol alone is not enough, as other risk factors may be missed; if your cholesterol is normal, it does not necessarily mean that your overall cardiovascular risk is normal.

Check your toenails once a month, but if you're diabetic be sure to check your feet every day.

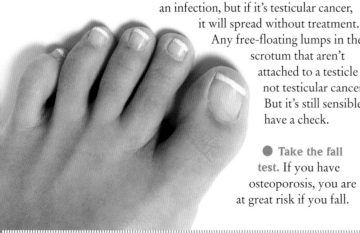

● **Check your toenails once a month.** Look for early signs of fungal infection or ingrown toenails – best treated early.

● **For women only: conduct a breast self-check every month just after your period,** or, if you're postmenopausal, on the first of the month. The Canadian Breast Cancer Foundation recommends the following five steps:
● Know what's normal for you.
● Know what changes to look for.
● Look and feel for changes.
● Report any changes to your doctor without delay.
● Get a free breast screening done if you're over 50 (or 40 in some provinces).

Here's what to look out for:
● **Size:** has one breast become larger or lower? Is there any change in the outline or shape of the breast, especially if caused by arm movements, or by lifting the breasts?
● **Nipples:** has a nipple become inverted or has it changed position or shape? Are there any rashes on or around the nipple, or moist reddish areas that don't heal easily? Is there any discharge?
● **Skin changes:** are there any dimples or is there any puckering?
● **Is there any pain or discomfort** in one breast, which is different from normal, particularly if it is new or persistent?
● **Is there a lump,** thickening or bumpy area in one breast or armpit that seems to be very different from the same part of the other breast or armpit? This is very important if it is new.

If you find any changes, remember that the majority will be normal changes or benign (non-cancerous) conditions, but it's important to see your doctor right away.

● **Get naked every two to three months.** Then, with your partner (or a close friend), conduct a head-to-toe

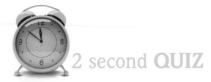

2 second QUIZ

Weight or waist size?
ANSWER: **WAIST SIZE.**

The circumference of your waist is a better predictor of heart disease risk than your body mass index (BMI). The reason is that it's belly fat – not the fat on the thighs or buttocks – that poses the most danger to your heart and arteries. Research shows that for women, health risk begins to rise with a waist circumference above 80 cm (32 in.); over 89 cm (35 in.) is a serious threat. For men, the risk rises above 94 cm (37 in.); over 102 cm (40 in.) is a serious concern. Wrap a tape measure around your skin at mid-abdomen, at or near the belly button. Keep it snug, but not tight – and don't suck in your stomach.

skin check, looking for any new moles, changed moles, suspicious spots or rashes. Be sure to check your scalp, between your toes and fingers, and even on the underside of your arms. If you find anything worrying, see your doctor.

Do the ABCD test when checking moles:
● **Asymmetry:** the two halves don't match.
● **Border irregularity:** the edges are jagged.
● **Colour:** it's uneven. Different shades of black, brown or pink may be seen.
● **Diameter:** it's more than 6 mm ($^1/_4$ in.) wide.

● **Know your body mass index, or BMI.** This measure relates weight to height. A normal BMI is 18.5 to 24.9. A BMI of 25 to 30 puts you in the overweight category, while a BMI above 30 means you are obese. To find out your BMI, divide your weight in kg by your height in metres squared or go to www.hc-sc.gc.ca and type BMI into the search box. Body fat percentage is also important. You can buy scales and handheld devices to measure this yourself, or have it done at a gym.

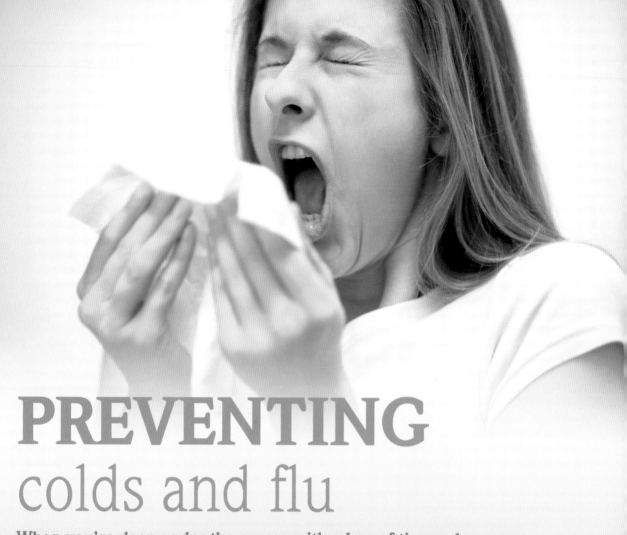

PREVENTING
colds and flu

When you're deep under the covers with a box of tissues by your bedside do you turn green with envy thinking of those people who never seem to get ill? Want to be one of them? While colds won't kill you, they can weaken your immune system, allowing other, more serious, germs to take hold. Given that most of us have two or three colds a year, that's a lot of opportunities for serious illness. Although it's impossible to promise that you'll never catch another cold or suffer from another bout of flu, you can increase your odds of staying well with these strategies. And if you do get sick, there are some tips on how to get better faster.

22 WAYS TO STAY HEALTHY ALL YEAR ROUND

Wash your hands and wash them often. A U.S. study of 40,000 naval recruits who were ordered to wash their hands five times a day found that the recruits cut their incidence of respiratory illnesses by 45 per cent.

● **Every time you wash your hands, do it twice.** Researchers who looked for germs on volunteers' hands found that one handwashing had little effect, even when using antibacterial soap. So wash twice if you're serious about fending off colds.

● **Use this hand-drying strategy in public toilets.** Studies find a shockingly large percentage of people fail to wash their hands after using a public toilet. And every single one of them touches the door handle on the way out. So after washing your hands, use a paper towel to turn off the tap. Use another paper towel to dry your hands, then open the door with that paper towel as a barrier between you and the handle. It sounds a bit crazy, but it could help to protect you from infectious diseases such as colds and flu.

☺ **Carry hand sanitizer with you.** Colds are typically passed not from coughing or kissing (although those are two modes of transmission) but from hand-to-hand or hand-to-object contact, since most cold viruses can live for hours on objects. You then put your hand in or near your mouth or nose and, voilà, you're infected. Carry hand sanitizer gel or sanitizing wipes with you and you can clean your hands at any time, even if the closest water supply is miles away. It works.

● **Use your knuckle to rub your eyes.** It's less likely to be contaminated with viruses than your fingertip. This is particularly important given that the eye provides a perfect entry point for germs, and most of us rub our eyes or nose or scratch our faces 20 to 50 times a day.

● **Put your toothbrush in the microwave** on high for 10 seconds to kill germs that can cause colds and other illnesses. Once you're finished brushing your teeth, your toothbrush is a breeding ground for germs. Sterilize it in the microwave before you use it or simply replace it every month when you change the page on your calendar and after you've had a cold.

☆ **Get a flu vaccination every autumn.** In some provinces, flu vaccination is offered free of charge to seniors or anyone with a long-term medical problem that makes them more vulnerable (for example, heart or lung disease, being on immunosuppressant drugs, having diabetes or no spleen). Employers often also offer the vaccine to health-care staff.

● **Stop blaming yourself when things go wrong at work.** Believe it or not, blaming yourself makes you more likely to catch a cold. At least, that's what researchers found when they studied more than 200 workers over three months. Even those who had control over their work were more likely to begin sneezing if they lacked confidence or tended to blame themselves when things went wrong. Researchers believe that such attitudes make people more stressed on the job, and stress, as everyone knows, can challenge your immune system.

Microwave your toothbrush to eradicate nasty germs.

😊 **Leave the windows in your house open a crack in winter.** Not all of them, but one or two in the rooms in which you spend the most time. This is particularly important if you live in a newer home, if fresh circulating air has been sacrificed to energy efficiency. A bit of fresh air will do wonders for chasing out germs.

● **Lower the heat in your house by a few degrees.** The dry air of an overheated home provides the perfect environment for cold viruses to thrive. And when your mucous membranes (of the nose, mouth and tonsils) dry out, they can't trap those germs very well. Lowering the temperature and using a room humidifier helps to maintain a healthier level of humidity in winter.

● **Speaking of which, buy a hygrometer.** These little tools measure humidity. You want the reading in your home to be around 50 per cent. A consistent measure

higher than 60 per cent means mould and mildew may start to grow on your walls, fabrics and kitchen; lower than 40 per cent and the dry air makes you more susceptible to germs.

● **Sit in a sauna once a week.** Why? Because an Austrian study published in 1990 found that volunteers who frequently used a sauna had half as many colds during the six month study period as those who didn't use a sauna at all. It's possible that the hot air you inhale kills cold viruses. Most gyms have saunas these days.

☆ **Take a garlic supplement every day.** When 146 volunteers received either one garlic supplement a day or a placebo for 12 weeks between November and February, those taking the garlic were not only less likely to get a cold, but if they did catch one, their symptoms were less intense and they recovered faster.

● **Eat a container of yogourt every day.** A study by an American university found that people who ate one cup of yogourt – whether live culture or pasteurized – had 25 per cent fewer colds than non-yogourt eaters. Start your yogourt eating in the summer to build up your immunity before the cold and flu season starts.

● **Once a day, sit in a quiet, dim room,** close your eyes and focus on one word. You're meditating, which is a proven way of reducing stress. And stress, studies find, increases your susceptibility to colds. In fact, stressed people have up to twice the number of colds as non-stressed people.

● **Scrub under your fingernails** every night. They're a great hiding place for all sorts of germs.

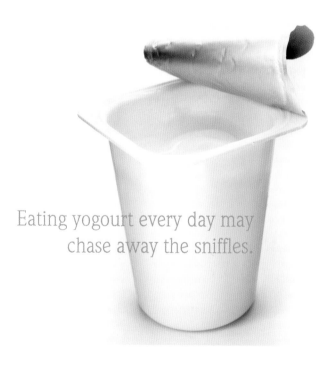

Eating yogourt every day may chase away the sniffles.

● **Change or wash your hand towels** every three or four days during the cold and flu season. When you wash them, use hot water in order to kill the germs.

✦ **At the very first hint of a cold, launch a preventive blitz. Here's how:**
● Suck on a zinc lozenge until it melts away. Then suck another every two waking hours. Or use a zinc-based nasal spray. Some studies suggest that zinc may help, but the jury is still out.
● Cook up a pot of chicken soup.
● Roast garlic in the oven (drizzle whole cloves with olive oil, wrap in foil, roast for an hour at 400°F/200°C), then spread the soft garlic on toast and eat.

Studies find that all either reduce the length of time you suffer from a cold or help to prevent a full-blown cold from occurring.

● **Sneeze and cough into your arm or into a tissue.** Whoever taught us to cover our mouths when we cough or sneeze got it wrong. That just puts the germs right on our hands, where you can spread them to objects – and other people. Instead, hold the crook of your elbow over your mouth and nose when you sneeze or cough if a tissue isn't handy. It's pretty rare for you to shake someone's elbow or scratch your eye with an elbow, after all.

● **Don't pressure your doctor for antibiotics.** Colds and flu (along with most common infections) are caused by viruses, so antibiotics – designed to kill bacteria – won't do a thing. They can cause harm, however, by killing off the friendly bacteria that are part of our immune defences. If you've used antibiotics a lot lately, consider a course of probiotics – the replacement troops for friendly bacteria.

● **Wipe your nose – don't blow.** Your cold won't hang around as long, according to a U.S. study. It turns out that the force of blowing not only sends the phlegm out of your nose into a tissue, but propels some back into your sinuses. If you need to blow, blow gently, and blow one nostril at a time.

● **Put a box of tissues wherever people sit.** In October, bulk buy boxes of tissues and place them strategically around the house, your workplace, your car. Don't let aesthetics thwart you. You need to have tissues widely available so that anyone who has to cough or sneeze or blow his or her nose will do so in the way that's least likely to spread germs.

Place a handy box of tissues wherever people sit and they're more likely to use them.

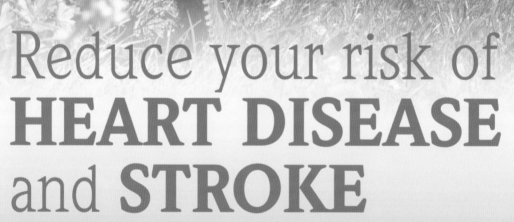

Reduce your risk of
HEART DISEASE
and STROKE

Death rates from cardiovascular disease (CVD) have been falling in Canada since the 1950s. And Canada's death rate from stroke is one of the lowest in the world. But that may change as the elderly segment of our population grows over the coming years. The good news is that modern medicine will help mitigate things. But is being pulled back from the brink by bypass surgery your idea of a healthy future? Or needing a vast array of medicines? It's better to avoid CVD altogether. Add these small changes to your life for a powerful dose of heart disease prevention.

25 SIMPLE SOLUTIONS

♥ **Ride your bike for 20 minutes a day.** When German researchers asked 100 men with mild chest pain, or angina, either to exercise for 20 minutes a day on a stationary bike or to undergo an artery-clearing procedure called angioplasty, they found that a year after the angioplasty, 21 men suffered a heart attack, stroke or other problem compared to only six of the bikers. Just remember: if you already have angina, you should begin an exercise program only under medical supervision.

☆ **Eat a piece of dark chocolate several times a week.** Believe it or not, several small studies suggest that dark chocolate could be good for your heart. The beneficial effects are probably due to chemicals in chocolate called flavonoids, which help the arteries to stay flexible. Other properties of the sweet stuff seem to make arteries less likely to clot and prevent the "bad" cholesterol, LDL, from oxidizing, making it less likely to form plaque. Dark chocolate is also rich in magnesium. But steer clear of milk chocolate, which is high in butterfat and thus tends to raise cholesterol.

♥ **Have a beer once a day.** A study published in the *Journal of Agricultural and Food Chemistry* found that men who drank one beer a day for a month lowered their cholesterol levels, increased their blood levels of heart-healthy antioxidants and reduced their levels of fibrinogen, a protein that contributes to blood clots. Of course, red wine might be even better (see page 225). Choose either beer or wine – don't have both.

♥ **Record yourself at night.** If you hear yourself snoring (or if your sleeping partner has been kicking you a lot), make an appointment with your doctor. You may have sleep apnea, a condition in which the breathing stops hundreds of times throughout the night. It can lead to high blood pressure and other medical problems, and even increase your risk of a heart attack or stroke.

♥ **Go to bed an hour earlier tonight.** A Harvard study of 70,000 women found that those who got less than 7 hours of sleep had a slightly higher risk of heart disease. Researchers suspect that lack of sleep increases stress hormones, raises blood pressure and affects blood sugar levels. Keep your overall sleeping time to no more than 9 hours, however. The same study found that women sleeping 9 or more hours had a slightly increased risk of heart disease.

☆ **Eat fish at least once a week.** Have it grilled, sautéed, baked or roasted. A study published in the *Journal of the American Medical Association* in April 2002 found that women who ate fish at least once a week were a third less likely to have a heart attack or die of heart disease than those who ate fish only once a month. Other studies show similar benefits for men. Another major study found that regular fish consumption reduced the risk of atrial fibrillation – rapid, irregular heartbeat – a major cause of sudden death.

♥ **Have a high-fibre breakfast cereal at least four times a week.** In a study published in the *American Journal of Clinical Nutrition* in September 1999, Harvard University scientists found that women who ate 23 g of fibre a day – mostly from cereal – were 23 per cent less likely to have heart attacks than those who consumed only 11 g of fibre. In men, a high-fibre diet slashed the chances of a heart attack by 36 per cent.

Keep your heart happy by eating fish at least once a week.

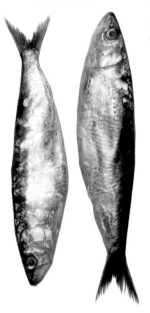

A strong case for **FISH OIL**

Consider, for a moment, the Inuit in the North and their cousins in Alaska and Russia. These hardy souls survive on diets of nearly pure fat, and yet they tend to be completely free of heart disease. How on earth is this possible? The answer is fish oil.

Every medical journal on heart health brings, it seems, another study demonstrating the cardiovascular benefits of the oil – specifically, its omega-3 fatty acids, a type of polyunsaturated fat found in few foods other than fish and flaxseeds. A primary reason it's so healthy: omega-3s are a natural anti-inflammatory. In recent years, scientists have discovered that inflammation within our arteries – triggered in response to damage done by plaque, high blood pressure and free radicals – is a major cause of heart disease. While inflammation is a healing response, in your blood vessels it only causes further damage, leaving them stiffer and working at far less then optimal capacity. Omega-3s cause this type of inflammation to recede.

There's more: omega-3 fatty acids also seem to make blood less sticky, so it's less likely to form clots that can block blood flow and trigger a heart attack. And they help to reduce levels of triglycerides, blood fats linked with heart disease.

The bottom line: get more omega-3 fatty acids into your body, either through foods or supplements. There are ideas for doing this throughout this book.

Here are the fish with the largest amounts of this crucial nutrient (amounts are per 100 g of fish):

- Fresh salmon: 2.3 g
- Sardines: 2.2 g
- Pilchards: 2.2 g
- Mackerel: 2.0 g
- Fresh tuna: 1.6 g
- Trout: 1.2 g

♥ **Drink at least two cups of tea a day.** Black or green, it doesn't seem to matter. At least, that's the result of a Dutch study which found that only 2.4 per cent of 5,000 healthy Rotterdam residents who drank two or more cups of tea a day had a heart attack within six years, compared with 4.1 per cent of those who never drank tea. Another major analysis of 17 studies on tea drinkers found that three cups a day could slash the risk of a heart attack by 11 per cent.

♥ **Stir a handful of nuts into a vegetable-and-chicken stir-fry.** Just 45 g of nuts a day can reduce your risk of cardiovascular disease. A good idea: crush unsalted nuts and use them to coat fish or chicken, then bake.

♥ **Include beans or peas in four of your dishes every week.** Researchers have found that people who did so slashed their risk of heart disease by 22 per cent compared to those who ate fewer legumes.

♥ **Have sex tonight.** It counts as physical activity, which, of course, is good for your heart. That may be why University of Bristol researchers found that men who have sex at least twice a week are less likely to have a stroke or other cardiovascular problems than men who have it less often. Women probably stand to benefit too.

☺ **Eat 15 cherries a day.** Studies find that the anthocyanins (plant chemicals), which give cherries their scarlet colour, also lower levels of uric acid in the blood, a marker for heart attacks and stroke. If it's not cherry season, try sprinkling dried cherries on your salad or use canned.

☆ **Choose a breakfast cereal fortified with folic acid in the morning.** Do that and you'll be getting at least 300 mcg of folate. A study in New Orleans found that people who consumed at least that much folate slashed their risk of stroke by 20 per cent and their risk of heart disease by 13 per cent more than those who got less than 136 mcg per day of the B vitamin. Other good sources of folate include Brussels sprouts, asparagus, peas, chickpeas, brown rice, oranges and orange juice, and bananas.

♥ **Eat an orange every day.** Or drink a glass of orange juice. Oranges are a great source of vitamin C. Studies suggest that diets high in this vitamin may reduce your risk of stroke, especially if you smoke. Strawberries, Brussels sprouts, broccoli and chopped red pepper are some other excellent sources of vitamin C.

♥ **Skip the soft drinks and have orange juice instead.** It's all to do with inflammation, the body's response to damage or injury. Chronic inflammation, linked to heart disease, is significantly affected by your diet. For instance, U.S. researchers found that drinking glucose-sweetened water triggered an inflammatory response in volunteers, but drinking the same calories in orange juice didn't. They theorize that the anti-inflammatory effects of vitamin C and various flavonoids in juice may provide some protection. Choose 100 per cent juice, not drinks that are mostly sweetened, flavoured water. Other studies on orange juice find that it can increase blood levels of heart-protective folate by almost 45 per cent and reduce levels of heart-damaging homocysteine by 11 per cent.

☺ Drink 1 cup (250 ml) of water every 2 hours. A study in California found that women who drank more than five glasses of water a day were half as likely to die from a heart attack as those who drank fewer than two. This is probably due to the fact that maintaining good hydration keeps blood flowing well; dehydration can cause sluggish blood flow and increase the risk of clots forming. Water works best when it comes to improving blood flow; soft drinks are worthless.

Just for **WOMEN**

Tell a woman that she's more likely to die of a heart attack or stroke than of breast cancer and she might not believe you. A 2003 survey of 204 women with heart disease found that many considered their condition a "man's disease." Not so. Every year about 35,000 women in Canada die from heart disease and disease of the blood vessels. In fact, cardiovascular disease claims more women's lives than all forms of cancer. So follow these health-boosting gender-based tips:

● **Remember who comes first: you.** One hospital study found that women rate poor self-esteem as the primary reason for not making changes to improve their cardiovascular health. Remember: if you're not around, it won't matter what you used to do for others.

● **Meditate or simply go into a dark, quiet room for 20 minutes when you get home from work.** Stress harms the heart directly and also indirectly – by preventing you from making lifestyle changes that could help your heart. And in a woman's life, the stress of work is often simply compounded by the stress of home. Give yourself a time-out period between your two worlds – it will do you a whole world of heart-healthy good.

● **Follow simple heart-healthy steps – not just for you but for your whole family.** As well as eating healthily and not drinking too much or smoking, encourage your children and grandchildren to be aware of the importance of looking after their hearts. That way you can help to prevent heart disease in future generations. Encourage them to be active along with you. Involve them in food preparation so that they know about "good" and "bad" foods.

● **Listen to your body.** Don't assume that if you're not having crushing chest pain you're not having a heart attack. Symptoms of a heart attack in women can include extreme weakness or a feeling similar to indigestion. So pay attention to your body. Surveys of women who have had heart attacks find that they may exhibit some unique symptoms in the month before the attack, such as feeling unusually fatigued, having problems sleeping, having indigestion and weakness in their arms.

♥ **Cook with ginger or turmeric twice a week.** They have anti-inflammatory properties, and inflammation is a major contributor to heart disease.

♥ **Go to the toilet whenever you feel the urge.** Research at Taiwan University found that a full bladder causes your heart to beat faster and puts added stress on the coronary arteries, triggering them to contract, which could lead to a heart attack in people who are vulnerable.

♥ **Ask for next Monday and Friday off.** American researchers analyzed data on more than 12,000 middle-aged men from the famous Framingham Heart Study and found that those who took regular vacations sliced their risk of death from heart disease by a third.

♥ **Drive with the windows closed and the air-conditioning on.** This reduces your exposure to airborne pollutants, which a Harvard study found reduces something called "heart rate variability" (HRV), or the ability of your heart to respond to various activities and stresses. Reduced HRV has been associated with increased deaths among heart attack survivors.

♥ **Call a friend and arrange dinner.** A study published in the journal *Heart* in April 2004 found that having a very close relationship with another person, whether it's a friend, lover or relative, can halve the risk of a heart attack in someone who has already had one.

♥ **Pay attention to the basics.** Two major studies found that nearly everyone who dies of heart disease, including heart attacks, had at least one or more of the conventional risk factors, such as smoking, diabetes, high blood pressure or high cholesterol levels.

☆ **Along with exercising every day, take a supplement** containing the antioxidant vitamins C and E. A study published in the *Proceedings of the National Academy of Sciences* found that while moderate exercise alone reduced the development of atherosclerosis, or hardening of the arteries, adding the vitamins (as well as L-arginine) to the mix boosted the effects astronomically. The two – exercise and the supplements – have a synergistic effect in enhancing production of nitric oxide, which protects against a variety of heart-related problems.

♥ **If you find you're having trouble getting out of bed in the morning,** have lost interest in your normal activities, or just feel really off-colour, call your doctor. You may be depressed, and untreated depression significantly increases your risk of a heart attack.

♥ **Adopt a dog.** The power of furry friends to improve heart health is proven. Not only will a dog force you to be more active (think about all the walks), but the companionship and unconditional affection a dog provides has been shown to reduce the risk of heart attack and other cardiovascular problems.

Man's best friend may also be your heart's best friend.

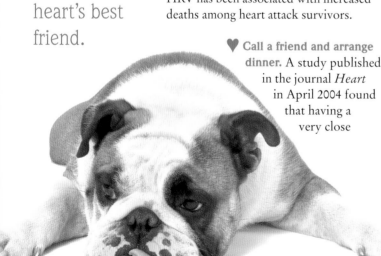

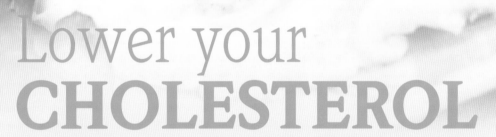

Lower your
CHOLESTEROL

According to the Heart & Stroke Foundation of Canada, an estimated 10 million Canadian adults have high cholesterol levels. If you're one of these people, it means that your body produces too much harmful low-density lipoprotein (LDL) but produces too little "good" high-density lipoprotein (HDL). "Bad" LDL carries cholesterol into your arteries, contributing to artery-clogging plaque and increasing the risk of heart disease and stroke, while "good" HDL carries cholesterol away to the liver and out of the body.

Even if you're taking cholesterol-lowering medication, you should pay special attention to the tips in this chapter because research suggests that by eating the right foods and taking good care of yourself, you could slash your risk of dying from heart disease by an incredible 80 per cent.

15 WAYS TO GET THE NUMBERS DOWN

Healthy INVESTMENT

A slow cooker

They're perfect for making bean-based soups and stews high in cholesterol-lowering soluble fibre. Slow cookers are also ideal for simmering lean cuts of meat, which are healthier due to their low fat content, but also tougher for the same reason.

disease (reduced blood flow to the hands and feet).

● **Down more orange juice.** Some studies suggest that drinking 2 glasses of orange juice a day helps to cut total cholesterol and a Canadian study found that drinking 3 glasses a day for four weeks raised healthy HDL levels by 21 per cent and improved the ratio of good to bad cholesterol by 16 per cent.

● **Use honey instead of sugar in your tea.** A study from Dubai in the United Arab Emirates found total and LDL cholesterol levels fell in healthy people after they drank a solution containing honey, but not after they drank solutions with glucose or artificial honey. After 15 days of the honey drink, participants' HDL levels rose and homocysteine levels dropped. Homocysteine is an amino acid linked to an increased risk of heart disease, stroke and peripheral vascular

● **Eat six or more small meals a day.** A large study of British adults found that people who ate more often had significantly lower cholesterol than those who ate twice a day, even though the grazers got more calories and fat. In fact, the differences in cholesterol levels were large enough to reduce the grazers' risk of heart disease by 10 to 20 per cent. Just be sure those six meals are truly small.

Make all your sandwiches from whole-wheat bread.

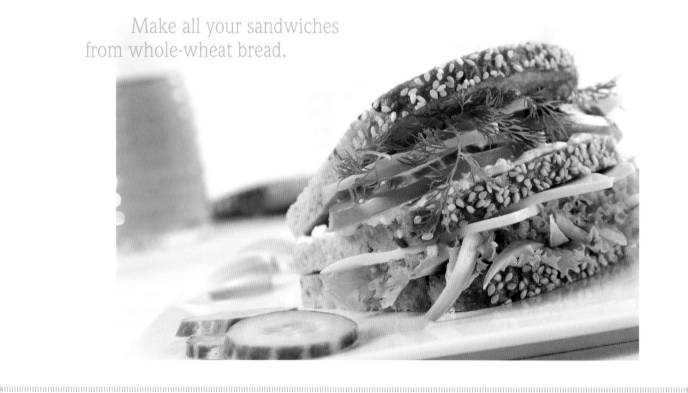

● **Have a small glass of wine most evenings with dinner.** Studies find a daily glass of wine or beer a day can boost levels of HDL cholesterol. Opt for red wine as it is three to ten times higher in plant compounds called flavonoids, believed to be responsible for much of wine's beneficial effects on cholesterol.

● **Eat whole-wheat sandwiches.** Cutting back on simple carbs such as white bread and eating more complex carbs, including whole-wheat bread and brown rice, can increase HDL levels slightly and significantly lower triglycerides, another type of blood fat that contributes to heart disease.

● **Use olive oil in your salad dressing.** A U.S. study found that diets rich in the kind of monounsaturated fat found in olive oil reduced LDL cholesterol in people with diabetes or metabolic syndrome – a cluster of risk factors including low HDL, high insulin levels and being overweight – just as effectively as following a low-fat diet.

● **Sip a cup of black tea every 4 hours.** Scientists found that drinking 5 cups a day of black tea for three weeks reduced cholesterol levels in people with mildly high levels.

☆ **Add half a tablespoon of cinnamon to your coffee maker.** A Pakistani study found that 6 g of cinnamon a day (about $1/2$ tablespoon) reduced LDL cholesterol in people with Type 2 diabetes by nearly 30 per cent and cut their total cholesterol by 26 per cent.

● **Have oatmeal for breakfast every morning.** There's a reason oat manufacturers are allowed to boast about the grain's cholesterol-lowering benefits:

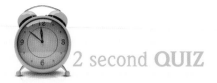

plenty of research has confirmed them. Rich in a soluble fibre called beta glucan, oatmeal can reduce your LDL by 12 to 24 per cent if you eat a bowl of oats every day, combined with other foods rich in soluble fibre such as beans and legumes. Choose quick-cooking or old-fashioned oats rather than instant.

☺ **This week, have a few glasses of cranberry juice every day** (mix it with water to reduce the sugar content). Cranberries are rich sources of anthocyanins, proanthocyanidins and flavonols, plant chemicals that prevent LDL cholesterol from oxidizing, a process that makes it more likely to stick to artery walls. These chemicals also keep red blood cells from getting too sticky. An added bonus: they initiate a complex chemical reaction that helps blood vessels

Get tested **IN THE AUTUMN**

Believe it or not, U.S. researchers found that cholesterol levels in healthy adults were higher in the autumn and winter than in the spring and summer – significantly higher. Why? We tend to have greater blood volume in the spring and summer, which will reduce cholesterol levels. So if you were tested in July and the reading was normal, check again before Christmas.

What causes
HIGH CHOLESTEROL?

One of the main causes of high cholesterol levels in Canada is eating too much saturated fat. Here are some other cholesterol facts to be aware of:

- Although cholesterol is found in some foods such as eggs, liver, kidneys and some seafood, such as shrimp, this type of cholesterol generally does not affect the cholesterol levels in your blood. It is more important to tackle the amount of saturated fat you consume, and to replace saturated and trans fats with healthier monounsaturated and polyunsaturated fats.

- Some people who eat a healthy diet have high cholesterol levels because of a condition called familial hyperlipidemia. Your doctor can advise you if this applies to you.

- Eating oily fish regularly is a great cholesterol buster. It provides the richest source of omega-3 fats, which help to reduce triglyceride levels (another fatty substance – high triglyceride levels lead to a greater risk of cardiovascular disease).

- Foods that are high in soluble fibre can help to lower your cholesterol. Think legumes, lentils, nuts and fibre-rich fruit and veggies.

- Being physically active also helps to raise your levels of "good" HDL cholesterol.

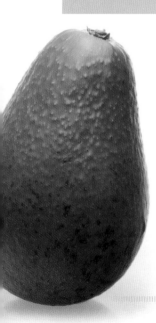

to relax. Plus they decrease "bad" LDL cholesterol levels. Not only that, but American researchers reported that three glasses of cranberry juice a day can raise "good" HDL cholesterol levels by up to 10 per cent.

● **Eat a grapefruit every other day.** Grapefruits are particularly high in pectin, a soluble fibre that can help to reduce cholesterol levels. Grapefruits

interfere with the absorption and processing in the liver of several medicines, however, so check with your doctor first. Other good sources of pectin include apples and berries.

● **Pour soy milk over your morning cereal.** A Spanish study of 40 men and women found that those who drank about 2 cups (500 ml) of soy milk a day for three months reduced their harmful LDL cholesterol levels, while at the same time increasing their beneficial HDL levels. Just make sure that you buy soy milk fortified with calcium.

● **Whip up some guacamole this evening.** Several studies find that eating one avocado a day as part of a healthy diet can lower your LDL by as much as 17 per cent while raising your HDL.

● **Spend 10 minutes a day doing strength-training exercises.** You don't have to do these at a gym – push-ups, squats, leg lifts, hip extensions – they all count. And they matter when it comes to counting your cholesterol levels: a study in the *British Journal of Sports Medicine* found that strength training lowered total cholesterol by 10 per cent and LDL cholesterol by 14 per cent among women who worked out for 45 to 50 minutes three times a week. If you can't manage that amount, start with 10 minutes a day, six days a week, and gradually work up.

● **Drink a glass of purple grape juice every day.** Rich in cholesterol-lowering flavonoids, grape juice is an extremely healthy drink, and an excellent alternative if you don't like red wine.

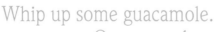

Whip up some guacamole.
One avocado a day can lower your LDL.

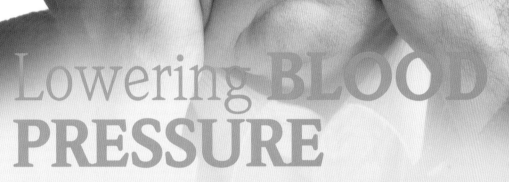

Lowering BLOOD PRESSURE

You can't see it, you can't feel it and, unless you get it checked, you won't even know you have it. That makes high blood pressure, or hypertension, a quiet killer, one that slowly damages your blood vessels, heart and eyes while simultaneously increasing your risk of heart disease, stroke, dementia and kidney disease.

According to the Heart & Stroke Foundation of Canada, five million Canadians have high blood pressure, but up to 42 per cent may not know it. The following tips will help keep your blood pressure at a healthy level. In addition, see "Cutting back on salt," page 110, to see how reducing your salt intake can also make a difference.

18 WAYS TO GO BEYOND LOW-SALT

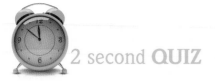
A good book or a good friend?
ANSWER: **A GOOD FRIEND.**

Perhaps not every night, but, in general, time spent with friends is time well invested in your health. Relationships are critical in terms of reducing the negative effects of stress hormones on blood pressure.

● **Every morning, take a brisk 15 minute walk.** Amazingly, you don't need a lot of exercise to make a difference to your blood pressure. When Japanese researchers asked 168 inactive volunteers with high blood pressure to exercise at a health club for different amounts of time each week for eight weeks, blood pressure levels dropped almost as much in those who exercised for 30 to 90 minutes a week as in those who exercised for more than 90 minutes a week.

● **Write "take medication" on your calendar every day.** Twenty-five per cent of the time, when your blood pressure hasn't gone down after you've been prescribed medication, the reason is that you've forgotten to take your pills.

Healthy INVESTMENT

A yoga DVD
The stress-reducing and blood-pressure-lowering benefits of practising yoga are well documented. A DVD is a great way to introduce yourself to this ancient practice in the privacy of your own home, with just a minimal investment.

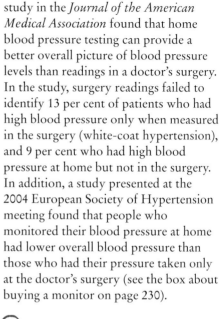

● **Buy a home blood pressure kit.** A study in the *Journal of the American Medical Association* found that home blood pressure testing can provide a better overall picture of blood pressure levels than readings in a doctor's surgery. In the study, surgery readings failed to identify 13 per cent of patients who had high blood pressure only when measured in the surgery (white-coat hypertension), and 9 per cent who had high blood pressure at home but not in the surgery. In addition, a study presented at the 2004 European Society of Hypertension meeting found that people who monitored their blood pressure at home had lower overall blood pressure than those who had their pressure taken only at the doctor's surgery (see the box about buying a monitor on page 230).

☺ **Sprinkle 2 tablespoons of flaxseeds on your yogourt in the morning** and mix 2 tablespoons into your ice cream, soup, spaghetti sauce or other food later in the day. One small study found that adding 4 tablespoons of the seeds significantly lowered systolic blood pressure (the top number) in postmenopausal women with a history of heart disease. Flaxseeds are rich in many nutrients and in fibre.

● **Drink tea instead of coffee.** An Australian study found that each one cup increase in daily tea consumption decreased systolic blood pressure by 2 points and diastolic pressure by 1 point. But the benefits ended after 4 cups.

● **Dip tortilla chips in guacamole.** Why? Avocados have more blood-pressure-lowering potassium than any other fruit or vegetable, including bananas. Canadian men and women should get 4,700 mg of potassium every day, but many get just half this amount.

● **Turn to dark chocolate when your sweet tooth asserts itself.** Unlike milk chocolate, dark chocolate is rich in flavonoids that keep your arteries flexible, preventing the increases in pressure that come with stiffer blood vessels. That's thought to be one reason for the normal blood pressure of a tribe of indigenous Panamanians who eat a high-salt diet but also consume massive amounts of cocoa. In addition, a study published in the *Journal of the American Medical Association* found that 85 g of dark chocolate a day helped to lower blood pressure in older people with isolated systolic hypertension (when only the upper number of a pressure reading is high). Other good sources of flavonoids include tea and wine, as well as many fruits and vegetables.

▐▌▶ **Snack on roasted soybeans** for a crunchy, nutrient-packed munch. Studies show that people with high blood pressure can lower their systolic readings by an average of 10 points by eating 30 g of roasted soybeans (also called soy

Do **THREE** things…

If you do only three things to lower your blood pressure, make it these three, many doctors agree:

1 **Quit smoking.** The nicotine in tobacco products constricts blood vessels and raises blood pressure in the short term.

2 **Get out every day for a walk.** And if you're overweight, make that two walks. Losing just a little weight will make a huge difference to your blood pressure readings.

3 **Follow a diet high in fruit and vegetables and low in high-salt, high-fat and high-cholesterol foods.** One of the quickest ways to lower your blood pressure is to reduce your salt intake. Combine this with hitting your daily fruit and vegetable target and reducing your fat intake and you're well on the way to getting your blood pressure down.

nuts) a day for two weeks. The beans are available at some supermarkets and health-food stores. Make sure you buy them unsalted.

● **Flavour food with lots of pepper.** Why? Pepper is a strong, dominant flavour that can help you to reduce your taste for salt. Without salt, meals may seem bland for a couple of days, but your taste buds can easily be retrained. Add more pepper and, if that doesn't appeal, try garlic, lemon, ginger, basil or other spicy flavours you enjoy. After a week, old favourite foods will taste extremely oversalted and your blood pressure will be singing your praises.

Snack on roasted soybeans. They make a crunchy, nutrient-packed munch.

Choosing a home BLOOD PRESSURE MONITOR

If you decide to monitor your blood pressure at home, you will need to get a home blood pressure monitor. But there's a wide range available, so how do you know which is the best? Talk to your doctor or pharmacist when you're choosing a monitor, as they'll be able to help you select the best model for you. Opt for a monitor that measures your blood pressure at your upper arm rather than at your wrist or finger in order to get the most accurate results. Here's some advice about other features to look for in a home blood pressure monitor:

- Get the right size of cuff. Measure around your bare arm halfway between your shoulder and elbow to find your size.
- Select a monitor that is endorsed by the Canadian Hypertension Society. The sentence "Recommended by the Canadian Hypertension Society" will appear somewhere on the box or in the manual. See www.hypertension.ca for a list of CHS-endorsed monitors.
- Choose a monitor you can afford. Monitors vary in price and some of the more expensive models may include features that you don't need.
- Keep your monitor calibrated to make sure the reading is accurate. Send it back to the manufacturer or take it in to your health-care provider every year to get it recalibrated.

☺ **Eat a handful of dried apricots every afternoon.** Like bananas, apricots are a particularly good source of potassium. Plus they have lots of fibre, iron and beta carotene. The drying process actually increases the concentration of these nutrients, which are all good for your circulatory system. And as a snack, dried apricots are low in calories: roughly eight total just 100 calories. Look out for an unsulphured brand.

● **Park in the Outer Mongolia of the car park.** All you need is an extra 4,000 to 5,000 steps a day and you could lower your blood pressure by 11 points. That's what U.S. researchers found when they tracked postmenopausal women.

● **Hold hands with your partner for 10 minutes.** That (plus a brief hug) is all it took in one study to keep blood pressure steady during a stressful incident.

● **Sleep with earplugs in tonight.** Studies suggest that being exposed to noise while you're sleeping may increase your blood pressure as well as your heart rate, so block out any noise.

● **Drink a glass of orange juice every morning and another at night.** One U.S. study found that this lowered systolic blood pressure by an average of 7 per cent and diastolic blood pressure by an average of 4.6 per cent – thanks to the high levels of potassium in orange juice.

● **Think about your sleep.** Are you waking up tired? Is your partner complaining that you snore a lot? Talk to your doctor. You may have sleep apnea. Studies find that half the people who have the condition, in which you stop breathing dozens or hundreds of times during the night, also have hypertension.

● **Find (and eliminate) at least one hidden source of salt a day.** For instance, did you know that many breakfast cereals contain salt? Who needs salt in their cereal? Find a brand that's salt-free.

☆ **Spend 5 minutes a day sitting in a quiet room repeating this mantra,** "One day at a time." Numerous studies show that meditation eases stress and lowers blood pressure. Other good mantras include: "This, too, shall pass," "Breathe" and "Calm, calm, calm."

● **Take these supplements daily:** garlic, fish oil, calcium, CoQ10. All have blood-pressure-lowering properties. Just check with your doctor first.

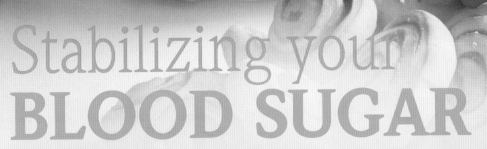

Stabilizing your
BLOOD SUGAR

Blood sugar, or glucose, has become one of today's most studied and discussed health topics. One important reason is that diabetes, a disease reaching epidemic proportions, is directly associated with blood sugar levels. Recent research has also linked blood sugar to heart disease, memory difficulties and even fertility problems.

Whether you already have diabetes, are overweight or want to prevent future problems, here are 19 ways to make sure your blood sugar and insulin levels are as healthy as can be. In addition, look at "Cutting down on sugar," starting on page 101, for more ideas on stabilizing your blood sugar counts.

19 TIPS FOR STABLE, STEADY GLUCOSE LEVELS

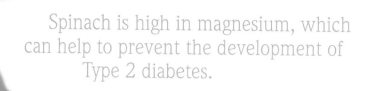

Spinach is high in magnesium, which can help to prevent the development of Type 2 diabetes.

😊 **Drink at least two servings of low-fat dairy products a day** (one serving is a 1 cup [250 ml] glass of skim or 1% milk, or a 175 g container of yogourt). A study of 3,000 people found that those who were overweight, but also ate a lot of dairy foods, were 70 per cent less likely to develop insulin resistance (a precursor to diabetes) than those who didn't. It turns out that the lactose, protein and fat in dairy products improves blood sugar by filling you up and slowing the conversion of food sugars to blood sugar.

😊 **Buy bread products with at least 3 g of fibre and 3 g of protein per serving.** Complex carbohydrates of this type slow down absorption of glucose and decrease possible insulin rises. Plus, the hearty dose of fibre and protein will keep your stomach feeling satisfied for longer.

😊 **Serve up a spinach salad for dinner.** Spinach is high in magnesium, which a large study suggests can help to prevent the development of Type 2 diabetes. One study in women found higher intakes of magnesium (also found in nuts, other leafy greens and fish) reduced diabetes risk by about 10 per cent overall, and by about 20 per cent in women who were overweight. Another great source of magnesium? Avocados.

➤ **Sprinkle cinnamon over your coffee, yogourt, cereal and tea.** Researchers from Pakistan (where cinnamon is widely used) asked volunteers with Type 2 diabetes to take either 1 g, 3 g or 6 g of cinnamon or a placebo for 40 days. Those taking the fragrant spice saw their blood glucose levels drop by between 18 and 29 per cent depending on how much cinnamon they took.

😊 **Eat soba noodles for dinner one night a week.** The "Japanese pasta" is made from buckwheat, a grain that lowered blood glucose levels by 12 to 19 per cent in one well-controlled study on rats. Of course, you're not a rat, but buckwheat is an excellent source of fibre, and the evidence on fibre and blood glucose improvement is unquestionable.

😊 **Include a glass of wine with your dinner.** One study found that women who had a glass of wine a day cut their risk of diabetes in half compared to teetotallers. Not a wine lover? The study found the same effects for beer. But cork

Healthy **INVESTMENT**

A vegetarian cookbook
Learn to use beans and lentils as alternatives to meat for some of your dinners. These foods are high in top-quality protein, but also rich in soluble fibre – which can help to improve blood sugar and insulin levels, assist with weight control and lower cholesterol.

the wine bottle once dinner is over. An Australian study found that drinking a glass of wine immediately after eating can result in a sudden drop in the insulin in your blood, meaning the glucose from your meal hangs around longer, eventually damaging the arteries.

☻ **Cut back on saturated fat.** The reason you want to avoid saturated fat is simple: American scientists evaluated 3,000 people and found that those with the highest blood levels of saturated fats were twice as likely to develop diabetes.

☆ **Walk about 2 kilometres a day.** That's all it took in one large U.S. study to slash the risk of dying from diabetes by more than a third. Believe it or not, if you walk 10 kilometres a week, you'll be nearly 40 per cent less likely to die from all causes and 34 per cent less likely to die from heart disease, the leading cause of death in people with diabetes. The reason? Walking makes your cells more receptive to insulin, which leads to better control of blood sugar. It also raises levels of "good" HDL cholesterol. See "Walking," page 140, for great ways to motivate yourself to walk.

☻ **Rent a comedy and watch it after dinner.** A Japanese study found that people with diabetes who laughed soon after eating (while watching a comedy) had significantly lower blood sugar levels than those who listened to a boring lecture. The connection held even for those without diabetes.

☻ **Have half a grapefruit with breakfast tomorrow morning.** American researchers asked 50 obese patients to eat half a grapefruit with each meal for 12 weeks and compared them to a group that didn't eat any. Those patients who ate the

grapefruit lost an average of 1.6 kg (3.6 lb). They also had lower levels of insulin and glucose after each meal, suggesting a more efficient sugar metabolism. (Make sure you talk to your doctor first before eating grapefruit if you are on any medication, as it can affect the way that medicines are processed in the liver.)

☻ **Add at least one day a week of resistance training.** You'll build more muscle than you will by walking, and the more muscle mass you have, the more efficiently your body burns glucose and the less that hangs around in your blood.

☻ **If you can't resist that cake, have a cup of decaffeinated coffee with it.** British researchers found that combining decaf with simple sugars (such as those in doughnuts, cakes and cookies) reduces the rise in blood sugar that such sweet things create. Standard coffee didn't have the same benefit. The reason? While plant chemicals in coffee slow the rate at which your intestines absorb sugar, caffeine delays sugar's arrival in the muscles, keeping it in the bloodstream for longer.

Do **THREE** things...

If you were to do only three things to maintain healthy blood sugar levels and prevent diabetes, here is what doctors recommend. Together, they can slash your risk of the disease by nearly 60 per cent:

1 **Lose weight.** If you're overweight, losing 3 to 3.5 kg (7 or 8 lb) is all it takes.

2 **Be physically active.** Thirty minutes a day is all you need.

3 **Add more fibre** to your diet by eating vegetables, fruits, whole grains, nuts, seeds, beans and lentils regularly.

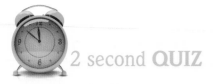

2 second QUIZ

Cut carbs or cut fat?
ANSWER: **NEITHER.**

It's more important to make sure you choose the right carbs and the right fats. Carbs from sugary foods and white breads and pasta raise blood sugar, while "good" carbs – whole grains, fruit, vegetables, beans, lentils, nuts and seeds – help to stabilize it. Similarly, some fats – the saturated fats in meats and full-fat dairy and trans fats such as hydrogenated oils – are bad for your health, while the polyunsaturated and monounsaturated oils in nuts, seeds, olives, avocados and fish reduce the risk of diabetes.

8 hours. Numerous studies find that sleep deprivation has a dramatic effect on your blood sugar and insulin levels. If you need help falling (and staying) asleep, see "The Sleep Routine," on page 72, for tips on getting a better rest.

☺ **Ask your partner if you snore.** Harvard researchers found that women who snored were more than twice as likely as those who didn't to develop diabetes – regardless of weight, smoking history or family history of diabetes. If you do snore, see your doctor. You may have a physical problem, or you may simply need to lose some weight and change the way you sleep.

Eat soba noodles for dinner one night a week. They are an excellent source of fibre.

☺ Prepare your breakfast, lunch and dinner, but then divide each meal in half. Eat half now, then the other half in a couple of hours. Eating several small meals rather than three large meals helps to avoid the major influx of glucose that, in turn, results in a blood sugar surge and a big release of insulin.

☺ **Don't skip a meal.** Your blood sugar drops like a rock when you're starving (hence the headache and shakiness). Then when you do eat, you flood your system with glucose, forcing your pancreas to release more insulin and creating a dangerous cycle.

☺ **Go to bed at 10 p.m., wake up at 6 a.m.** Adjust the hours accordingly so that you're always getting a consistent

☺ **Spend 10 minutes a day tensing then relaxing each muscle in your body,** from your toes to your eyes. The technique is called progressive muscle relaxation, and a study of 100 people with high blood sugar levels found that this kind of stress-relief significantly improved their blood sugar levels. For other tips, see "Defusing Stress," on page 270.

☺ **Eat 75 g of beans a day.** These high-fibre foods take longer to digest, so they release their glucose more slowly. Studies find just 75 g a day can help to stabilize blood sugar and insulin levels.

☺ **Sprinkle a few walnuts over your salad.** Walnuts are great sources of monounsaturated fat, which won't raise your blood sugar as many other foods do. And some researchers suspect that this fat even makes cells more sensitive to insulin, helping to combat high blood sugar.

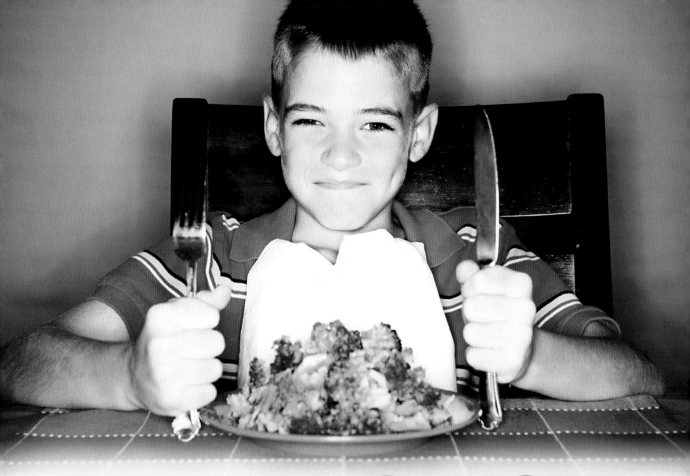

Preventing **CANCER**

Consider this number: 10 million. That's how many cases of cancer are diagnosed worldwide each year. Now consider this number: 15 million. That's how many cases of cancer the World Health Organization estimates will be diagnosed in the year 2020 – a 50 per cent increase – if we don't take some preventive action.

The truth is, most cancers don't develop overnight or out of nowhere. Cancer is largely predictable, the end result of a decades-long process, rather like heart disease. And, like heart disease, just a few changes in your daily life can significantly reduce your risk of developing the dreaded "Big C." Here are 27 of the best pieces of advice.

27 WAYS TO HELP PROTECT YOURSELF AGAINST THE BIG C

Cook some salmon on the grill tonight.

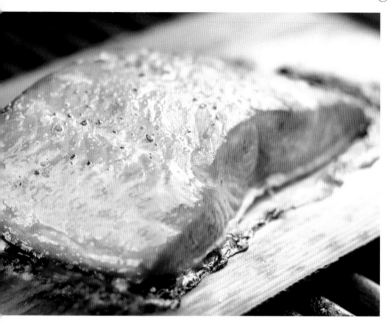

● **Take a calcium supplement with vitamin D.** A U.S. study suggests that these supplements reduce colon polyps (a risk factor for colon cancer) in susceptible people. And make sure that all the dairy products in your diet are fat-free – you'll get all the calcium benefits with none of the detriments of saturated fat.

● **Add garlic to everything you eat.** Garlic contains sulphur compounds that may stimulate the immune system's natural defences against cancer, and may have the potential to reduce tumour growth. Studies suggest that garlic can reduce the incidence of stomach cancer by as much as a factor of 12.

☺ **Sauté two cloves of crushed garlic in 2 tablespoons of olive oil, then mix in a can of chopped tomatoes.** Stir gently until heated and serve over whole-wheat pasta. The lycopene in the tomatoes protects against colon, prostate and bladder cancers; the olive oil helps your body to absorb the lycopene; the fibre-filled pasta reduces your risk of colon cancer; and see above for garlic. Plus, it tastes good – a perfect combination.

☺ **Introduce your family to sauerkraut.** Not only does cabbage contain cancer-protecting plant compounds called flavonoids but, also, a Finnish study has found that the fermentation process involved in making sauerkraut produces several other cancer-fighting compounds, including ITCs, indoles and sulphoraphane. Rinse canned or bottled sauerkraut to reduce the salt.

● **Steam rather than microwave broccoli.** Broccoli is a cancer-preventing superfood, one you should eat frequently. To preserve its nutrients, steam it, eat it raw or add it to soups and salads.

● **Sprinkle Brazil nuts over your salad.** They're a rich form of selenium, a trace mineral that convinces cancer cells to commit suicide and helps cells to repair their DNA. A Harvard study of more than 1,000 men with prostate cancer also found that those with the highest blood levels of selenium were 48 per cent less likely to develop advanced disease over 13 years than men with the lowest levels.

● **Every week, buy a cantaloupe from the supermarket** and cut it up after you put away your groceries. Store it in a container and eat several pieces every morning. Cantaloupe is a great source of carotenoids, plant chemicals shown to reduce significantly the risk of lung cancer.

● **Mix a handful of blueberries into your morning cereal.** Blueberries rank highly in terms of their antioxidant power. Antioxidants neutralize free radicals, which are unstable compounds that can damage cells and lead to diseases including cancer.

● **Learn to eat artichokes tonight.**
Artichokes are a great source of silymarin, an antioxidant that may help to prevent skin cancer. To eat these delicious veggies, peel off the tough outer leaves on the bottom, slice the bottom and cut off the spiky top. Then boil or steam until tender, about 30 to 45 minutes. Drain. Dip each leaf in a vinaigrette or garlic mayonnaise, then gently tear the fibrous covering off with your front teeth, working your way inwards to the tender heart. Once there, gently scoop the bristles from the middle of the heart, dip in a little butter or lemon juice, and enjoy.

● **Whenever you go to the bathroom, drink a glass of water.** A major U.S. study found that men who drank six 250 ml glasses of water every day cut their risk of bladder cancer by 50 per cent. Another study suggests that women who drink more water reduce their risk of colon cancer by up to 45 per cent.

● **Take up a tea habit.** The healing powers of green tea have long been valued in Asia. Now new research reveals that it protects against various cancers as well as heart disease. Some scientists believe that a chemical in green tea called EGCG could be one of the most powerful anticancer compounds ever discovered.

● **Have a beer tonight.** Beer protects against the bacterium *Helicobacter pylori*, known to cause ulcers and possibly linked to stomach cancer. But don't overdo it. Drinking more than one or two alcoholic drinks a day may increase your risk of mouth, throat, esophageal, liver and breast cancer.

☆ **Grill some salmon tonight.** Australian researchers studying Canadians found that those who ate four or more servings of fish a week were nearly a third less likely to develop the blood cancers leukemia, myeloma and non-Hodgkin's lymphoma. Other studies show a link between eating fatty fish (mackerel, salmon, sardines and tuna) and a reduced risk of endometrial cancer in women – again attributed to omega-3s.

● **Consider taking a multivitamin every morning.** Many studies suggest that getting optimum levels of vitamins and minerals can improve immune system function and help to prevent a variety of cancers. If you're not eating a balanced, healthy diet, a multivitamin could help.

☺ **Get about 15 minutes of sunlight on your skin each day.** You've heard of the sunshine vitamin, vitamin D – it turns out that many of us aren't getting enough of this valuable nutrient – possibly because we are always advised to protect against sun damage. Researchers find that getting too little vitamin D may increase your risk of multiple cancers, including breast,

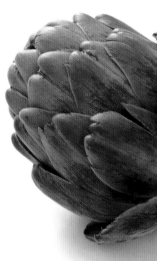

Learn to cook artichokes.

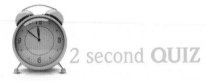

2 second QUIZ

Fresh tomatoes or tomato sauce?
ANSWER: **TOMATO SAUCE.**

Tomatoes are rich in lycopene, an antioxidant believed to reduce the risk of prostate cancer and possibly several other cancers. But only by cooking it will you release the lycopene from the tomato cell walls so that your body can absorb it. What's more, lycopene is fat-soluble, meaning your body is better able to absorb and use it when you get it with a bit of fat – such as the olive oil found in most tomato sauces.

Cancer screening

Getting the relevant cancer screening is the best way to catch cancer at a treatable stage. Here are some guidelines from the Canadian Cancer Society.

● **Breast cancer.** Women over 40 should get a clinical breast exam every two years, between 50 and 69, it's recommended to also have a mammogram every two years.

● **Cervical cancer.** Cervical screening is not a test for cancer as such – it is rather a method of preventing cancer by detecting early abnormalities (like the human papillomavirus, or HPV) that could lead to cancer if left untreated. Sexually-active women should get a Pap test done every 1 to 3 years, depending on their province's guidelines.

● **Colorectal cancer.** Men and women over 50 should get a fecal occult blood test (or FOBT) done every 2 years. This test is aimed at identifying polyps that may become trouble. Anyone whose test comes back positive will be sent for further testing, including double contrast barium enema, a colonoscopy or a sigmoidoscopy. Higher risk people should plan a personalized screening program with their doctor.

● **Prostate cancer.** Men over 50 usually get a digital rectal exam (DRE) as part of a regular checkup, but there is also another test called the Prostate Specific Antigen test, which is a blood test. High levels of PSA don't always mean cancer, so the PSA test is not a good replacement for a DRE.

● **Use a condom and stick to one partner.** The more sexual partners a woman has, the greater her risk of contracting human papillomavirus, or HPV, which causes cervical cancer. Having an unfaithful partner also increases a woman's risk.

● **Cut out high-fat animal protein.** A Yale University study found that women who ate the most animal protein had a 70 per cent higher risk of developing non-Hodgkin's lymphoma, while those who ate diets high in saturated fat increased their risk by 90 per cent. So switch to low-fat or fat-free dairy products, have poultry or fish instead of beef or pork, and use olive oil instead of butter.

● **Ask your partner to feed you grapes.** They're great sources of resveratrol, the cancer-protecting compound found in wine, but without the alcohol of wine, which can increase the risk of breast cancer in women. Plus, the closeness such an activity engenders strengthens your immune system.

☆ **Sprinkle green onions on your salad.** A diet high in onions may reduce the risk of prostate cancer by 50 per cent and the effects are strongest when they're eaten raw or lightly cooked. Try green onions, shallots or chives for a milder taste.

● **Squeeze a fresh lemon or lime.** A daily dose of citrus fruits may cut the risk of mouth, throat and stomach cancers by half, Australian researchers found. So squeeze in some lemon or lime juice to add a bit of zing to your meals.

● **Take a 30 minute walk after dinner every evening.** That's all it takes to reduce your breast cancer risk, according to a study conducted in Seattle. It turns out

colon, prostate, ovarian and stomach cancers, as well as osteoporosis, diabetes, multiple sclerosis and hypertension. UVB rays in natural and artificial sunlight are the best source. About 15 minutes a day is enough. To protect against skin cancer, always avoid over-exposure.

● **Eat a kiwi.** Kiwi is a little powerhouse of cancer-fighting antioxidants, including vitamin C, vitamin E, lutein and copper. You can also rub a couple of cut kiwis on a low-fat cut of meat as a tenderizer.

that moderate exercise reduces levels of estrogen, a hormone that contributes to breast cancer. When 170 overweight, inactive women, aged between 50 and 75, did some form of moderate exercise for about 3 hours a week, their levels of circulating estrogen dropped significantly after three months. After a year, those who lost at least 2 per cent of their body fat had even greater decreases in estrogen. Another study suggested that 4 hours a week of walking or hiking could halve the risk of pancreatic cancer. The benefits were probably related to improved insulin metabolism as a result of the exercise.

● **Buy clothes that don't need to be dry-cleaned.** Many dry-cleaners still use a chemical called perc (perchloroethylene), found to cause kidney and liver damage and cancer in animals repeatedly exposed through inhalation. Buying clothes that don't require dry-cleaning, or handwashing them yourself, can reduce your exposure to this chemical. If you must dry-clean your clothes, take them out of the plastic bag and air them outside or in another room before wearing.

● **Choose cucumbers instead of pickles, fresh salmon instead of smoked.** Studies find that smoked and pickled foods contain various carcinogens.

Healthy INVESTMENT

A pepper grinder
But don't fill it with pepper. Instead, fill it with organic flaxseeds. This makes it easy to add a sprinkle of the disease-fighting seeds (which contain important phytochemicals, fibre and omega-3 fatty acids) to cereal, yogourt, soups and stews. Studies find that ground flaxseeds reduce levels of hormones linked to breast cancer.

☺ **Switch from fries and potato chips to mashed potatoes.** A potential cancer-causing compound called acrylamide forms as a result of the chemical changes that occur when foods are baked, fried or roasted. Many of the foods with the greatest amounts of acrylamide are also the least healthy, such as fries and chips.

● **Go for a spray-on tan.** They're available in most tanning salons and, unlike sunbeds, there's no evidence that they increase your risk of skin cancer.

● **Phone a friend and go bowling.** A U.S. study found that men with high levels of stress and few family or social contacts had higher levels of prostate-specific antigen (PSA) in their blood, a marker for the development of prostate cancer. Bowling reduces stress and gives you quality time with a friend.

Reminder

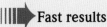 **Fast results**
These are tips that deliver benefits particularly quickly – in some cases, immediately.

 Easy gains
These are health boosters that offer the best value for the least amount of effort.

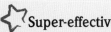 **Super-effective**
This is advice that scientific research or widespread usage by experts has shown to be particularly effective.

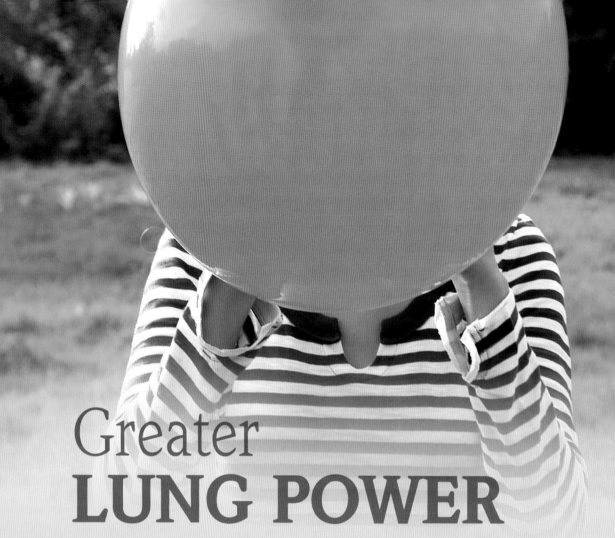

Greater
LUNG POWER

If you want to be able to blow out all the candles on your cake when you're 75 (assuming your family dares to put on a candle for every year), not to mention climb three flights of stairs without needing oxygen, now is the time to take action. What, you're wondering, could you possibly do beyond quitting smoking to get your bellows in better shape? The answer: plenty. Although stopping smoking is at the top of any list, here are another 15 tips that will have you doing less huffing and puffing, as well as protecting your lungs from damage and disease. In addition, read about proper breathing technique on page 273, part of the discussion on managing stress.

15 WAYS TO BREATHE EASIER

Have a heart-to-heart with your sleeping partner. The key question to ask: do I snore? If the answer is yes, make an appointment with your GP and ask for a referral to a sleep centre to get checked for sleep apnea. This condition, in which someone stops breathing dozens or even hundreds of times during the night, can actually damage the lungs nearly as much as smoking. Fortunately, it's treatable.

Make several trips up and down stairs every day. The kind of exercise that makes your heart beat faster, such as climbing stairs, riding a bike or walking briskly, is very important for keeping your heart and lungs in good shape. For instance, studies find that walking for about 15 minutes at a time, three to four times a day, improved breathing in people with the lung disease emphysema.

Make sure you get enough omega-3. Most airway problems, including asthma, are related to inflammation. Omega-3 fatty acids reduce inflammation.

Breathe from your abdomen for at least 5 minutes every day. This kind of breathing, called diaphragmatic breathing, involves training and strengthening your diaphragm so that it requires less effort to take in each breath. To do it, inhale deeply through your nose, filling your lungs from the bottom up. If you're doing it right, your stomach will push out. Exhale and repeat.

Expand your chest like a cocky rooster. To help your chest to expand and boost your lung capacity, lie on your back with your knees bent and your feet flat on the floor. Place your hands behind your head and bring your elbows together so they're nearly touching. As you inhale, let your elbows drop to the sides slowly so your arms are flat on the floor when your lungs are full. As you exhale, raise your elbows again.

Make spaghetti sauce tonight, tomato and basil salad tomorrow night and roasted tomatoes over the weekend. British researchers found that people who ate tomatoes three times a week had improved lung function and experienced less wheeziness and fewer asthma-like symptoms.

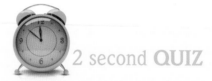

2 second **QUIZ**

Apple or orange?
ANSWER: **APPLE.**

The old adage is true after all. A study from the University of Nottingham found that people who ate more than five apples a week had improved lung function, less wheeziness and fewer asthma-like symptoms. Eat them raw, try them baked, add them diced into a salad or sauté an apple with onions as a side dish for chicken or fish.

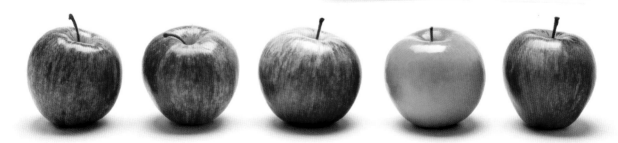

Read the fine print on household cleaners. Some products, such as oven cleaner, can be toxic if inhaled. If the instructions say to open a window or use in a well-ventilated space, make sure you do so. And wear a face mask when working around toxic dust or fumes. Even simple household tasks such as sanding paint could send damaging fragments into your lungs.

Work in 10 to 20 crunches a day. Your abdominal and chest muscles allow you to suck air in and out. Strengthen them, as well as practising your deep breathing, to get the breathing power of a professional opera singer (or at least close).

Take your medicine and listen to your doctor if you have asthma. There's some good evidence that people with asthma eventually develop chronic obstructive pulmonary disease, or COPD, a lung disease that strikes people aged 65 and older. There's also evidence that keeping your asthma under control can prevent the disease from developing.

Look on the bright side. When Harvard researchers followed 670 men with an average age of 63 for eight years,

they found that the optimists had much better lung function and a slower rate of lung function decline than the pessimists.

Get at least seven servings of fruit and vegetables a day. A 1998 study found that the high amounts of antioxidants they contain, including vitamin C, vitamin E, selenium and beta carotene, meant better lung function – even in smokers.

Have a glass of wine tonight. Drinking wine, particularly white wine, both in the recent past and over your lifetime, seems to help your lungs, possibly because of wine's high antioxidant levels. It has to be wine, though; researchers found no such correlation when they looked at the effects of other forms of alcohol.

Brush your teeth twice a day and floss after every meal. American researchers found that patients with periodontal – gum – disease were $1^1/_2$ times more likely also to have COPD. The worse the gum disease, the worse the lung function, suggesting a direct correlation between the two.

Say no to dessert. A 2004 study has revealed that carrying extra weight makes your respiratory muscles work harder and less efficiently. This results in shortness of breath, making it hard to exercise, which makes it hard to lose the weight ... To break out of this depressing cycle follow the tips in "Losing Weight," page 199.

In hot, dry or very cold weather, or in dusty or polluted air, breathe in through your nose and out through your mouth. Our nasal passages are designed to filter the air and regulate its temperature and humidity. If you breathe in through your mouth, everything – dust, coldness, etc. – goes straight on into the lungs.

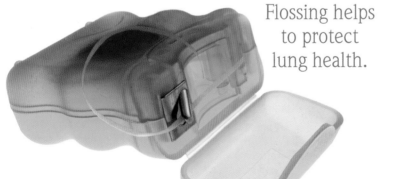

Flossing helps to protect lung health.

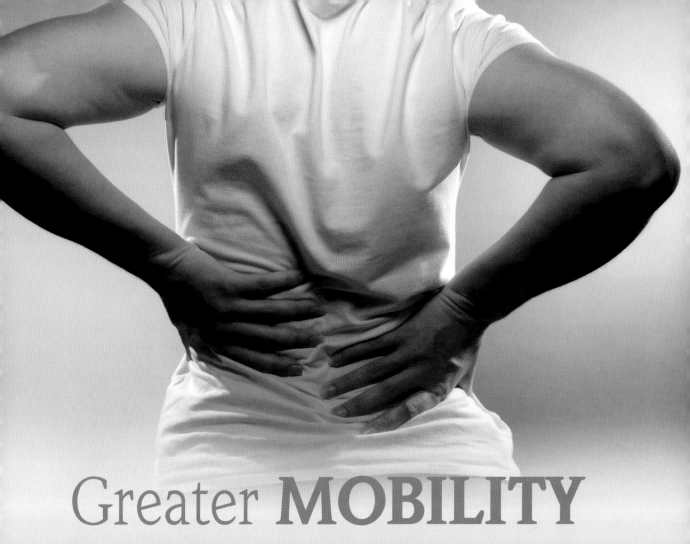

Greater **MOBILITY**

If you've ever crawled out of bed in the morning aching as if you'd played a mean game of football in your sleep, heard your knees creaking as you descended the stairs or needed two ibuprofen before you could even bend over to tie your shoelaces, then this chapter is for you.

Making some simple changes to your diet and daily activities – even just to the way you sit – coupled with taking a few key supplements a day, can save a lot of wear and tear on your joints and ligaments as well as reduce your pain. Here are the top tips to help you where you hurt.

17 WAYS TO KEEP YOUR JOINTS AGILE AND ARTHRITIS AT BAY

Add spice to your life when your arthritis flares up. It's easy to do if you always have a bottle of hot sauce on your table.

● **Sip a cup of green tea in the morning.** Polyphenols called catechins in green tea prevent arthritis in mice and significantly reduce cartilage damage in human beings.

● **Empty out any kitchen cupboard below waist level (or better still, ask someone else to empty them for you).** You'd be surprised at how much unnecessary bending people do to get at low cupboards. If you have mobility problems, fill the empty cupboards with less-used items, such as the turkey roasting pan that comes out only at Christmas, or dishes that you use only when you are entertaining.

☺ **When you sit, keep both feet on the ground.** Crossing your legs cuts off your blood circulation and pulls your back out of alignment.

Healthy INVESTMENT

A bottle of glucosamine/chondroitin
Even the most conservative orthopedic surgeon admits that this supplement, derived from animal products, can not only provide pain relief, but may even slow the degeneration of cartilage. Glucosamine doesn't fight pain right away in the way that drugs such as ibuprofen do. But, over time, it becomes an effective pain reliever and anti-inflammatory. More importantly, it can actually help to repair damaged cartilage – something ibuprofen can't do at all. In fact, drugs like ibuprofen may even interfere with normal cartilage repair. So if you have pain and need relief right away, use a drug such as ibuprofen for prompt pain relief, but start taking glucosamine at the same time. After about a month, you should be getting enough pain relief from the glucosamine to allow you to stop the ibuprofen. Then continue the glucosamine indefinitely for its anti-inflammatory and cartilage-repairing effects.

● **Switch over to spicy foods when your arthritis flares up.** Spices such as cayenne pepper, ginger and turmeric contain compounds that reduce swelling and block a brain chemical that transmits pain signals. So buy yourself some Mexican, Indian and Thai cookbooks, or keep a bottle of hot sauce on your table at all times.

● **Use a wrist rest to keep your wrists straight, not to rest your wrists on.** Resting your wrists on the pad when typing can compress soft tissues – such as tendons, nerves and blood vessels – in your forearms, reducing blood flow to your wrists and fingers. This, in turn, can increase pressure in the carpal tunnel located inside your wrists and ultimately lead to nerve damage. Instead, use the pad only for support during typing breaks. Even then, most experts recommend resting the palms of your hands, rather than your wrists, on the pad to reduce the risk of injury.

☺ **Keep a small rubber ball on your desk and in your car.** Every time you get up to go to the toilet (at work) or come to a red light (when you're in the car) squeeze the ball 20 times in each hand. This helps to strengthen your hands and improves flexibility.

● **Prevent tennis elbow by icing your arm after play.** The easiest way is to put water in a paper cup before you start, freeze it, then peel back the top of the cup to expose the ice. Now you can hold the ice against your arm without freezing your hand off. If, however, the tennis elbow arrives despite the ice, try this exercise: bend your arm at 90 degrees, keeping your elbow at your side, palm facing up. Hold this pose for 5 to 10 seconds, then slowly lower your arm. Do this ten times.

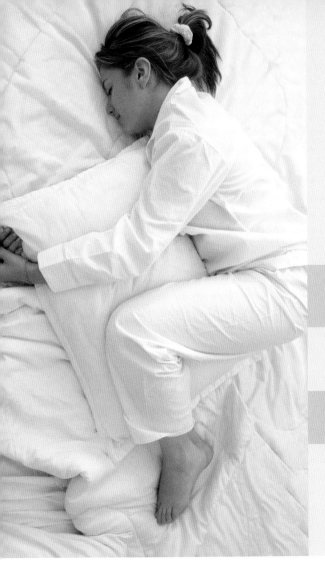

Proper
SLEEPING POSITIONS

If you're waking up sore and achy every morning and your mattress is new, you may need to re-evaluate how you're sleeping. Lying flat on your back forces your spine into an unnatural position, which can strain your muscles, joints and nerves. Your spine isn't meant to be straight – it has three natural curves: one in your lower back, one in the middle of your back and one near your neck. Following this advice may help:

● Lie on your side in the fetal position with your knees bent and a pillow tucked between your legs. This will take the most stress off your back.

● If you must sleep on your back, prop a big, fluffy pillow under your knees to reduce the pressure on the sciatic nerve in your lower back.

● Use a small pillow or a rolled-up towel under your neck as long as it doesn't push your chin too far forward.

● Don't sleep on your stomach. Sleeping face down can exaggerate the arch at the base of your spine and cause strain. Try sewing or taping a tennis ball to the front of your nightgown or pyjama top. It will put an end to your stomach-sleeping days.

You may need to re-evaluate your sleeping position.

☆ **Think about taking these supplements:**
● **Ginger extract twice a day.** U.S. researchers found that ginger reduced knee pain significantly in patients with osteoarthritis of that joint, as well as improving knee movement. It turns out that ginger has some anti-inflammatory effects, just like ibuprofen.
● **Fish-oil capsules.** A British study found that 86 per cent of people with arthritis who took cod liver oil had far fewer enzymes that cause cartilage damage compared to those who got a placebo. Plus, they had far fewer pain-causing enzymes. Cod liver oil is a fish oil, so taking a basic fish-oil supplement is fine.
● **Glucosamine/chondroitin.** See the Healthy investment box opposite for more on this topic.

● **Wash your dishes by hand and give the dishwasher the night off.** The combination of warm, running water and light exercise, requiring complex movement of the wrist and hand, is an

Do **THREE** things...

If you do only three things for back pain, doctors concur that these make the most sense:

1 Get up and go. The old idea of lying around when your back hurts just makes things worse. As soon as the acute stage of back pain is over, you need to get up and move. Walking is great. So are stretching exercises.

2 Make sure you're sleeping on the right mattress. One study of 313 men with lower back pain found that those who slept on a medium-firm mattress were twice as likely to get some pain relief. If your mattress is more than ten years old, it's time to go mattress shopping.

3 Wear soft-soled shoes with low heels. High heels throw your entire body out of alignment, contributing not only to back pain but also to knee and hip pain and injuries as well, not to mention what they do to your feet.

effective and low-cost way of rehabilitating the hand and wrist after injury or surgery. It will also keep your wrists and hands flexible with good blood circulation if you have arthritis or other painful problems.

● **Enhance the range of motion in your wrist with this exercise.** Slowly bend your wrist backwards and forward, holding for a 5 second count in each position. Do three sets – ten times for each hand – twice a day.

● **Always bend from the knees, not the back, when lifting.** Also, keep the weight you're carrying close to your body, as if carrying a baby, for less risk of back strain.

● **Crunch your way through 20 modified sit-ups every morning.** These strengthen the abdominal muscles while stretching and relaxing the back. To do a modified sit-up, bend your knees or place your feet on a small stool or chair as you complete the crunch.

▶ **On long drives, take a break every hour,** get out of the car and walk around for 5 minutes, stretching like a cat. Your back will thank you later.

● **For back relief, get on your hands and knees** (on a padded surface) and round your back, again like a scared cat. Hold for 5 seconds, then let your stomach relax and sag for 5 seconds. Do two sets of ten each any time you've been sitting for more than an hour.

● **Serve up some pickled herring for lunch or supper.** It's rich in omega-3 fatty acids, shown to reduce inflammation and alleviate pain from arthritis.

● **Play a computer game, read a book or watch a film when your joints are hurting.** Researchers find that concentrating on what you're doing distracts you from your pain.

● **Quit smoking.** Smoking narrows the arteries and reduces your circulation and that, according to a study in the medical journal *Spine*, increases your risk of back pain and slows healing.

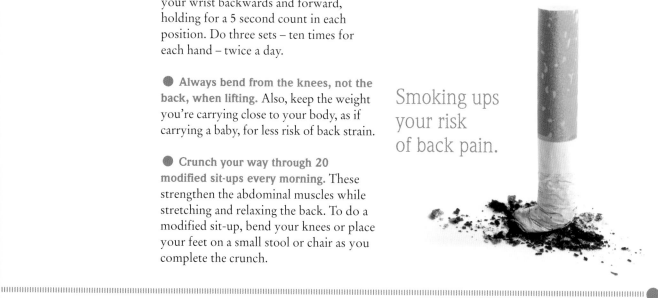

Smoking ups your risk of back pain.

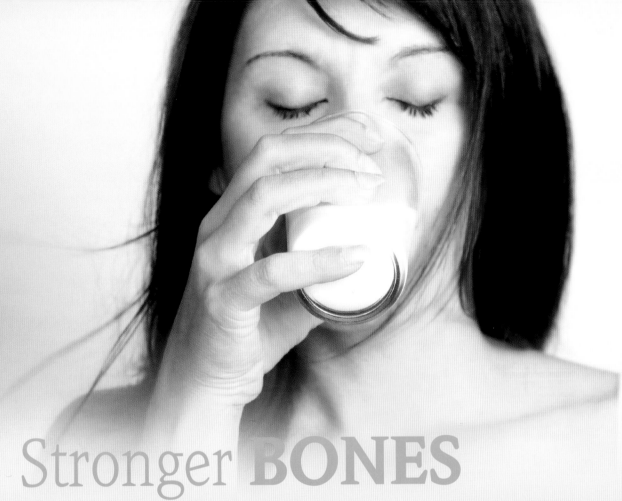

Stronger BONES

Drink your milk! Surely you remember your mother admonishing you with those very words when you were a child. And she was right: children who drink plenty of milk (or who get plenty of calcium from other sources) grow up to have less risk of osteoporosis, the disease that causes bones to become thin and brittle. It appears that many of us didn't take the advice, though; almost two million Canadians – one in four women and at least one in eight men over age 50 have osteoporosis. Yet even as an adult there's plenty you can do to protect yourself, from increasing your calcium intake to getting the right exercise. Pay special attention to this advice if you're over 50, have a family history of osteoporosis or are a woman who has gone through menopause, because your bones may be more vulnerable.

20 WAYS TO HELP TO PREVENT OSTEOPOROSIS

☺ **Add almonds to everything.** They're packed with bone-strengthening calcium. Just 25 g of the sweet nuts provides 60 mg of calcium. Try them toasted and sprinkled over salad or yogourt, crushed and mixed into meat or turkey for meatballs, used in place of pine nuts for homemade pesto, or as a topping for ice cream or frozen yogourt.

● **Drain a can of sardines,** mash the fish with a tablespoon of reduced-fat mayonnaise, add some salt and pepper, and spread over whole-wheat crackers. Another packed-with-calcium food, sardines (the kind with the bones) make a great substitute for tuna. Pair this snack with a glass of milk and your bones have got it made!

● **Drink one cup of tea a day.** That's all it took in a study of 1,256 women aged 65 to 76 to increase their bone density by 5 per cent. That translates to a 10 to 20 per cent reduction in fracture risk. Another

study found that among more than 1,000 Chinese men and women, those who regularly drank tea (usually green tea) had denser bones than those who didn't.

☺ **Make two of your daily glasses of water mineral water.** Mineral water contains calcium, and a study published in *Osteoporosis International* in 2000 found that your body absorbs the mineral just as well from water as it does from milk. Make sure the water is labelled "mineral water," not just "spring water." If you live in a hard-water area, rather than a soft-water area, you will get some calcium from tap water too.

● **Do 12 to 16 squats every day just before you get into bed.** Squats are particularly beneficial for your hips, which are especially prone to fracture. Pretend you're about to sit in a chair, but without a chair behind you. As you "sit," try to lower yourself enough so that your thighs are parallel or nearly parallel to the floor, but don't let your knees extend beyond your toes.

● **Skip for 10 minutes every day.** It's one of the best all-around exercises for building bone. Some skipping ropes measure not only the number of jumps you complete, but how many calories you burn. Be careful when you start, though. This exercise requires coordination, and if your bones already happen to be thin, the last thing you want to do is fall.

● **Turn your face up to the sun every day.** Aim for about 15 minutes a day of sun exposure, without sunscreen. That's how much your body needs to make vitamin D, the "sunshine vitamin" important to bone health. And exposure to sunlight enhances mood because sunlight affects levels of the hormone

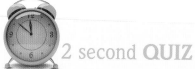

2 second QUIZ

Cheese or calcium tablets?
ANSWER: **CHEESE.**

A study of pre-teen girls found that those getting 100 g of low-fat cheese a day increased their total bone mass more than girls who took calcium tablets containing the same amount of calcium. Researchers speculate that the calcium in the cheese is better absorbed. Still, there is a trade-off. The cheese has calories and saturated fat, the supplements none. So the advice is to include plenty of fat-free dairy produce in your diet, occasional cheese as a treat, and a calcium supplement as an insurance policy.

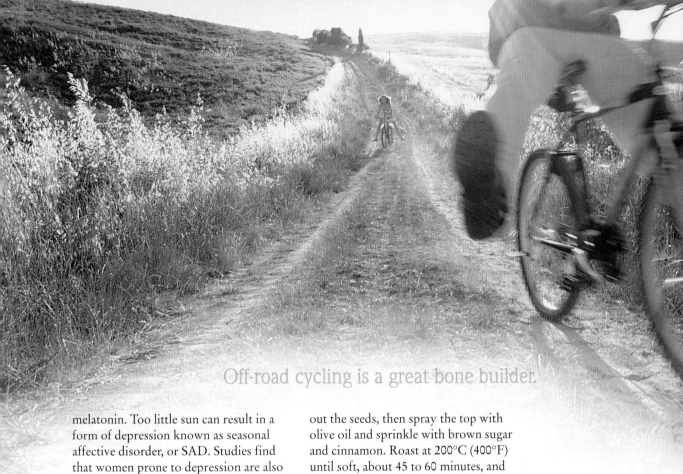

Off-road cycling is a great bone builder.

melatonin. Too little sun can result in a form of depression known as seasonal affective disorder, or SAD. Studies find that women prone to depression are also more likely to have lower bone density.

● **Try some coleslaw or stuffed cabbage rolls for dinner once a week.** Cabbage is rich in vitamin K, a vitamin that helps to turn on a bone-building protein called osteocalcin.

● **Ride your bike off-road this weekend.** A study published in the journal *Bone* found that cyclists who spent part of their time off-road had above-average bone density, while those who stuck to the streets had slightly below-average bone density. They speculate that the bouncing you do over rough terrain helps to stimulate bone growth.

● **Roast a butternut squash tonight.** Butternut squash is not only a tasty treat any time of the year, but it is a great source of calcium. Slice one open, scoop out the seeds, then spray the top with olive oil and sprinkle with brown sugar and cinnamon. Roast at 200°C (400°F) until soft, about 45 to 60 minutes, and scoop out the flesh. Voilà!

● **Take the right kind of calcium at the right time.** Calcium citrate, for instance, is more expensive, but can be absorbed on an empty stomach. Calcium carbonate, the cheapest and most common supplement, is absorbed best with food, particularly acidic foods such as citrus juice or fruit.

Healthy INVESTMENT

A pair of 2 kg (5 lb) hand weights
Weight-bearing exercise is critical for staving off bone loss. Keep the weights on the floor in your living room and use them for the duration of a commercial break.

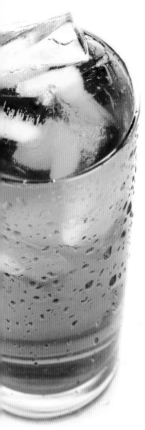

● **Have a pizza topped with sardines and spinach.** Not only is it delicious (go on, give it a try), but you'll get bone-protecting calcium in every bite.

● **Have four dried figs for a midafternoon snack.** Dried figs are a great source of calcium. Sprinkle a few diced figs over your yogourt.

● **Sip water or iced tea instead of soft drinks.** An American study found that women who drank at least one 355 ml can of cola every day for four years had up to 5 per cent lower bone mineral density than women who drank fewer than one a week. All the women were drinking the same amount of milk, so researchers think the phosphoric acid in soft drinks affects the body's absorption of calcium.

● **Hang room-darkening shades in your bedroom.** You'll sleep much better without ambient light, and sleep is important for bone. Much of your bone remodelling, in which old bone is replaced by new, occurs during sleep.

☆ **Walk for 30 minutes a day.** Most women lose 3 to 6 per cent of their bone mass every year during the five years before and after menopause. But women who walked regularly (about 12 kilometres/7.5 miles a week) took four to seven years longer to lose the same amount of bone as women who didn't walk at all. Walking briskly, you should be able to cover 3 kilometres (2 miles) in 30 minutes; walk for 30 minutes just four days a week and you'll get the 12 kilometres (7.5 miles) in. Add an extra day, just for good measure.

☆ **Start a vegetable and flower garden.** U.S. researchers found that gardening (and weight training) were strongly associated with reducing the risk of osteoporosis in 3,310 women aged 50 and older. It turns out that pushing a lawnmower, thrusting a shovel into the ground, lifting heavy wheelbarrows filled with mulch, raking, carrying and pulling weeds are all great weight-bearing exercises. Would you rather lift weights in a sweaty gym or plant and harvest your own ruby-red tomatoes?

● **Sign up for a tai chi class at your local sports centre.** Several studies have found that tai chi cut the risk of falling by nearly a half and reduced the rate of fractures even in people who had falls. Ideally, you should practise tai chi for 10 to 15 minutes at a time, once or twice a week, to gain the benefits.

● **Make low-fat yogourt a daily snack.** With 300 mg of calcium in a 175 g low-fat yogourt, you're taking in at least a quarter of the daily calcium required (1,000 mg per day for 19 to 50 year olds, and 1,200 mg for people 51 years and older).

● **Swap peas for frozen fresh soybeans this evening.** The science is still evolving, but it seems that the natural plant estrogens in soy help to strengthen bone in the same way that our own hormones do.

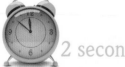

2 second QUIZ

Swimming or walking
ANSWER: **WALKING.**

While swimming is a great exercise for your lungs and heart, it doesn't do anything for your bones, because there's little resistance in water.

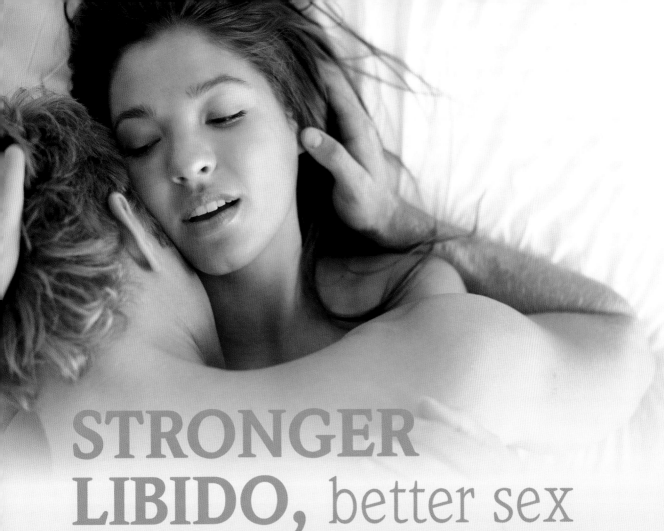

STRONGER
LIBIDO, better sex

Your parents probably never told you this, but it's true: sex is good for you! Plenty of studies show it: regular sex increases immunity from viruses, relieves stress and even helps to protect the health of a man's prostate gland by emptying the fluids held there. It also triggers the release of chemicals that improve mood and ease pain. While menopause in women does affect sexual drive and function somewhat, there is no reason why healthy men and women can't experience sexual pleasure throughout their lives. The nature and intensity of the sex may change, but the love and pleasure don't. So if your sex drive has stalled, try a couple of health-boosting tips to get your engine ticking over again in no time.

26 WAYS TO GET THERE

● **Have sex tonight!** Having intercourse regularly helps to keep your sex drive in high gear by increasing the production of testosterone, which is the hormone mainly responsible for libido in both men and women.

● **Men: if you smoke, ask your doctor to prescribe you nicotine patches.** Why? Because it's scientifically proven that smoking can clog the blood vessels in the penis in the same way that it clogs the arteries in your heart. Ever heard of a better reason to quit?

● **Women: purchase at least one item of sexy lingerie.** The feel of soft silk against your skin will help to wake up those sensuality nerve endings. And who knows what will result if that happens?

☺ **Write down a list of all the medicines you're taking, then check for party-poopers.** More than 200 medicines can cause erection problems and diminished sex drive, including drugs used to treat high blood pressure, heart disease, depression and stomach problems. Check

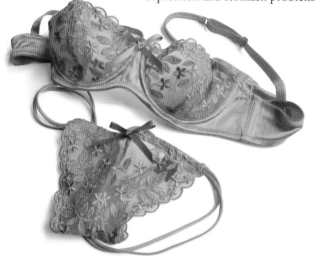

Enjoy the feel of silk against your skin.

the Internet or ask your pharmacist or doctor if any of the drugs on your list could be culprits. Of course, you can't stop taking a drug that you need, but you can talk to your doctor about possibly changing the brand, dose or timing of your medication.

● **Women: practise pelvic-floor exercises.** These are the squeezing exercises your doctor may have told you to do after pregnancy or because you were having a bit of a problem with leaking urine. What your doctor may not have told you is that they're also great for strengthening the pubococcygeus muscle, essential for orgasm. To do pelvic-floor, or Kegel, exercises, take note of the muscle you use to stop urinary flow, then practise contracting that muscle, gradually releasing it. Work up to doing 20 contractions three times a day.

● **Men: start taking supplements of ginkgo biloba every day.** The herb promotes better blood flow, getting more blood to the brain and … other organs. It doesn't take much imagination to figure out how that might help you. Follow the instructions on the bottle, but check with your doctor first.

● **Make pesto and serve it over pasta tonight.** Pesto contains pine nuts, which are a great source of arginine. This is the precursor for nitric oxide, a main ingredient in drugs such as Viagra. Arginine helps to open blood vessels so that blood flow improves.

● **Go to the movie theatre with your partner,** sit in the back row and kiss like you used to when you were teenagers. You'll be combining the forbidden with the frustrating – a sure bet to recall forgotten feelings.

☺ **Every time you pass your partner, reach out to touch or kiss him or her.** Don't allow these moments to go beyond a kiss or hug. Simply increasing the amount of physical contact you have with your partner will help with desire.

● **Sprinkle 1 tablespoon of wheat germ** on every bowl of yogourt and cereal that you eat. Wheat germ is rich in zinc, which is important to the production of that all-important hormone, testosterone. You can also get your fill of zinc from beef, eggs and seafood – especially oysters.

● **When you're at a party or out** in public with your partner, take a moment to stare at him or her across the room as if you were still wooing one another. Sex falls out of a relationship if you take one another's presence for granted. So don't!

● **Read a sexy bodice-ripper out loud to your partner.** Play-act the parts of the ravishing heroine and her handsome, yet dangerous lover.

● **Open your eyes when you kiss and when you're having sex.** Looking into your partner's eyes during such times sends an incredible message of trust and honesty.

▮▮▮▶ **Say exactly what's on your mind – sexually, that is.** If you're watching your partner pull out the tree stump in the backyard and you get a certain weakness in your legs watching the sweat roll off his back, tell him. If the sight of your partner comforting your teenage son after his first-ever girlfriend dumped him makes you glad all over again that you're with her, tell her. Simply expressing how everyday things make you feel deepens your intimacy when said out loud.

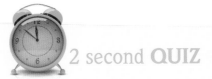

2 second QUIZ

Chocolates or flowers?
ANSWER: **CHOCOLATES.**

Particularly if the goal is to spark your sex life. Flowers are a great way to declare "I love you" to your partner and the world, and so are always a great gift. But chocolates are more sensuous and interactive, making them perfect for foreplay – feeding each other, feeding yourself off each other. Choose dark chocolates and they're even healthy for your heart.

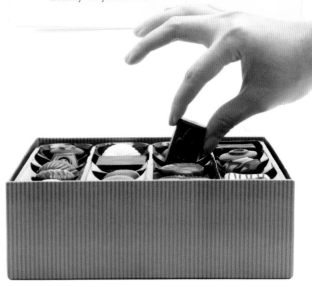

Flowers are a thoughtful gift, but chocolates offer more possibilities.

● **Pretend you've just met.** Remember that weak-in-the-knees, shivers-up-your-back feeling you used to get when you first met? You can have that again. Call her and ask her out on a date. Dress up for lunch with him. Buy new underwear.

☺ **Create your own intimate rituals.** That doesn't mean sex. What about waking your partner up with a cup of steaming coffee instead of the alarm every morning? What about having a hot

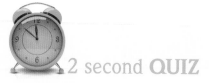

Cream cake or an orange
ANSWER: **ORANGE.**

A U.S. study of 32 obese women found that more than half of those who lost weight said their sex lives improved.

Lose weight for more vitality.

bath ready in the evening? How about a meal out every Tuesday – when most couples are slumped in front of the TV? Or massaging your partner's feet while you watch a DVD together? The key is consistency. These are not things you do just once, but over and over again.

● **Get a massage.** Or a pedicure, or a facial, or whatever makes you feel better about yourself. If you take care of your own body, you're much more likely to enjoy it. Another good way to take care of yourself is to exercise. An extra benefit is better blood flow to crucial organs.

● **Turn the timer on for 15 minutes and talk to him (or her)** about anything other than children, money problems or work issues. Talk about the dream you had last night, an article you read, the great presentation you made. When the timer goes off, it's your partner's turn.

● **Go away for a couple of days – by yourself.** While you're away, make a list of all the things you love and like about your partner. Close your eyes and picture yourself making love.

Call him or her and have an erotic phone conversation. By the time you get home, you'll be greedy for each other.

● **Send the children away and stay at home together.** Make love in a different part of the house, be it your bath or a blanket in front of the fireplace.

● **Before you go to bed, take a few minutes** to write out a to-do list and a list of your worries. This gets rid of the anxieties that can often interfere with your ability to relax and become aroused.

● **Spend an hour touching every part of your partner's body – without using your hands.** Use other parts of your body instead. Conversely, caress one another, with your hands touching every part of the body except the genital zones. This can remove any pressure you might feel to "get right to it" after a hectic day and is a wonderful way to relax and escape from the daily grind and transition from other (oh-so-non-sexual) roles.

● **Stop at one (or two) drinks.** A small amount of alcohol can set the mood; more can drown the flame of desire, or lessen your ability to see your desire through.

● **Create a romantic CD.** Have it playing when your partner returns home. Light a few scented candles while you're at it.

☺ **Tell your partner two things you love about him or her every day.** Love, affection and mutual respect are the bases for a steamy sex life.

● **Do something physical together,** for example, skiing, a long country walk, a stroll along a beach, canoeing. Such activities create a sense of physical vitality that readily translates into intimacy.

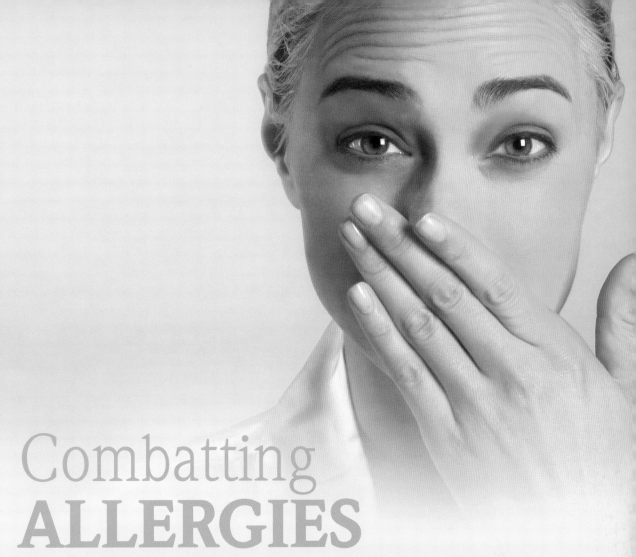

Combatting
ALLERGIES

If the constant drip, sniff, sneeze and itch of allergies make you think of buying shares in the company that makes Kleenex, dry your eyes and prepare to take action. You're going to wage battle inside your house and even inside your body to reduce the number of allergy attacks you suffer and minimize those annoying symptoms. Allergies may not be life-threatening, but they're nothing to sneeze at either. Here are 16 of the best ways to protect yourself. Plus, turn to "The cleaning routine," on page 68, for more on safe, healthy ways to purge your home of allergens.

16 WAYS TO STOP BEING SNEEZY

Choose chicken instead of beef. A two year study of 334 adults with hay fever and 1,336 without found that those who had the most trans oleic acid in their diets, a form of monounsaturated fat found primarily in meat and dairy products, were nearly three times as likely to have hay fever as those who ate the least. Olive oil is OK; although it's got a lot of oleic acid, it's not the "trans" form.

● **Eat one orange every morning.** They're rich in vitamin C, which acts as a natural antihistamine. Some studies link low levels of vitamin C with allergies. When your allergies are flaring up, consider taking a vitamin C supplement.

● **Clean out your eavestroughs and make sure they're not clogged.** Clogged eavestroughs can result in water seeping into the house, leading to mould growth, which can exacerbate allergies. Next time it rains, check your eavestroughs. If you see water leaking out of the end caps, flowing on the outside or dripping behind them, it's time to get out the ladder.

● **Always run the exhaust fan and/or leave the window and door open** when taking a shower or bath. Another option is to run a small portable fan (away from water sources) during and after showers.

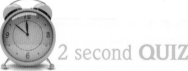

2 second QUIZ

Fresh air or recycled?
ANSWER: **RECYCLED.**

Pressing the recycled air button in your car ensures the air will be filtered so you'll breathe in fewer allergens.

Again, you're trying to keep surfaces dry and prevent mould growing. Also, check to see that the outside vent where the exhaust fan exits isn't blocked by leaves.

● **Wash the shower curtain in hot water and bleach every month.** Or use a shower liner that you can replace every couple of months for just a few dollars.

● **Keep your thermostat set above 18°C (65°F) in winter.** If you set it too low, you're encouraging the growth of mould in damp air. The heat dries out the air, preventing mould growth. Of course, air that's too dry can also irritate your lungs and sinuses. The perfect humidity in a home is around 50 per cent.

● **Follow your clothes dryer vent and make sure it's vented to the outside.** For every load of laundry that you dry, 9 kg of moisture has to go somewhere. If your dryer is vented to the garage or basement, you're just asking for mould build-up.

● **Clean the tray under the fridge with a bleach solution and sprinkle with salt.** The tray is a veritable mould magnet. Adding salt reduces the growth of mould and bacteria. Also, clean under the refrigerator occasionally; food can get trapped there, become mouldy and the mould spores are blown into the kitchen every time the compressor kicks in.

Wash all your bedding in very hot water every week. It's the best way to kill those nasty microscopic dust mites that love your bed even more than you do.

Spend this weekend decluttering. Get rid of coats and other clothing you haven't used in the past year. Put sports equipment in the garage or attic where it belongs. When you finish, give everything a good vacuum to reduce significantly the amount of dust in your house.

● **Water your plants sparingly and put pebbles on top** of the dirt to discourage mould spores from getting into the air. Overwatering houseplants can contribute to the growth of mould. Also, water might leak through onto the carpet.

● **Choose a doormat made of synthetic material.** Doormats made of natural material (wicker, etc.) can break down and become feeding grounds for mites, mould and fungus, which then get tracked into the house. Wash mats weekly.

● **Clean all dead insects from your porch lights.** As they decompose, they can become an allergen source.

● **Put a shelf by the front door for shoes** and encourage your family and guests to remove their shoes before entering to reduce the amount of allergens carried in.

● **Keep your bedroom door shut so that your dog and/or cat can't get in.** Let him or her bark or meow. You spend more time in your bedroom than in any other room of the house, and this should keep it free of cat and dog dander, to which many people are allergic.

● **Avoid foods containing the additive monosodium benzoate.** An Italian study found that it triggered allergy-like symptoms, including sneezing and nasal itching, in adults without allergies. The preservative is often found in juices, pie fillings, pickles, olives and salad dressings.

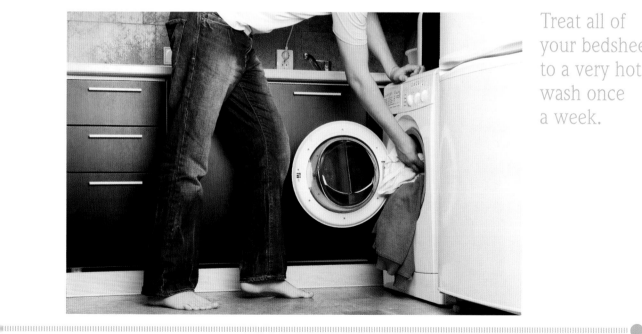

Treat all of your bedsheets to a very hot wash once a week.

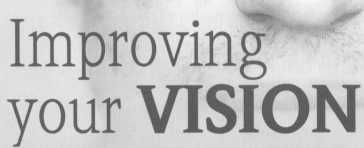

Improving your **VISION**

Chances are you take your eyes for granted. Most of us do. So imagine if you couldn't gaze at your family or even navigate your way safely around the kitchen. A well-balanced diet can protect against age-related macular degeneration (AMD), the leading cause of blindness in people over 50 in the Western world. Every year almost 100,000 new cases are reported in Canada. The good news: the most common diseases are all preventable to some extent. The first step, if you smoke, is to stop. Smoking increases your risk of major eye conditions.

21 WAYS TO SEE CLEARLY FOR EVER

Mix a handful of blueberries with a cup of yogourt for breakfast this morning. Blueberries are one of the richest fruit forms of antioxidants. A study published in *The Archives of Ophthalmology* found that women and men who ate the greatest amount of fruit were the least likely to develop age-related macular degeneration (AMD), the leading cause of blindness in older people.

😊 Have spinach or kale twice a week. It could be a spinach quiche, steamed kale or maybe Tuscan spinach – sautéed in some olive oil with garlic and raisins. Regardless, be sure to get as much of both as you can. Studies find that lutein, a nutrient that is particularly abundant in spinach and kale, may prevent age-related macular degeneration (AMD) and cataracts. Ideally, get your lutein in combination with some form of fat (olive oil works well) for the best absorption.

● Cook with red onions, not white. Red onions contain far more quercetin, an antioxidant that is thought to protect against cataracts.

● Aim your car vents at your feet – not your eyes. Dry, air-conditioned air will suck the moisture out of the eyes. Aim the vents in your car away from your eyes, or wear sunglasses as a shield. Dry eyes can be more than an inconvenience; serious dryness can lead to corneal abrasions and even blindness if left untreated.

● Walk at least four times a week. Some evidence suggests that regular exercise can reduce the intraocular pressure, or IOP, in people with glaucoma. In one study, glaucoma patients who walked briskly four times a week for 40 minutes lowered their IOP enough for them to stop taking medication for the condition.

Healthy INVESTMENT

Sunglasses
Make sure they're close-fitting, preferably wraparound, and block out 99 to 100 per cent of UVA and UVB rays. Step outside while wearing them before you buy to make sure they do a good job of blocking glare and yet aren't too dark.

Move your computer screen to just below eye level. Your eyes will close slightly when you're staring at the computer, minimizing fluid evaporation and the risk of a condition called dry eye syndrome.

● Twice a week, walk away from greasy or sweet snacks. A 2001 study found that people whose diets were high in omega-3 fatty acids and low in omega-6 fatty acids (found in many fat-filled snack foods such as pre-prepared pies, cakes, cookies and chips) were significantly less likely to develop AMD

Red onions may keep cataracts at bay.

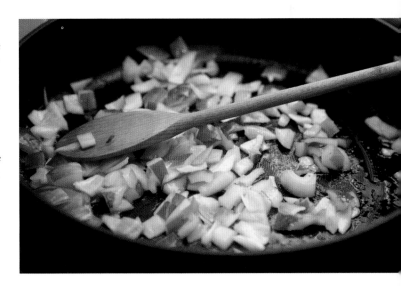

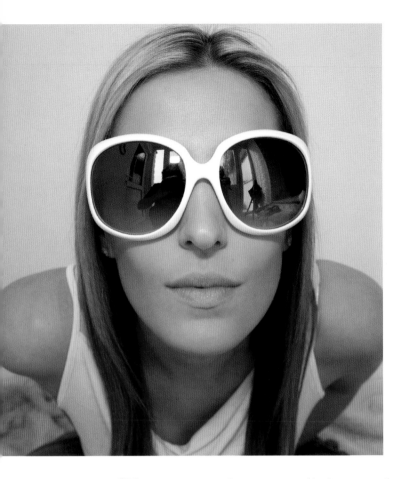

If you can't stand fish, or are worried about mercury consumption, try fish-oil supplements to get your omega-3s.

● **Have sweet potatoes for dinner tonight.** Since they're rich in vitamin A, these sweet spuds can help to improve your night vision.

☺ **Wear sunglasses whenever you leave the house.** When researchers examined the relationship between exposure to sunlight and cataracts or AMD in fishermen, they found that those who protected their eyes from the harsh glare of the sun and its damaging UV rays were significantly less likely to develop these conditions than those who went bare-eyed. Wear sunglasses even when it's not sunny outside to protect your eyes from the drying effects of wind. See the Healthy investment box on page 259 for tips on choosing the right sunglasses.

Wearing sunglasses at all times when outside, even when it's not sunny, protects your eyes from wind as well as sun.

than those whose diets were high in omega-6 fatty acids and low in omega-3 fatty acids. In fact, if someone's diet was high in omega-6 at all – even if he or she still ate plenty of fish – the protective effects of the omega-3 fatty acids disappeared.

● **Eat fish twice a week.** A study by Harvard researchers presented at the annual meeting of the Association for Research in Vision and Ophthalmology in 2003 evaluated the diets of 32,470 women and found that those who ate the least amount of fish (thus getting the smallest amount of omega-3 fatty acids) had the highest risk of dry eye syndrome.

● **Turn down the heat in your house.** Heat dries out the air and this dries out your eyes. In winter, you might also try adding some humidity with a humidifier or even grouping a few plants together in the room in which you spend the most time.

● **Wear a broad-brimmed hat along with your sunglasses.** A wide-brimmed hat or cap will block roughly 50 per cent of the UV radiation, as well as reducing the UV radiation that may enter your eyes from above or around the glasses.

● **Roast some fresh beets for an eye-saving side dish.** Beets get their deep red colour from phytochemicals

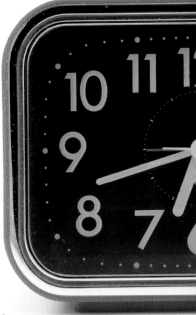

Remind yourself to tear your eyes away from your computer screen every 30 minutes by setting an alarm.

called anthocyanins, powerful antioxidants that protect the smaller blood vessels in your body, including those in your eyes.

● **Switch to "low" sodium or use spices and herbs instead of salt.** Studies find that high-salt diets increase your risk of certain types of cataracts, so stay away from the salty stuff. And while you're de-salting your diet, don't forget the salt in processed foods. Check labels for "no-sodium" or "low-sodium" tags when buying canned and other prepared foods.

● **Dab essential oil of jasmine, peppermint or vanilla on your arm and sniff.** Jasmine, says scent researcher Dr. Alan R. Hirsch, of the U.S. Smell & Taste Treatment Research Foundation, increases the beta waves in the frontal lobes of your brain, promoting wakefulness and enabling you to focus better and see things more acutely. All three scents stimulate the limbic system in your brain, which, in turn, stimulates the rods in your eyes, helping you to see in dim light.

☺ **When you're working or reading, set your alarm to beep every 30 minutes.** Use this as a reminder to look up and away from your computer or look to some distant point for 30 seconds. This helps to prevent eye fatigue and eye strain.

● **Check your blood pressure every month.** You can do this yourself with a home blood pressure kit (see page 228), at your GP's office or at some pharmacies. Two leading causes of blindness are high blood pressure and diabetes, both of which damage blood vessels. For more on controlling blood pressure, turn to page 227. For more on maintaining healthy blood sugar levels, see page 231.

● **Replace your mascara every three months** and other eye make-up once a year. Eye make-up is a great repository for bacteria, which can easily be transferred to your eyes and cause infections.

● **Use eye make-up remover every night before going to bed.** This prevents small pieces of mascara from ending up in your eye and possibly scratching your cornea.

● **Wear goggles when you're doing carpentry or even gardening.** Debris in the eye can lead to corneal abrasions, which can ultimately damage your vision. Also use protective goggles when you're swimming to protect your eyes from chlorine.

● **Stick to your own washcloth for wiping your face.** Sharing washcloths is liable to spread conjunctivitis.

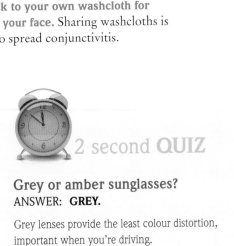

2 second QUIZ

Grey or amber sunglasses?
ANSWER: **GREY.**

Grey lenses provide the least colour distortion, important when you're driving.

Improving your
HEARING

If you spent your youth at rock concerts, or were frequently exposed to any other loud noise, the chances are you're paying for it now with a bit of age-related hearing loss. Do visitors casually mention that your TV is blaring? Do you keep asking people to repeat themselves? You're not alone. One in four Canadians has some degree of hearing loss. Although most are over the age of 60, that still means plenty of younger adults have hearing problems too. Unfortunately, once you lose your hearing, you can't get it back without help from hearing aids, so here's how to protect what you have left. (If you're worried, ask your GP to refer you for audiology testing.)

15 WAYS TO HEAR A PIN DROP

● **Go for a walk in the woods.** Not only will the silence help you to focus better on sounds, but researchers find that physically fit people tend to have better hearing than those who aren't in good shape. The reason? Aerobic exercise brings more oxygen into your system and improves blood flow to your ears.

● **Scoop up the guacamole at your next picnic.** Guacamole is rich in magnesium. Studies find that low levels of magnesium might make you more susceptible to noise-induced hearing loss.

☺ **Switch to decaf coffee and low-sodium soups.** Caffeine appears to hamper blood flow to the ears, while sodium can lead to fluid retention, which can cause swelling and interfere with ear functioning. Plus, studies find that people with high blood pressure are more likely to have age-related hearing loss than those with normal blood pressure.

● **Quit smoking and stay away from other smokers.** A study published in the *Journal of the American Medical Association* found that the more exposure you receive to cigarette smoke, the more likely you are to experience age-related hearing loss.

● **Sip a beer or glass of wine, but don't overdo it.** Believe it or not, moderate drinking can protect against age-related hearing loss. But excessive amounts may actually contribute to hearing loss.

● **Brush your teeth at least twice a day and floss after every meal.** For some reason, there's a link between the number of teeth you've lost and your hearing, with researchers finding that the more of your own teeth you still have in your mouth in old age, the better your hearing.

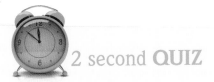

2 second QUIZ

Turn up the sound or move closer?
ANSWER: **MOVE CLOSER.**

Also, listen more closely. Any effort you can make to listen at quieter levels should help to preserve your hearing. If you cannot comfortably hear another person talking to you in the same room within a couple of metres (six feet), the TV or music is probably too loud.

☆ **Serve whole-grain bread and split-pea soup for lunch.** Whole grains and legumes are great sources of B vitamins, which studies find protect the neurons and blood vessels connected to the cochlea, the tiny bone found in your inner ear. Also, one study published in *The American Journal of Clinical Nutrition* found that women with hearing problems had low blood levels of vitamin B_{12} and folate.

● **Drink a glass of skim milk every morning.** The calcium and vitamin D in milk are critical for keeping the bones in your ear, especially the cochlea, healthy. One study of 70 healthy women found that those with hearing loss had much lower spinal density (a measure of bone strength) and calcium intake than women with normal hearing.

● **Bake a sweet potato for dinner tonight.** A wonderful source of vitamin A, it can also help your hearing because, according to animal studies, too little of this nutrient may increase the inner ear's sensitivity to noise, thus potentially increasing the risk of noise-induced hearing loss.

Sweet potato is rich in vitamin A – a great hearing protector.

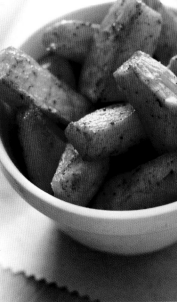

How loud IS TOO LOUD?

Exposure of just 1 minute to sounds of 110 decibels or higher can damage your hearing.
No more than 15 minutes of unprotected exposure is recommended for noises of 100 decibels, as well as several hours' exposure to noises of 90 decibels or higher. Here's the decibel level of some common noises:

- **140 decibels:** rock concerts, fireworks
- **110 decibels:** chainsaw
- **100 decibels:** woodworking equipment
- **90 decibels:** lawnmower, motorcycle
- **80 decibels:** city traffic noise
- **60 decibels:** normal conversation
- **40 decibels:** refrigerator humming
- **20 decibels:** whispered voice
- **0 decibels:** threshold of normal hearing

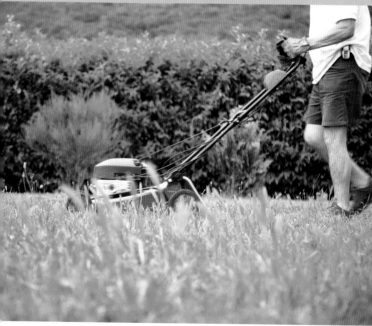

● **Get five servings of vegetables a day.** When researchers explored the connection between a variety of lifestyle factors and sudden deafness in 109 patients, comparing their deaf patients to those with normal hearing, they found that those who ate the most fresh veggies had the lowest risk of sudden deafness. See page 83 for ways to eat more.

☺ **Ask your doctor to clear the wax from your ears.** It's often all that's needed to improve your hearing. Just don't try it yourself; sticking pointed objects into your ear canal is a no-no. If you want to de-wax at home, try wax-softening ear drops, sold at pharmacies. If the wax doesn't liquefy and find its way out, see your GP to request ear syringeing.

● **Go to bed and rest when you have a cold.** That gives your body the strength to fight off the infection and reduces the risk that it will develop into something more serious, such as an ear infection, which could eventually affect your hearing.

● **Make earplugs a standard part of your wardrobe.** Keep a pair in your bag, in your car, in the garage with the gardening tools and by the lawnmower. That way, if you find yourself unable to escape from loud noise, you're always prepared to protect your hearing.

● **Get a friend to stand next to you while you're plugged into your iPod** (or MP3 player). If your friend can hear it through your earphones, it's too loud.

● **Try a ginkgo biloba supplement.** Some studies suggest that the herb might not only help with ringing in the ears (tinnitus), but may also benefit hearing loss by improving blood flow to the ears. The herb takes weeks to work, so be patient.

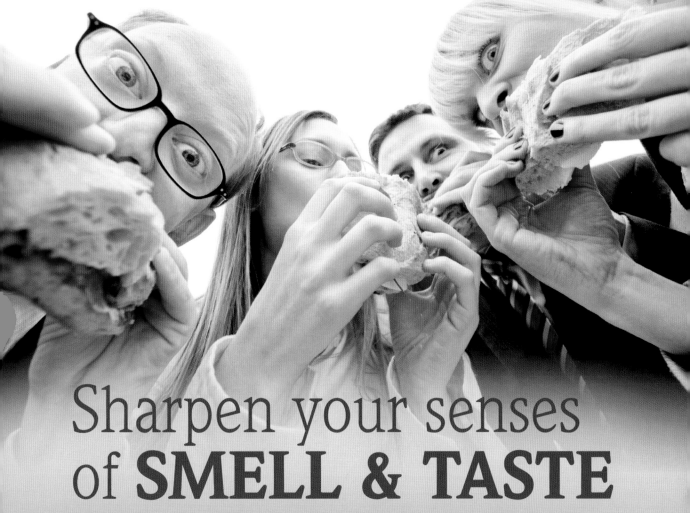

Sharpen your senses of **SMELL & TASTE**

We all know that feeling of having a bad taste in the mouth, or the way a stuffy nose makes even the most fragrant garlic pizza taste like cardboard. But did you know that your senses of smell and taste naturally decline as you age? Often the change is so gradual that you barely notice it. That wouldn't be a problem, except that it can affect your health – studies find that people with an impaired ability to smell and taste tend to follow less healthy diets. It also puts you in danger: your sense of smell serves as an early-warning system for things like rotten food and gas leaks.

Here's how to sustain your senses of smell and taste so that every bite (and sniff) tells you what you need to know.

19 SENSIBLE STRATEGIES

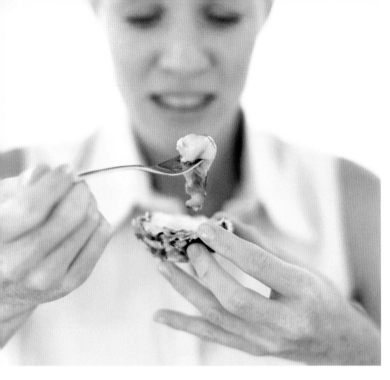

Get a healthy dose of zinc by indulging in a dozen oysters.

● **Serve food that looks like itself.** Forget fancy presentation. If you're serving fish, keep it looking like a fish. Your sense of taste is stronger if your brain can connect what you're eating with how it looks.

● **Go for a brisk 10 minute walk or run.** Our sense of smell is higher after exercise. Researchers suspect it might be related to additional moisture in the nose.

☆ **Drink a glass of water every hour or so.** Dry mouth – whether due to medication or simply dehydration – can adversely affect your sense of taste.

● **Make a list of any medicines you're taking and ask your doctor about their effect on smell and taste.** Hundreds of medications affect taste and smell, including statins, antidepressants, high blood pressure medicines and chemotherapy drugs such as methotrexate,

also used to treat rheumatoid arthritis. If your medicines are on the list, talk to your doctor about possible alternatives or lower doses. Don't, however, stop taking your medication or cut the dosage yourself.

● **Indulge in a dozen oysters.** Among their other benefits, oysters are one of the highest food sources of zinc, and zinc deficiencies contribute to a loss of smell as well as taste.

● **Stub out that cigarette and make it your last.** Nothing messes up the smell receptors in your nose and the taste receptors on your tongue like cigarettes. Long-term smoking can even permanently damage the olfactory nerves in the back of your nose.

● **Eat only when you are hungry.** Our sense of smell (and thus taste) is strongest when we're hungriest.

● **Humidify your air in the winter.** Our sense of smell is strongest in the summer and spring, most likely because of the higher moisture content in the air.

● **Eat in a restaurant or with other people.** Studies find that eating in the presence of other people makes food taste better than eating alone.

● **Stay away from the diaper bin and other bad smells.** Prolonged exposure to unpleasant smells tends to wipe out your ability to smell. So if you must be exposed to such odours on a prolonged basis, wear a mask over your nose and mouth that filters out some of the bad smells.

● **Add spices to your food.** Even if your senses of smell and taste are a little jaded, you should still retain full function in your "irritant" nerve, the nerve that makes you cry when you cut an onion. So use spices such as hot chili powder to liven up your food.

● **Blow your nose and clean it out with saline spray.** A simple thing, but it can help, because a blocked nose means blocked nerve receptors.

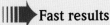 **Chew thoroughly and slowly.** This releases more flavour and extends the time that the food lingers in your mouth so that it spends more time in contact with your taste buds. Even before you start chewing, stir your food around – this aerates the molecules in the food, releasing more of their scent.

● **Stick to one glass of wine or beer.** Some research finds that the sense of smell declines as blood alcohol levels rise.

 Eat a different food with every forkful. Instead of eating the entire steak at once, then moving on to the potato, take a bite of steak, then a bite of potato, etc. Varying the scents and tastes as you eat keeps your olfactory nerves from getting bored.

● **See an allergy expert.** If you suffer from hay fever and over-the-counter products bring no relief, ask your GP if he or she can prescribe a suitable medicine or refer you to an allergy expert.

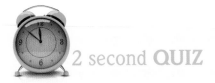 2 second **QUIZ**

Airline food or bring your own food?
ANSWER: **BRING YOUR OWN FOOD.**

And put some hot peppers on whatever you bring. The dry air of an airplane affects your senses of smell and taste, making anything you eat while airborne taste worse. That's one reason airline food is often heavily salted and sugared – to compensate for the blandness.

● **Reset your taste for sugar and salt.** Processed foods have so much sugar and salt that you practically stop tasting them if you eat them often. Try this experiment: check the salt content of your cereal; if it has more than 200 mg of sodium per serving, switch to a low-salt brand for two weeks. Once you switch back, you'll taste all the salt you were overlooking. The same goes for sugar.

● **Avoid very hot foods and fluids.** They can damage your taste buds.

● **Try sniff therapy.** It's possible to train your nose (and brain) to notice smells better. Start by sniffing something with a strong odour for 2 minutes a few times a day. Do this for three or four months and you should notice your sense of smell getting stronger – at least for that item.

Reminder

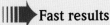**Fast results**
These are tips that deliver benefits particularly quickly – in some cases, immediately.

Easy gains
These are health boosters that offer the best value for the least amount of effort.

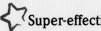**Super-effective**
This is advice that scientific research or widespread usage by experts has shown to be especially effective.

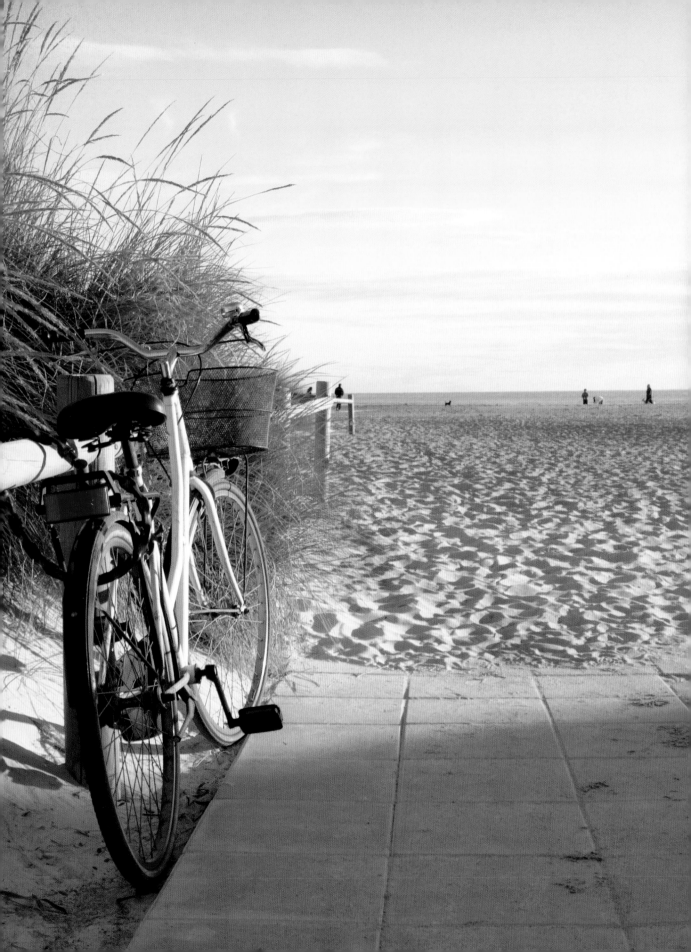

part 6

STEALTH HEALTHY MENTAL RELIEF

Attitudes can harm, and attitudes can heal – science has proven both beyond question. For better health, here's how to replace stress and worry with calm and happiness.

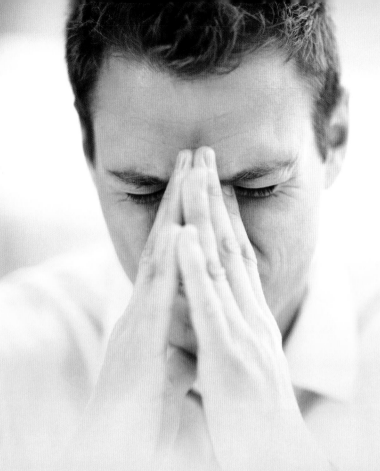

Defusing **STRESS**

Some days it seems as if life throws stress at you from all directions.
It can drain your energy, destroy your good mood and challenge your outlook. But science
has shown that stress also causes your body to release hormones that raise blood pressure,
speed up your heart and breathing, halt digestion, cause a surge in blood sugar and more.
When stress is ongoing, this constant physical reaction can significantly raise your risk of
colds, diabetes, heart disease, back troubles and almost every other major health concern.
Yet stress can be relatively easy to manage. All it takes is mental commitment – and an
open mind. So give some of these approaches to stress management a try.

34 WAYS TO CALM YOURSELF DOWN

Embrace the number one truth about stress: only you create it. Stress isn't defined as a large workload, a difficult child or a rise in terrorism. Stress is your physical and mental reaction to these external stimuli. Consider the saying about alcoholism – that admitting to being an alcoholic is more than 50 per cent of the cure. The same is true for stress: embracing the fact that stress is your reaction to external stimuli – and not the stimuli themselves – is half the battle towards managing it. You can't change a crazy world. But you can learn to handle it with humour, humility and hope. So it should come as no surprise that virtually every stress-relief method that follows is about how to improve your reaction to external factors.

● **Give your partner a hug every day before work.** It's so simple, yet so often overlooked when you're trying to make your lunch, find your shoes and keys and get on the road before rush hour. American researchers discovered that the few seconds it takes to hug your partner can help you to remain calm as chaos unfolds around you.

● **Buy yourself flowers once a week and display them prominently on your desk.** Women who sat near a bouquet of flowers were found to be more relaxed during a typing assignment than women who didn't have flowers, according to a U.S. study.

● **Take a deep breath, then try to see yourself in someone else's shoes.** Consider for a minute that your boss and others who annoy you may be experiencing just as much inner turmoil as they are creating around them. When people are rude, they are often suffering in one way or another.

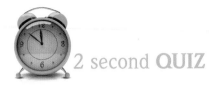

2 second QUIZ

Needlework or cooking?
ANSWER: **NEEDLEWORK.**

At least for most people. Research shows that repetitive tasks such as embroidery and crochet can reduce stress just as effectively as meditation or yoga. Many people find cooking relaxing, but unless you are preparing a very familiar dish with no margin for error, it does take mental energy and it can be stressful.

● **See the time waiting in a line as a chance to relax.** When you make a split decision about which line to join at the supermarket, chances are some other line will move more quickly. In a worst-case scenario, a customer in front of you has to have the price of one or more items checked by an assistant who takes a little time to get back. Rather than sending your stress hormones into the stratosphere as you steam over your bad luck, think about how busy you usually are and recognize this – in reality, usually just a few minutes – as a gift, as a time when you can just relax. As you wait, think about the things in life for which you are grateful, meditate on your breath, talk to one of the other customers or look at a magazine.

▶ **Develop a ritual in the morning** that focuses on calmness, beauty and the people who support you, or anything that helps you to feel a sense of peace. You might, for example, spend a few moments reminding yourself of your blessings. Your ritual might involve sitting outside (weather permitting), taking in your surroundings and appreciating the sounds of the birds and the sights of the sun glistening off the leaves and grass.

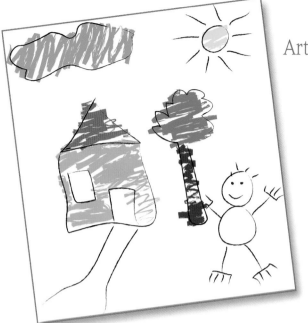

Art, children's drawings included, reduces stress.

to your ankles, then to your knees, on up your legs to your torso, chest, upper back, neck, head and face. As you get used to the technique, you can bring your awareness inside your body and focus on relaxing each body part whenever you start to feel stressed.

● **Decorate your office walls with your children's or grandchildren's pictures.** Studies find that viewing works of art – and yes, children's pictures are art – lowers stress hormones.

☺ **Designate one person to whom you can vent your frustrations.** Complaining widely about your work or family frustrations is not a healthy hobby to have – not only does it keep you in a negative frame of mind, but it's not very good for your professional or personal relationships either. The solution: designate one trustworthy friend or family member to be your confidant. Someone who is discreet and knows just to listen and not to attempt to solve all of your problems. Use that person to listen as you openly voice your stresses and how they are affecting you. Then, to the rest of the world, present yourself as positive and in control.

If you can't sit outdoors, go to a room in your home that you find calming. Settle down, take a few deep breaths, and call to mind three people or things that make life worth living. As your inner gratitude increases, pledge to commit one small act during the day to help someone else – somebody you know or a perfect stranger.

● **Twice a day, breathe deeply for 3 to 5 minutes.** As you breathe, focus your mind on your breath and push all other distracting thoughts from your consciousness.

● **Walk the stress off.** Stress hormones prepare your body for a physical response. So a healthy way to respond to a rush of stress is to get physical. Go for a brisk 15 minute walk and burn off your nervous energy. Use the time to think through the issue and return to a positive, peaceful frame of mind.

● **When you get out of bed in the morning,** spend a few minutes consciously sensing your body from toes to head. Focus on the feet first. Notice how they feel from the inside out and mentally relax them. Then move upwards

● **When you're ready to rip out your hair, phone a friend.** People who have strong social ties live longer. A diversionary conversation with a close romantic partner, friend or family member helps to prevent stress hormones from triggering high blood pressure and other health complications.

▐▐▐▶ **Don't take the bait.** If you really wanted to, you could spend your entire life angry at the world – at rude salespeople, bad bosses, crazy drivers, self-serving politicians, the rising cost of food. Happy, low-stress people choose not to get angry. Practise this: the next time someone does something that could – maybe even should – anger you, smile instead and say to yourself, "I'm not going to take the bait." And if you suddenly find yourself on the receiving end of aggression, don't automatically respond with the same. Take a breath, pause, then respond calmly and honestly, without undue defensiveness. If the other person won't engage constructively, smile and excuse yourself, with the message that you'll be happy to discuss the issue when the person regains his or her reason.

● **Every night before you go to bed, take 5 minutes to look over your day.** Instead of asking "How did my day go?," ask "How did I handle my day; how did it compare with six months ago?" Focusing on what you can handle – your response to stress – helps you feel more in control.

☆ **Decompress with a single alcoholic drink at the end of the day.** Not only will it help to prevent heart disease – one of the side effects of stress – but it will also disable your psychological inhibitions. When you let your guard down a bit, you can vent some of the feelings that you would otherwise harbour within you. Just be sure to stop at one drink.

☺ **Each Sunday, plan out your meals for the week.** Studies show that as late as 4 p.m., most people don't know what they're going to have for dinner. Planning ahead prevents the end-of-day stress of trying to figure out what to eat. Knowing what's for dinner when you come in from work cuts down on stress and encourages better eating habits and family time.

In PERSPECTIVE

Learn to breathe

Of course, you already know how to breathe. You do it every moment of every day without even thinking about it. Chances are, though, your breathing technique is not as healthy as you might think. Most of us breathe too shallowly, too quickly. Our lungs and hearts would greatly prefer longer, slower, deeper breaths. This is true for our general health, and it is also true for managing stress. Deep breathing helps to dissipate the fight-or-flight reaction that so many of us experience when we're stressed. It sends a signal to your brain to slow down, which results in hormonal and physiological changes that slow your heart rate and lower your blood pressure.

You might be surprised to find that there are lots of books on breathing method. That's because proper breathing technique is crucial for everyone from athletes to people with asthma to yoga experts. But for most of us there are only a few things you need to keep in mind:

● In general, inhale slowly and deeply through your nose. A healthy inhale takes about 5 seconds.

● In general, exhale slowly through your mouth. Empty your lungs completely. Good breathers focus more on thorough exhalation than on inhalation.

● For good deep breathing, engage your diaphragm – the sheet of muscle along the top of your abdomen that pulls your lungs down to draw in air, then pushes your lungs up to expel carbon dioxide. With a good inhalation, your lungs inflate as your diaphragm contracts and flattens. As you exhale, your diaphragm relaxes and rises. You may not feel the muscle moving but you can tell if you're using it as your abdomen will swell a little as you inhale.

● Work towards taking just six or eight deep breaths a minute. Most of us breathe more than 20 times a minute.

● **If exercise isn't helping to lower your stress levels,** switch from a repetitive type of exercise to a type that engages your mind. Sometimes workouts are not effective at reducing stress because we use the time to think about all the stressful things going on. Step aerobics, very active spinning classes (where you change positions a lot) and circuit or interval training (where you alternate different

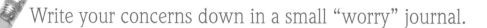

activities) prevent your mind from drifting, providing the mental break you need. A good option at home is dancing. Involve your whole family to benefit one and all.

● **Relax with a cup of basil tea.** Thought to help to induce a state of calm, this herb is easy to grow in a container garden and is widely available at supermarkets. Place three washed fresh basil leaves in a cup of hot water. Steep for 10 minutes, then sip.

● **Carry a small notebook with you.** This is your "worry" journal. When you feel stressed, get it out and scribble down everything on your mind. Close the notebook. Shut your eyes. Take ten deep breaths. Now open the journal and read what you've written. You'll find your worries are not nearly as stressful as you thought now that you've got them out of your head and onto the page.

● **Go somewhere blue or green.** Cool colours, such as light blues and greens, help people to relax and feel calm, relieving stress. When you're at the end of your tether, sit in a room where you can surround yourself with cool colours or find a bench in a park. Having lush green plants in your home or office can provide similar colour-related benefits.

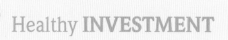

Healthy INVESTMENT

A yoga, Pilates or stretching book
For about 20 bucks, you can learn all types of moves that soothe your muscles, calm your spirit and improve your health. Doing 5 to 10 minutes of stretching or yoga positions each day can go a long way towards defusing stress.

● **Take on just one new activity at a time.** Try to master too many new things at once and you can easily feel overwhelmed. So at work and at home, take on new commitments with care. If you're particularly stressed at work, for instance, don't do more at home. Don't buy a new house and simultaneously take on higher car payments.

☆ **Schedule 6 to 8 hours of free time each week.** Use the time to daydream, read a novel, take a nap, see a film or generally relax in whatever way feels best to you. This is your time. Guard it well.

● **Drop in on a yoga class.** Just one class is all you need to lower levels of the stress hormone cortisol according to U.S. researchers. When they took blood samples from 16 beginners doing their first week of yoga classes, they found that levels of cortisol (the "stress hormone") dropped after the very first class.

● **Several times during the day, immerse yourself fully in the task at hand.** Chew your food slowly and taste every bite. Notice the sensation of the water as you wash the dishes. Even just sit and breathe, noticing the temperature of the air as it travels in and out of your nostrils. This will help you to let go of stressful thoughts and rest in the present.

● **Count your blessings once a day.** Once every day, say to yourself (or to someone else), "I feel lucky to have — in my life" or "I feel privileged to have —." Fill in the blanks with the names of family or friends, or with other positives, such as good health or a fulfilling career.

▸ **Have a really good cry.** By crying tears you were holding in, you can eliminate depression, make it easier to think clearly, heal old pain and hurt and achieve a sense of inner peace. Plus, studies find that crying boosts the immune system and reduces levels of stress hormones.

● **When you're stressed or tired and someone wants more of you than you can give,** tell him or her that you have only a few minutes to talk or that you are tired and not really able to listen right then. Believe it or not, the other person will trust you more because you're honest.

● **Practise some difficult assertiveness skills** such as declining a project, telling someone that you cannot talk now, expressing disagreement or disapproval or recommending an alternative. Increasing your assertiveness skills can greatly reduce your feelings of stress at work and increase your sense of self-confidence. Be assertive in a friendly but firm way.

● **Put Post-it notes** on your bathroom mirror, on your car dashboard and on your office computer that say "Slow down" and "What's the rush?" Your brain takes many cues from your body, and sometimes it misinterprets the cues, so use that to your advantage. Slowing everything down – by walking instead of running, say, or listening to slow music and speaking more slowly – will trick your brain into calming down your stress levels, too.

● **Think of your children or your pet.** Sometimes diverting your thoughts momentarily to those who love you, who matter most to you and who bring you pleasure helps you to put things instantly in perspective during very stressful moments. If you don't have a pet, get one. Studies find that pets, particularly dogs, are some of the best stress-relievers and health promoters around.

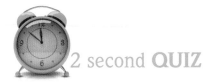

2 second QUIZ

Get mad or get even?
ANSWER: **NEITHER.**

Instead, get satisfaction by being a communicator. Let other people know when you're angry, and why. But be prepared to listen to their side, too, and try to find common ground. Reaching an understanding is less dangerous than holding in anger or expressing it aggressively.

● **Spray lavender scent into the air** (don't forget to spray yourself). Studies find the scent is instantly relaxing.

▌▌▶ **Unclench your muscles.** Until you do this exercise, called progressive relaxation, you won't even know how tense you really are. It works like this: starting with your toes and working your way up, clench each muscle for 10 seconds, then thoroughly relax them. You'll feel as if you've just undergone a massage.

● **Deprive your senses.** We've all heard of sensory deprivation. That's the theory behind flotation tanks in which you float in body-temperature water in a dark, enclosed capsule. To mimic one, find the darkest room in your house or office. Turn off all the lights, close the curtains or blinds and shut the door. Slip an eye mask over your eyes and stuff earplugs into your ears. Then lie back on the couch or a few pillows, get comfortable and let the relaxation take you away.

● **Slip in a CD of solo piano music from Chopin.** Or Enya, Ella Fitzgerald, Marvin Gaye – any soothing music, researchers find, actually produces slower brain-wave patterns, like those in people about to fall asleep or who are taking certain medicines.

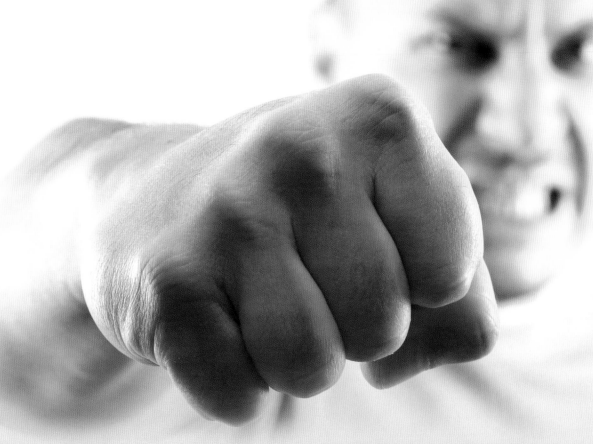

Defusing **ANGER**

Furious. Annoyed. Enraged. Outraged. Irate. Maddened. Raging. Riled. Wrathful. All synonyms for one of the most common human emotions: anger. There's no way to get through life without getting angry. The key is to learn how to defuse that anger constructively so that it doesn't end up destroying your health. Bottling up anger can increase your levels of homocysteine, a chemical linked to heart disease. It can also raise your cholesterol levels and heart rate, suppress your immune system, lead to depression and even give you a heart attack. But by defusing your anger you can reduce your risk of these health conditions. Here's how to let off steam safely and protect your health.

24 WAYS TO RELEASE YOUR EMOTIONAL STEAM

● **If you are angry with a politician, policy or some public injustice, do something about it.** In one American study, researchers tracked the brainwave patterns of students who had just been told the university was considering big tuition increases. They all exhibited brain patterns signifying anger, but signing a petition to block the increases seemed to provide satisfaction. Put simply, working to right a wrong is life-affirming and positive. Stewing in a bad situation without taking action has the opposite result.

● **Forget about punching a pillow, a wall or the object of your anger.** Contrary to popular belief, these common reactions don't decrease your anger. In fact, studies find, they only increase your hostility.

▐▐▶ **Take three deep breaths.** When you're angry, your body becomes tense. Breathing deeply helps to lower your internal anger meter.

● **Know why you feel angry.** Think like a detective and track down clues about the kinds of situations, people and events that trigger your anger. Once you're aware of them, try to avoid them if possible. If you can't avoid them, at least you'll know to anticipate them, which will give you more time to prepare for them so that they don't affect you so negatively.

☺ **Keep in mind that whoever loses it, loses.** Losing your temper makes you look like the bad guy to everyone else, no matter who is really at fault. To get better at controlling your anger, visualize a scene in which you got angry and replay the tape several times, each time imagining yourself responding in a different way. You're actually rehearsing different reactions and giving yourself

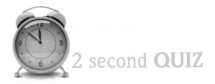

2 second QUIZ

Hold in anger or express it?
ANSWER: **EXPRESS YOUR ANGER.**

The real damage of a type A personality (see page 279) doesn't come from ambition, but from repressed anger. If you're angry, get it under control, then express it. But don't fixate on the anger; instead, concentrate on the underlying causes and issues. Try to be fair, but also be honest.

new options. The next time you're close to losing your temper, one of these options will pop into your mind, providing you with a better response.

● **Picture a red stop sign in your mind** or wear a rubber band on your wrist and snap it whenever you find your anger beginning to boil. Then take a few minutes to put the issue into perspective and ask yourself if it's worth the humiliation that comes from becoming overtly angry.

● **Recognize your own personal signs of escalating anger.** These might be clenched fists, trembling, flushing, sweating. Then use deep breathing to regain control of yourself before your anger erupts. If you're not sure about your own anger warning signs, ask a friend or family member. It's pretty likely they'll know!

☆ **Pinch yourself every time you hear yourself using the words "never," "always," etc.** Such thinking leads to a black-and-white, all-or-nothing mentality and that, in turn, shortens your fuse. Instead, look at things in shades of grey. Acknowledge that life can be unfair and that sometimes people do the wrong

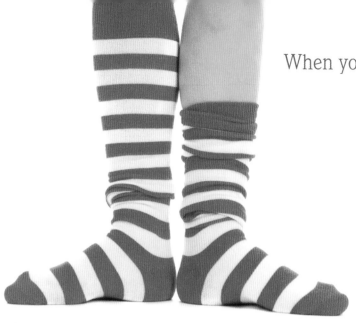

When you feel anger taking over, walk away.

- Relax your shoulders so that the muscles around them are neither tight nor tense.
- Breathe deeply in through your nose and exhale through your mouth to help your body to relax into this position.
- Close your eyelids lightly and continue breathing deeply.
- When using self-control time as a regular part of your day, it should last for approximately 3 minutes. When using it as a way to help you to regain self-control, it should last for approximately 1 minute.

thing. But don't fuel the fires with phrases such as "always disappoints" or "never comes through."

● **Take "self-control" time.** It works to get children to calm down, so it should work with angry grown-ups too. Here's how to do it:

- Sit up straight and relaxed wherever you are (a couch, the floor, a chair, etc.).
- Place your feet flat on the floor in front of you.
- Extend your hands palm down and place them gently in your lap. Make sure your elbows are naturally back by your sides.

▶ **When you get really angry, walk away from the source.** Then take a 5 minute walk to get some fresh air, or do something else that provides calm and relief. If your anger stems from the traffic jam you're stuck in, for example, turn up the radio and sing at the top of your voice. The idea is to create a mental and/ or physical escape from the situation.

● **When dealing with angry family members, find a way to make them laugh.** This is a trick family therapists often use. So, for instance, take a quick digital photo of yourself with a silly or contrite expression, print it out and put it on a family member's pillow. Or do some silly dancing together, or hide a gift in the mashed potatoes served at dinner. The point is to do something together that is lighthearted and fun. Not only does this defuse the anger, but it reminds everyone that you are in this family together, for ever.

● **Remember that anger is really a messenger.** So ask yourself exactly what is bothering you right now. Use the anger as a simple indication that something can and should be changed to improve things in the future.

Healthy INVESTMENT

An iPod (or any other portable music player with headphones)
Whenever you're in a situation in which you feel yourself beginning to get angry, pull out your iPod (which you've stocked with your favourite songs), put on your headphones, and mentally take yourself out of the situation.

● **Remember, too, that displays of anger don't accomplish anything except to anger or intimidate others.** It is not a disciplinary tool, a communication method or an emotional weapon. Anger is a damaging, personal, emotional state that is symptomatic of an underlying problem. So don't ever let yourself use anger as a threat – particularly with your children. Your anger should be your problem, not theirs.

● **When you're angry, look at your watch.** Let the second hand sweep around the dial for at least 2 minutes before you take any action. By then, you'll have had time to think and you can act in a more appropriate way.

● **Write a forgiveness letter or e-mail.** You don't even have to send it. Just the act of writing down your feelings will lighten the load of anger you've been carrying. If you want to resume your relationship with the person or people with whom you've been angry, however, do hit the send button. One major American study found that when volunteers thought about a person they were angry with, their blood pressure, heart rate and muscle tension leaped. But when they imagined themselves forgiving the other person – just imagined it – their blood pressure, etc. didn't rise nearly as much.

● **Embrace empathy.** True empathy means getting into another person's head and heart both to understand and feel that individual's experience. You can do this in numerous ways: by visualizing the situation through the other person's eyes; by writing a story from the other person's perspective of the situation; by telling the story to a friend but taking the other person's perspective.

In PERSPECTIVE

Type A vs. hostility

Have you ever taken one of those personality tests? The ones where you answer a set of questions, add up your score and come up with a category into which your personality fits?

If you took one and you have what's known in the literature as a "hostile" personality, then you're more likely to have insulin resistance or pre-diabetes than someone with a different form of personality. Hostility is also thought to be the culprit behind the link between so-called type A personalities – time-conscious, competitive individuals – and heart disease.

Put simply, hostile people are impatient and aggressive. That differs from the type A personality, however, in that type A behaviour itself – being driven, always in a hurry, a mega multi-tasker—isn't detrimental.

The hostile element, on the other hand – being quick to anger, aggressive and easily irritated – seems to be the heart-damaging part of the equation. Hostile people are also more cynical, quicker to think the world is out to get them, and less willing to trust other people. They're also more likely to have heart disease.

In one U.S. study, researchers found that doctors who scored in the top half on a hostility questionnaire administered at the age of 25 were four to five times more likely to have heart disease than low scorers by the time they reached the age of 50.

● **When you're angry with your parents, think about your children.** How do you want them to feel about you when they're your age? Wouldn't you want them to understand that you were only doing the best you could at the time?

☆ **Acknowledge some core truths about people:**
● Most people act out of the belief that they are doing the right thing.
● Most people are not malicious, mean-spirited or backstabbing.
● Most people are more sensitive and insecure than they let on.

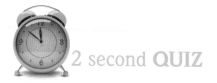

2 second QUIZ

Plane, car or train?
ANSWER: CAR OR TRAIN.

Flying might seem to be the fastest option but, if your destination is less than 500 km away, just think of the time spent driving to an airport, parking, getting through security and boarding – not to mention delays and even overbooked flights. So catch a train, if it's convenient, or drive. A direct train can be very relaxing, especially if you don't need transport at the other end. But in a car, you have more control over the situation, you're in your own environment and, if you check the traffic situation first and adjust your route accordingly, fewer things can go wrong (such as delays and cancellations).

● Most people aren't very good judges of how their actions affect others. In other words, we're neither villains nor saints. We're all just people – struggling to lead happy, healthy, meaningful lives in a complicated world. Yes, even the people who anger you. With this in mind, forgiveness comes much easier.

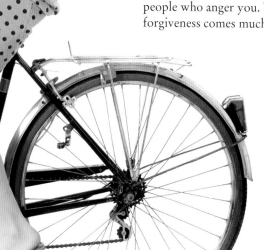

▶ **Get angry with the person who can make a difference.** There's nothing to be gained by becoming angry with the poor soul who is simply caught in the crossfire. This advice is particularly important when you're dealing with people who work in the service industries. Is it the fault of the salesperson that something you need is out of stock? No, but his or her manager could probably fix things.

● **Understand that someone, somewhere,** is gossiping about you, because that's what people do, but understand also that it has absolutely no impact on your life.

● **Take responsibility for your anger.** Recognize that it's your choice whether or not you become angry.

● **Talk about your anger.** This is different from expressing it; talking about it means unloading and decompressing with a friend, going over the situation with a neutral observer who can bring some perspective to the situation, or even talking out loud to yourself about it (preferably when no one else can hear you).

● **Get on your bike and go for a half-hour ride.** Or jump up and down on a trampoline. Or go for a vigorous swim. Or attack the weeds in your garden. Any kind of vigorous, intense physical activity helps to dissipate anger.

● **Get some perspective.** Is this person or situation really worth spending your emotional energy on? Risking your health over? Putting your dignity and peace of mind at risk?

If you want to lose your anger, get on your bike.

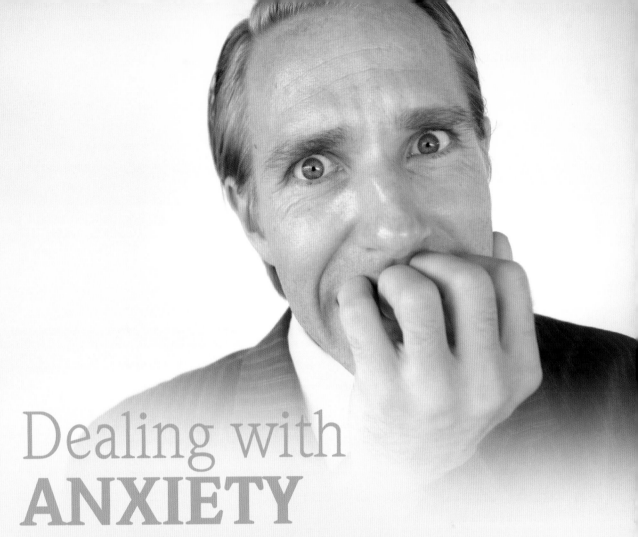

Dealing with
ANXIETY

You know the feeling. You're doing fine, then your son announces that he's dropping out of university, and you discover you need a new roof. Suddenly, you can't breathe. Your chest hurts and you're convinced it's a heart attack. It's more likely you're having an anxiety attack. According to the Public Health Agency of Canada, an estimated 12 per cent of Canadian adults experience anxiety disorders of some sort, including generalized anxiety, phobias, Post Traumatic Stress Disorder, Obsessive Compulsive Disorder and panic attacks. Sometimes the answer is medication and therapy, but quite often learning to cope with anxiety can make a big difference. Here are 17 ways to do it.

17 WAYS TO STOP WORRYING

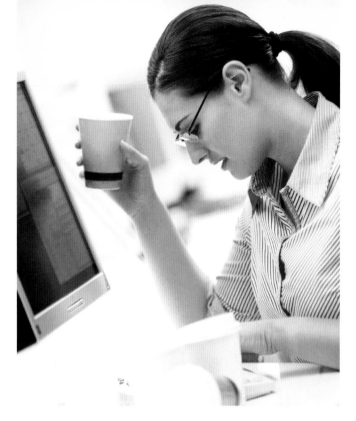

Cut out the caffeine – it increases that tense, jittery, anxious feeling.

● **Get out your bike, put on your walking shoes or grab your gym bag.** There's no better therapy for the "I can't breathe" feeling of an anxiety attack than to escape the situation quickly and get your blood moving and endorphins pumping through exercise.

● **Cut out all caffeinated drinks, foods and medicines.** The caffeine only adds to that tense, jittery, anxious feeling. Sources of caffeine include chocolate, beverages such as coffee, tea and soft drinks and some prescription and over-the-counter medicines.

☺ **Avoid conversations likely to increase your anxiety** when you're tired, overwhelmed or stressed. For instance, tell your children you're not available for problem solving after 8 p.m. Try to maintain a "trouble-free" time, especially before bed, when you don't address difficulties but focus on pure relaxation.

● **Buy a white-noise machine and use it when you go to sleep.** The soothing sound will help you to fall and stay asleep. A good night's sleep is critical when you're stressed, since sleep deprivation fuels anxiety even as anxiety leads to sleep deprivation. See "The sleep routine" (page 72) for more tips on getting a good night's sleep.

● **Choose one thing that is making you anxious.** Now sit down and write out all the fears you have about that one thing. If it's money, write down what would happen if you lost your job, if you couldn't pay your bills. What is the absolute worst thing that could happen?

In **PERSPECTIVE**

Coping with disappointment

When you're middle-aged or younger, stress and anxiety are often born out of career issues, a too-busy schedule and the struggle to achieve a balance between work, family and self. But for those past their career peaks, past having young children at home, past having to worry about how to get everything done in a day, stress often comes in different shapes and forms. And one of those forms is disappointment – in how life turned out, how children turned out, how the fanciful dreams of youth never quite became reality.

Too often, people skim over the discomfort associated with disappointment, yet it's a normal emotion. So don't ignore it. Understanding what you're disappointed about and why you're disappointed can be a valuable learning experience. For instance, if you're disappointed in other people's behaviour, perhaps you need to examine your expectations.

Ultimately, experts say, the trick is to forgive the past and have hope for the future, but to live in the present. Make today an outstanding day. Make tomorrow even better.

Now look at each item and mark it on a scale of 1 to 10, with 1 being highly unlikely that it would ever happen, 10 being likely that it would happen. You'll be surprised at how few items rank above a 5. This understanding should help to reduce your anxiety. If something does rank higher than a 5, you may want to develop a contingency plan for it. Nothing works better to calm anxiety than turning from pure worry to an action plan.

● **Rent a comedy and watch it.** Let yourself laugh out loud. The act of laughter stimulates endorphins that help to blow stress hormones (which contribute to that feeling of anxiety) out of your system the way that a good thunderstorm can blow away hot, humid weather.

☆ **Relax, detach and focus.** Try the following routines:
● Relax your body from the toes up.
● Detach from your thoughts.
● Centre yourself in the moment (for example, feel your head upon the pillow or your feet on the ground, etc., depending on where you are).
● Focus on who you want to be and how you want to feel.

● **Turn on the news and watch the disasters unfurl.** It will help you to put your own problems into perspective and realize it's a big world, filled with both triumph and disaster. The challenges in your life that make you anxious may not seem as great when you put them in the context of the whole world.

☺ **Don't borrow future problems.** Many people get into a cycle of predicting and worrying about future concerns. Ask yourself, "Is this something I know will happen and is it something I can do

Breathe away ANXIETY

In "Defusing stress," there's information on healthy breathing (see page 273). But proper breathing is particularly important during moments of great anxiety. At times like these, many people resort to chest breathing – the type of big, desperate inhales and exhales that make you rapidly puff up and deflate your chest.

To regain healthy breathing during periods of anxiety, lie on the floor and place your hand on your chest. Using your hand as a gauge, try to reduce the amount of chest movement, while continuing to breathe normally. You don't want your chest to move; you want the other parts of your body to take over the breathing – using your diaphragm instead of the big chest inhales and exhales. Do this for 5 minutes.

Be aware that chest breathing still has a purpose, but only in times of extreme emotional arousal or physical challenge. Most people use chest breathing because of instincts developed from fight-or-flight conditions. It's in those types of physically dangerous situations that it is still necessary – not for everyday stress or anxiety.

anything about right now?" If the answer to either of these questions is no, tell yourself you will revisit it later.

● **Simply experience your anxiety for 45 minutes.** That's usually all it takes for you to become used to it and for the anxious feeling to dissipate. The worst thing to do is ignore it, because anxiety tends to fight back if you push it down.

● **Talk to yourself.** Remind yourself of how you handled similar situations in the past, your strengths and how long you will need to get through it. Show yourself that this anxiety is manageable as well as time-limited.

● **Keep a journal noting what makes you anxious.** Then revisit these same items when you're feeling calm and develop plans to deal with them.

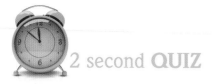

Laugh or cry?
ANSWER: CRY.

When life is so challenging that you're having anxiety attacks, it's a serious business. While laughing off the situation may seem like a mature, "I'm in control" response, it may be masking or denying some very unhealthy issues. Crying is a more honest, anxiety-releasing response, with positive physiological effects. It also signals to you and your loved ones that all is not well and that change may be in order.

Name your fears. The most anxiety-producing thing of all is the unknown. So make a point of dragging your worries out of the shadows. If you're worried about your son/daughter/partner getting hurt or killed in a car crash, for example, discuss it – at least with yourself. Look up the statistics on driving and injury to relieve your mind. Do the same for whatever else makes you worry, whether it's Ebola virus, bioterrorism, cancer or plane crashes. Once you name your fears and learn more about them, you can take steps to minimize your risk. You'll also find that the fears you name and tame are far less menacing than the fears left to lurk in the shadows of your imagination.

● **Make sure you're getting several servings of whole grains, fruit and vegetables every day,** along with healthy protein sources such as fish, poultry, lentils, soy or lean meats. The combination of healthy foods helps your brain to make serotonin, a chemical that induces a state of calm relaxation.

A good diet that includes plenty of fish and vegetables helps your brain to make serotonin, a chemical that induces relaxation.

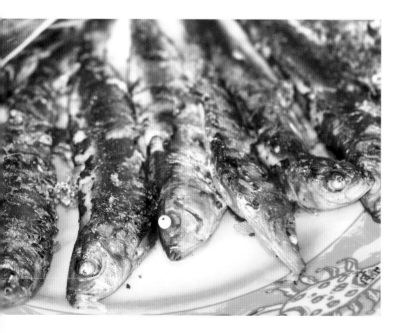

● **Go to the museum, see a film, read a good book or take up oil painting** (or some other hobby). People who are bored tend to score higher on tests designed to measure levels of anxiety.

● **Rent a meditation, tai chi or yoga DVD from the library.** They are all effective, non-medical ways of dealing with anxiety.

● **Share your anxieties with a confidant.** It's a good idea to find someone who can help you to understand why you worry too much. If appropriate, try to play the same role for that person. We are usually better at putting someone else's worries in perspective than we are our own.

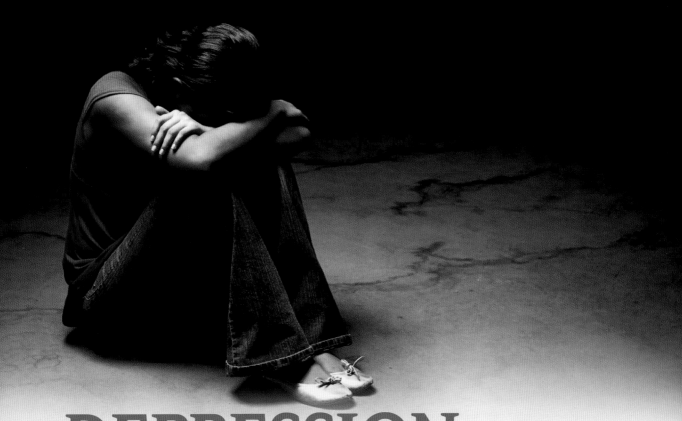

DEPRESSION

There comes a point when most of us realize: life sometimes isn't much fun. It may have been an eye-opening adventure in our youth, our teens, even our 20s, but, as time passes, the glee of living gets harder to sustain. Most of us cope just fine with this. With age, exuberance and excitement get replaced by a more subtle but deeper joy. We have families and friends we love, meaningful jobs, hobbies and vacations that provide real pleasure, accumulated wisdom that gives us a sense of value. But for millions of people, the path of life occasionally leads to depression. The point here is not to give you a diagnosis or treatment – that's for professionals to do. But even if you are taking medication for depression, the following lifestyle tactics may increase the drug's effectiveness. If you're simply feeling low, the tips may give you the boost you need to pull you up without the need for prescription drugs.

16 WAYS TO BANISH THE BLUES

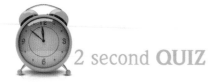

Exercise or antidepressants?
ANSWER: **EXERCISE.**

A study of older adults found that ten weeks of standard exercise was 20 per cent more effective at reducing depressive symptoms than medication. However, because depression may make you want to do anything but exercise, many doctors recommend combining the two treatments. With your doctor's approval, start taking an antidepressant until you feel energetic enough to begin exercising. Then, once you get into a regular exercise routine, talk to your doctor about possibly reducing the dosage of your medication or weaning yourself off it altogether.

Spend at least 1 hour each week with a close friend. In a British study, when 86 depressed women were paired with a volunteer friend, 65 per cent of the women felt better. In fact, regular social contact worked as effectively as antidepressant medication and psychotherapy. Regular contact with a close friend may boost self-confidence and encourage you to make other positive changes that will help to lift depression, such as starting an exercise program.

Eat seafood twice a week or more. A Dutch study found that people who consume diets rich in omega-3 fatty acids, a type of fat found in cold-water fish such as salmon and mackerel, were less likely to suffer from depression than people whose diets were low in this important fat. One reason researchers think the rate of depression has skyrocketed is that we get so few omega-3 fatty acids in our diets. While pregnant women are advised to eat one portion of oily fish a week, they should avoid eating shark, swordfish and marlin or more than 280 g cooked or canned tuna a week because of potentially dangerous mercury levels. Another way to get your omega-3s is from ground flaxseeds. Keep a container in the fridge and sprinkle them on everything from ice cream to yogourt to cheese omelettes.

● **Play with a dog for a few minutes every day.** When non-pet owners played with a dog for just a few minutes a day as part of a U.S. study, blood levels of the brain chemicals serotonin and oxytocin – both mood elevators – rose. You don't need to own a dog to experience these feel-good effects (although dogs are great antidotes to the kind of chronic stress that can result in depression). Pet your neighbour's dog, offer to take it for walks, or volunteer at an animal shelter for some furry one-on-one therapy.

● **Eat a bowl of fortified breakfast cereal or take a multivitamin every day.** This will ensure you consume the recommended amount (400 mcg) of folate, an important B vitamin that may help to lift depression. Folate and other B vitamins help to maintain nerve and blood cells, used in brain reactions and essential for the production and function of a number of mood-boosting brain chemicals. In a Finnish study published in the *Journal of Nutrition*, participants with the lowest folate consumption were at the highest risk of depression. Another study, published in the *Annals of Clinical Psychiatry*, found that this vitamin helps to enhance the effectiveness of antidepressant medication. Another good source? Avocados. They're one of the richest plant sources of B vitamins.

● **Get a 12 minute massage three times a week.** It doesn't have to cost a lot. Whether you pay a professional or ask

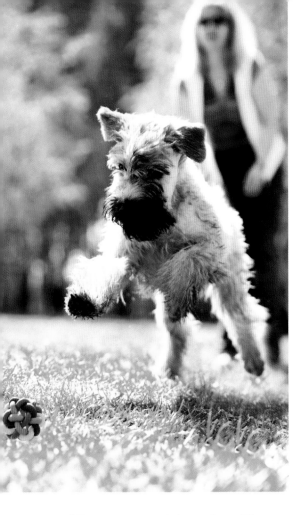

Diagnosing **DEPRESSION**

How do you know if you're just feeling blue or if you're truly depressed? Everybody has a day or two when they feel some sadness. Perhaps you're a little under the weather; maybe something unpleasant has happened. But this tends to pass.

Depression, on the other hand, drags on for weeks or months. It affects your mood and thoughts, and impacts on you physically, acting on the way you eat and sleep. Studies find that people with depression are also more likely to develop such serious diseases as heart disease and diabetes.

Classic symptoms of depression include:
- Difficulty concentrating
- Short-term memory loss
- Pessimism
- Loss of enjoyment in activities you once found pleasurable
- Fatigue
- Irritability
- Changes in appetite
- Lack of sexual desire
- Difficulty sleeping

If your symptoms last for two weeks or more, you may need more than home remedies. Make an appointment to see your doctor.

Hang out with a dog if you want to lift your spirits.

a partner or friend to rub your back, the result is the same: a natural mood boost. In a study of depressed dialysis patients, participants who received a 12 minute massage three times a week were less depressed than those who didn't get the soothing rub. Another study of 84 depressed pregnant women found that those who received two 20 minute massages a week from their partners reduced their incidence of depression by 70 per cent. Researchers suspect that massage boosts serotonin levels (which jumped by 17 per cent in the women who received twice-weekly massages) and reduces levels of the stress hormone cortisol.

● **Pull an all-nighter.** Staying up all night for one night – and therefore depriving yourself of sleep – has been shown to lift depression for as long as a month. Although researchers aren't sure why it works, they speculate that one night of sleep deprivation may reset the sleep clock, enabling people who are depressed to sleep better.

● **Eat a bowl of whole-grain cereal.** When you consume high-carbohydrate foods – such as cereal – you encourage the amino acid tryptophan to flood your brain, boosting serotonin levels. A slice of whole-wheat bread and honey will also produce the same effect. Why the

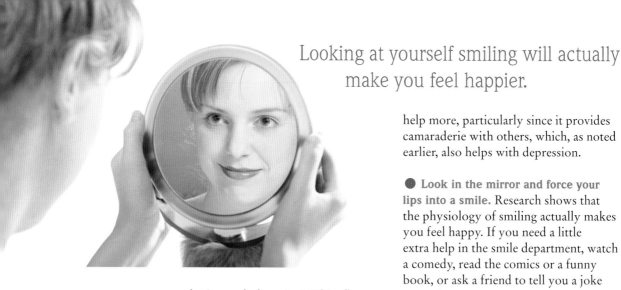

Looking at yourself smiling will actually make you feel happier.

help more, particularly since it provides camaraderie with others, which, as noted earlier, also helps with depression.

● **Look in the mirror and force your lips into a smile.** Research shows that the physiology of smiling actually makes you feel happy. If you need a little extra help in the smile department, watch a comedy, read the comics or a funny book, or ask a friend to tell you a joke every day.

● **First thing in the morning,** lie on your back with your head hanging over the edge of your bed. Grip a 2 kg or 4 kg (5 lb to 10 lb) dumbbell with both hands and extend it behind your head, letting your arms hang down towards the floor. Take ten deep breaths, trying to expand your ribcage as much as possible. Bring the weight back and place it on the bed beside you. Shift yourself onto the bed so that your head is supported, and take another ten deep breaths. Repeat three times. The stretch will open your ribcage and chest, making it easier to take a deep breath. Apparently the most common unrecognized source of mild depression is restricted trunk flexibility, which interferes with full breathing. Most people with mild depression are shallow breathers because their chest and stomach are too tight to allow full, easy breathing.

emphasis on whole grains? White flour provides similar benefits, but the effects wear off quickly, taking you from peak to trough in an hour or so.

● **Just bang on something.** People at a retirement community who took a drumming class felt more energetic and less depressed six weeks after the class than before they started it. Researchers speculate that drumming helps to relax your body. Whacking a few beats out on your desk may help, but joining or starting a weekly drumming circle may

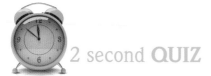

2 second QUIZ

Work or sex?
ANSWER: SEX.

A group of economists found that going from having sex once a month to having it at least weekly is equivalent to the amount of happiness that an enormous pay raise would bring to the average person. The findings hold regardless of age or gender. The reason? Probably the fact that people with good relationships and healthy sex lives tend to be happier overall than those without.

● **Drink 1 or 2 cups of coffee or tea each morning.** Regular, modest caffeine intake decreases the risk of depression by more than 50 per cent.

● **Sleep in a different bedroom.** Many people with depression also have insomnia. Changing your sleep location can help. You can also reduce insomnia by getting up at the same time every day, never napping for more than 20 minutes, shunning caffeine after 3 p.m. and relaxing for an hour before bed.

▐▐▐▶ **Break out of your routine.** Sometimes being stuck in a rut is just that. Get out of it and your mood may come along with you. Book a day off from work to explore a town nearby. Go out to a restaurant for dinner – even though it's a Tuesday night. Take a different route as you drive to work, wear something that is totally "not you," or take your camera and go on a photography walk. For a major blue mood, it might be time for a vacation.

Healthy INVESTMENT

A light box
Bright light therapy has been shown to relieve depression during pregnancy as effectively as antidepressant medication. Additional research shows that it can also ease seasonal affective disorder, a type of depression some people experience during the winter months when sunlight is in short supply. It may ease other types of depression as well. The therapy involves sitting in front of a specially designed light box shortly after waking each morning for 20 minutes to an hour. You can purchase a light box for home use from a variety of sources, many of them online.

Walk out in winter to get your quota of daylight.

☺ **Take a 10 minute walk three times a day during winter.** Many people feel depressed during the winter months, when they travel to and from work in darkness and don't get enough natural sunlight. Physical exercise, however, encourages the release of hormones and neurochemicals that boost mood. Walking outside during the day will give you a few short doses of sunlight, also shown to improve mood, particularly in winter.

● **Go easy on yourself.** When something goes wrong, resist the urge to beat yourself up mentally. When you catch yourself berating yourself for some supposed failing, replace your negative thoughts with the phrase, "I am doing the best I know how to do. When I know a better way and can do it, I will."

● **Plan a day of vigorous outdoor recreation,** such as hiking, canoeing or cycling. Let the combination of nature and physical activity work their magic on your mood.

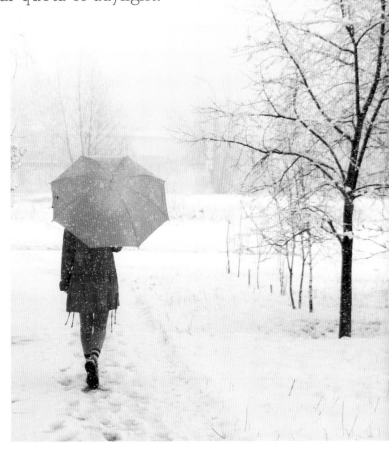

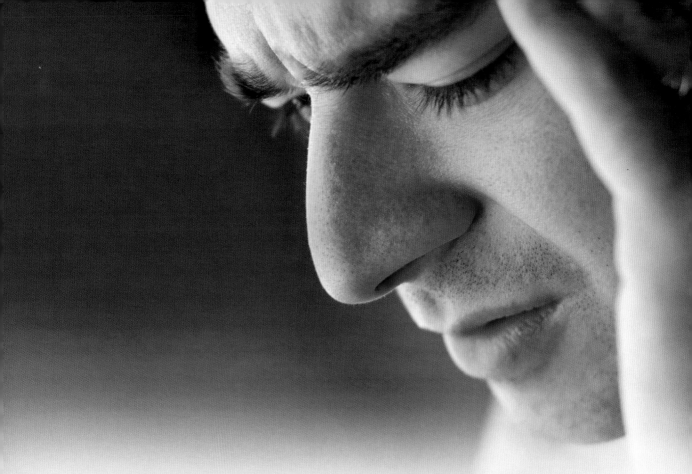

Dealing with **GUILT**

Ask anyone to define "guilt," and they'll hum and haw. It's hard to describe, a feeling of "I should have done something or should not have done something." The *Canadian Oxford English Dictionary* defines it as "a feeling of having committed a specified or implied offence." It's a revealing definition – it's a *feeling* of having committed an offence rather than *committing* an offence. Of course, sometimes you should feel guilty (if you've committed a crime, say, or intentionally hurt someone). But if you're like most of us, you feel guilty because of all the "shoulds" in your life. That's bad for your mental and physical health, so read on to find out how to shed some of that guilt.

19 TIPS FOR A CLEARER CONSCIENCE

☆ **Above all else, learn to forgive yourself.** If feelings of guilt haunt you, take some concrete steps to end this self-inflicted punishment. First, list the things you feel guilty about. It could be something stupid you said recently, an act of cruelty against a sibling in your childhood or a detrimental personal habit that has hurt your relationship with a loved one. Then ask, "How can I forgive myself and let it go?" Perhaps it's saying a prayer, writing a letter, having a talk, making a charitable donation or committing to personal change. Often it's merely having the courage to say, "I'm sorry." Then do what it takes so you can honestly, finally forgive yourself. You'll be amazed at the lightness this can bring.

● **Set a no-guilt-allowed rule whenever you go on vacation or do something just for yourself.** Often people, particularly women, do not experience vacations, breaks and other relaxing activities as stress-relieving because they feel guilty that they're not doing more productive things. Tell yourself that you are taking a break and doing it for a reason (improved health, decreased stress, etc.), so there is no reason to feel guilty. As soon as you hear yourself say, "I should be …" remind yourself why you are choosing not to do that. Make sure anyone you're travelling with knows about the no-guilt rule, too.

● **Take 5 minutes in the morning to feel guilty.** Then either resolve what's triggering the guilt (for example, call your mother) or forgive yourself for what you did that you shouldn't have done, knowing that you've learned your lesson and won't do it again.

▌▌▶ **Correct a mistake rather than feeling guilty about it.** For instance, if you're

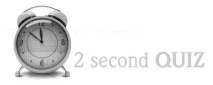

2 second QUIZ

Letter or phone call?
ANSWER: **LETTER.**

When an apology is due, sit down and write a letter. Not only will it give you a better opportunity to think through your thoughts, but you always have the option of sending it or not sending it. Sometimes the simple act of writing is enough to give you peace of mind. If you do send it, the person to whom you're sending it has a lifetime reminder of your apology.

feeling guilty because you went shopping on Saturday instead of going to see a relative in hospital, take time out of your schedule for a midweek visit. Many times, the things we feel guilty about are relatively easy to put right.

▌▌▶ **Recognize that a feeling of guilt doesn't always mean that what you did was wrong.** For instance, if you're feeling guilty because you decided it was more important to relax with a book than to have coffee with your always-in-a-crisis friend, that means you're learning to set limits and take time for yourself. In cases like this, have the confidence to admit that you made the right choice.

● **Commit to saying no** at least once a day – no guilt allowed.

● **Start a guilt journal.** When you feel guilty about something, write it down. Write the time, the day, why you feel guilty. Go back and reread this journal every couple of weeks to find the trends in your guilt. This will help you deal better with its underlying roots.

● **Stop asking, "What if?"** Instead, start asking, "What now?" Put another way, stop thinking about things you've already done and can't change, and instead focus on the present – what you can do today to make your life and the world around you better.

● **Recall all the healthy benefits of some of the most guilt-inducing foods.** For instance, dark chocolate is full of heart-healthy antioxidants. Red wine has fabulous benefits for your heart, cholesterol and other health markers. A handful of mixed nuts will give you a

2 second QUIZ

Gift or no gift?
ANSWER: **GIFT.**

If you've had a fight with your partner, particularly a bad fight, a peace offering goes a long way towards restoring, well, the peace – as long as it's delivered with a sincere apology or message of reconciliation. But be careful never to try to win back favour with a gift alone – that's called a bribe. It's the apology that matters; the gift reinforces the message of love and commitment.

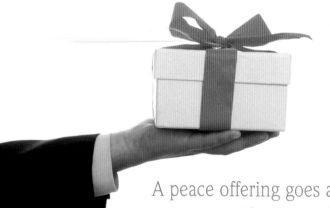

A peace offering goes a long way if tempers have been frayed.

healthy dose of monounsaturated fat and vitamin E. A serving of popcorn supplies a good portion of fibre. Just remember: moderation in all things.

● **Talk to a relative or friend** who recalls the incident about which you're feeling guilty. Often our own memories are not the most accurate; your feelings of guilt may be coming from something that really didn't happen the way you remember it.

☺ **Don't get caught up in blaming.** For some reason, many people feel compelled to assign blame (often to themselves) for anything that goes wrong, big or small. But that's a bad approach to a complex world. Instead, take a more forgiving view of the world and recognize that sometimes things just happen as a result of a cascade of events that cannot be blamed on any one person.

● **List ten things that you like about yourself.** Most of us are highly critical of ourselves, without acknowledging the good, the funny, the right choices, the successes. Guilt becomes less of an issue when we're happy and secure in who we are. Keep this list in your bag, in your pocket or on your computer. Look at it whenever you're feeling guilty about what you should or should not have done.

● **Recognize that you can do only your best.** Nothing more. So perhaps you weren't the kind of mother who got down on the floor to play with her children, but you were the kind of mother who took her children on outings to museums and parks. Maybe you aren't the kind of person to surprise your partner with romantic gestures and gifts, but you do provide a perpetually open ear, helping hand and unconditional support.

● **Write a cheque to a charity.** That's doing something concrete with your guilt. If you're feeling guilty about eating that chocolate cake last night, go for a long walk today. If you feel guilty about the long hours you've been spending at work, organize a day off and spend the time with your children and/or partner doing what they want.

● **Determine your priorities,** write them down, then stick the list on your fridge and in your office. Next time you start feeling guilty about something you didn't do, check the list. If it's not in the top three priorities, you're off the hook.

● **Accept some selfishness.** It really is OK to look out for yourself.

● **Don't leave guilt unresolved,** particularly if it relates to an older relative such as a parent. Address the issues that matter to you so that you're not left with regrets you can't address.

Politely decline other people's guilt. Parents have an amazing capacity for making children feel guilty – even when

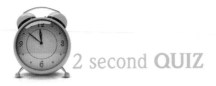

2 second QUIZ

Short or long apology?
ANSWER: **SHORT.**

The person you wronged doesn't want to hear about the kind of day you had, the idiot who cut you off on the road, the ketchup someone squirted on your tie or any other reasons for your foul mood. He or she just wants to know that you realize that barking angrily at him or her the minute you walked in the door was wrong. So say simply that you're sorry and that you know it was wrong. Then let the other person talk.

the "child" is aged 60. Some partners, bosses, children and religious leaders are also masters at making others feel bad about what they have (or haven't) done or said. The fact is, they have no right to do that, and you have no obligation to listen. Only you are accountable for your actions. Assuming you haven't broken a law or a solemn promise, only you can judge whether you did something wrong.

● **Ask yourself,** "Would I forgive someone else for doing/not doing what I did/didn't do?" If the answer is yes, then (to paraphrase the golden rule) do unto yourself as you would have yourself do unto others.

Reminder

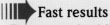**Fast results**
These are tips that deliver benefits particularly quickly – in some cases, immediately.

☺ **Easy gains**
These are health boosters that offer the best value for the least amount of effort.

☆**Super-effective**
This is advice that scientific research or widespread usage by experts has shown to be especially effective.

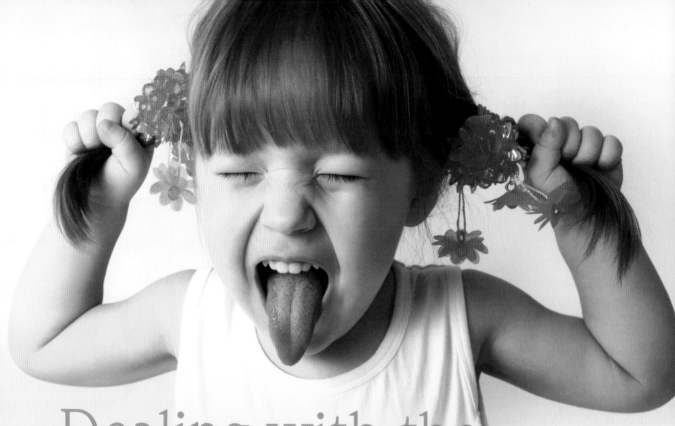

Dealing with the
UNCONTROLLABLE

You just have to turn on the news nowadays to realize how out of control the world is. First there are the big events – war, terrorism, famine. But then there are the smaller things that are out of your hands, ranging from the weather to your job to your son or daughter. And if you're an ordered person – someone who has to have everything just so – then feeling out of control is one of the most stressful things that could ever happen to you. But the golden rule of life hasn't changed, and never will: stuff happens. Much of it you can't influence. What you can influence is how you react to it and how much it affects you. Here are 12 ways to gain back a bit of control.

12 WAYS TO MAINTAIN A HEALTHY PERSPECTIVE

☺ **Above all else, distinguish what you can't control from what you can.** Then direct your energies to influencing the latter, and accepting the former. This might sound simplistic, but you'd be amazed at how many people still think they can control the traffic, the weather, their boss's mood or the stock market. Make a list of all the things in your life that you can't control, no matter how hard you try, and stick it on your fridge and your computer. Then accept it. Of course you can care about these things and try to influence their outcome. But it's essential that you untie your emotional well-being from those things that you cannot alter.

● **When things feel out of control,** clean a closet or a drawer. It puts you back in charge of at least some aspects of your life.

● **Take up a new hobby.** Mastering a new skill, whether it's paddling a kayak or learning to knit, will return a sense of control to your life.

● **When bad things happen,** sit down and write out what you might have done differently. This self-assessment is not aimed at blaming yourself or beating yourself up; it's a chance to say, "I may not control everything, but I do control me." What can I do with myself to make this work better and turn out more to my liking? So, if you get a bad evaluation at work, say, don't respond to it by blaming your boss or your bad luck. Instead, be honest with yourself about what you could have done differently that year – getting into work on time, meeting all your deadlines, etc. – to get a better result. Understanding your role in the situation will help you to realize that the world is actually a fairly controllable place.

Healthy INVESTMENT

A "mudroom"
The idea here is that there is one place in your house in which chaos can be contained, and you don't care how messy it gets. So designate a "mudroom" for all the coats, shoes and backpacks, or choose another room as the official house "chaos room." It can be the basement, garage, playroom, even a child's room (just close the door). At the same time, create a "sanctuary" room in your house that is kept orderly at all times. Use it to regain peace during those times when the mayhem of life overspills its boundaries.

● **When things feel chaotic, pick one thing in your life to work on** where you can make a difference. For example, start an exercise program, write in your journal one day a week, balance your bank account or make sure you take your car in for a scheduled tune-up.

● **Build in contingencies.** For instance, if you have an outdoor party planned for 20 people but it rains on the day. You can't control the weather, but you can control where you hold it (move it inside), when you hold it (postpone it) and how it's held (if you were planning a barbecue, prepare a couple of big lasagnas instead).

● **Make a list.** Nothing puts more control back into your hands than taking all the "to-dos" swirling through your head and writing them down. Now plan how you will accomplish each one. If one of the things on your list is Christmas shopping, say, set yourself a date, a time and a time limit to do it. If another item on your list is to clean the whole house, break it down into smaller, more manageable parts. So on Monday you clean the kitchen, on Tuesday the bathroom and so on.

Coping with **GRIEF**

There's nothing more uncontrollable than the death of someone you love. But there are ways to cope. The following tips can help you to move through what may seem like endless grief. Note the pattern in the suggestions – maintaining your love for the person and honouring his or her memory, while still moving on with your life:

● Think of your grief as a certain number of tears you must shed before the intensity of the sadness, anger and guilt subsides. The more opportunities you take to grieve and feel all the related feelings, the sooner you will reach your magic number of tears.

● Create a special place in your house, with a picture, a candle and perhaps some small mementos of your loved one. When you feel sad, spend some time there, and "talk" to the person you lost about how you're feeling.

● Get a scrapbook and make a memory album of the good times you had together. Put in photos, greeting cards, menus or postcards. You can also write in it. Refer back to it in times of sadness.

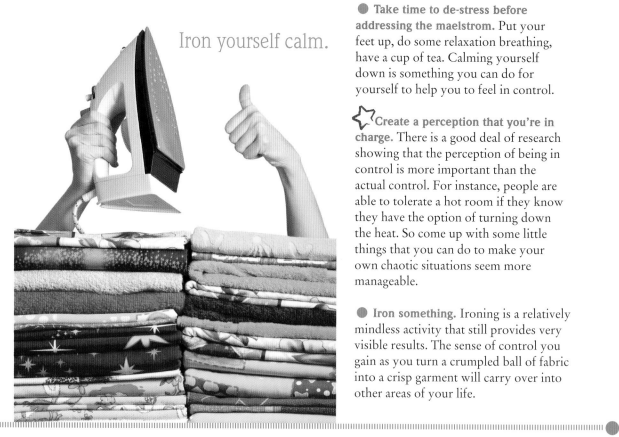

Iron yourself calm.

● **Build up tolerance to chaos** by giving yourself small out-of-control experiences. For instance, if you are typically the main driver of the family car, ask your partner to take the wheel next time you all go out together. Ask someone to interrupt you periodically, invite your partner to make the weekend plans without your input, turn over the bill paying to your partner. These will help you to learn to accept being out of control.

▶ **Practise positive self-talk.** It would be great if someone else did this for you, but often you have to do it for yourself. Self-talk means saying things like, "I'm going to be OK," "I'll get through this" or "Right now, I have to give myself a few minutes, then I can begin coming up with a plan to handle this."

● **Take time to de-stress before addressing the maelstrom.** Put your feet up, do some relaxation breathing, have a cup of tea. Calming yourself down is something you can do for yourself to help you to feel in control.

☆ **Create a perception that you're in charge.** There is a good deal of research showing that the perception of being in control is more important than the actual control. For instance, people are able to tolerate a hot room if they know they have the option of turning down the heat. So come up with some little things that you can do to make your own chaotic situations seem more manageable.

● **Iron something.** Ironing is a relatively mindless activity that still provides very visible results. The sense of control you gain as you turn a crumpled ball of fabric into a crisp garment will carry over into other areas of your life.

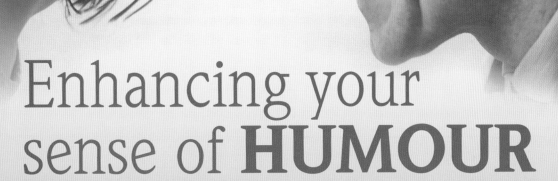

Enhancing your sense of HUMOUR

What is the greatest reward of being alive? Is it chocolate, sex, ice cream, exotic vacations, hugs, a perfect night's sleep or the satisfaction of a job well done? A thousand people, a thousand different answers. But one supreme pleasure that everyone shares is laughter. Little can compare to the feeling of a deep, complete, heartfelt bout of laughter. No matter your age, wealth, race or lifestyle, things are good when laughter is frequent. Life is also healthier. Research finds that humour can help you to cope better with pain, enhance your immune system, reduce stress and even help you to live longer. Here are our 17 tips for getting – or developing – your sense of humour.

17 WAYS TO BRING OUT THE LAUGHTER INSIDE YOU

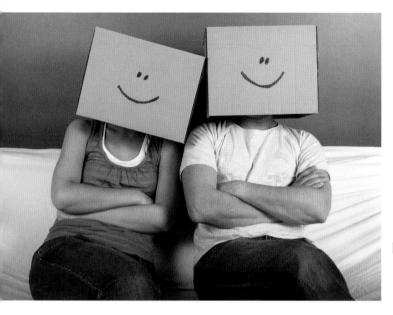

Find someone to be funny with.

First, regain your smile. A smile and a laugh aren't the same thing, but they are related. Be sure to smile at simple pleasures – the sight of children playing, a loved one or friend approaching, the successful completion of a task, the witnessing of something amazing or humorous. Smiles indicate that stress and the weight of the

world haven't overcome you. If your day isn't marked by at least a few dozen, then you need to explore whether you are depressed or overly stressed.

● **Find a humour buddy.** This is someone you can phone just to tell him or her something funny; someone who will also call you with funny stories of things he or she's seen or experienced.

▶ **Treat yourself to a comedy festival.** Rent films such as *Meet the Parents*; *Young Frankenstein*; *Monty Python and the Holy Grail*; *This is Spinal Tap*; *Some Like it Hot*; *Four Weddings and a Funeral*; *Dr. Strangelove*; or *Shrek*. Reward yourself frequently with the gift of laughter.

● **Recall some of the most embarrassing moments in your life.** Then find the humour in them. Now practise telling stories describing them in a funny way. It might take a little exaggeration or dramatization, but that's what good storytelling is all about. By revealing your vulnerable moments and being self-deprecating, you open yourself up much more to the humorous aspects of life.

● **Any time something annoying and frustrating occurs,** turn it on its head and find the humour. Of course, you can be angry at getting splashed with mud, stepping in dog poo or inadvertently throwing a red towel in with the white wash. In fact, that is probably the most normal response. But it doesn't accomplish anything other than to put you in a sour mood. Better to find a way to laugh at life's little annoyances. One way to do that: think about it as if it happened to someone else, someone you like – or maybe someone you don't. Laugh at him or her, then laugh at yourself.

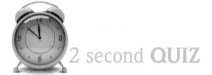

2 second QUIZ

To tease or not to tease?
ANSWER: **TEASE.**

But there are rules. One, do it with love, not hostility. Two, both teaser and teasee must be in on the fun. Third, you must be willing and able to reverse roles. Teasing is a way of highlighting the humour in our idiosyncrasies. Get used to being teased as a way of seeing the humour in yourself. But if someone's feelings get hurt, it's time to re-examine the ground rules.

● **Read the comics every day** and cut out the ones that remind you of your life. Post them on a bulletin board, the fridge or anywhere else you can see them.

● **Sort through family photographs and write funny captions** or one-liners to go with your favourites. When you need a pick-me-up, pull out the album.

● **Every night at dinner,** make family members share one funny or even embarrassing moment from their day.

● **When a person offends you or makes you angry,** respond with humour rather than hostility. For instance, if someone is always late, say, "Well, I'm glad you're not running an airline." Life is too short to turn every personal affront into a battle. However, if you are constantly offended by someone in particular, yes, take it seriously and take appropriate action. But for occasional troubles, or if nothing you do can change the person or situation, take the humorous route.

● **Spend 15 minutes a day having a giggling session.** Here's how you do it: you and one or more people (partner, child, friend, etc.) lie on the floor with your head on someone's stomach, and his or her head on another person's stomach and so on (the more people the better). The first person says, "Ha." The next person says, "Ha-ha." The third person says, "Ha-ha-ha." And so on. You'll be laughing in no time.

● **Read the activity listings page** in the newspaper and choose some laugh-inducing events to attend. It could be the circus, a film, a stand-up comedian or a funny play. Sometimes it takes a professional to get you to regain your sense of humour.

Do you even *have* a SENSE OF HUMOUR?

To evaluate your own sense of humour, consider these questions:

● Do I see the existence or possibility of funny stories in the absurd moments in my life?
● Do I spontaneously laugh out loud when I notice something funny?
● Am I able to share my amusing insights with others?

If all you're doing is answering no, then you need to spend some extra time working through the advice in this chapter.

● **When you run into friends or colleagues,** ask them to tell you one funny thing that has happened to them in the past couple of weeks. Become known as a person who wants to hear humorous true stories as opposed to an individual who prefers to hear gossip.

● **Add an item to your daily to-do list:** find something to laugh at. Don't mark it off until you do it.

☺ **Exaggerate and overstate problems.** Making the situation bigger than life can help us to regain a humorous perspective. Cartoon caricatures and slapstick comedy are all based on exaggeration.

● **Develop a silly routine to break a dark mood.** It could be something as silly as speaking with a comic voice or doing a funny dance.

● **Experiment with jokes.** Learn one simple joke each week and share it.

● **Focus humour on yourself.** For example, if you're a bit thin on top, tell people you're a former expert on how to cure baldness.

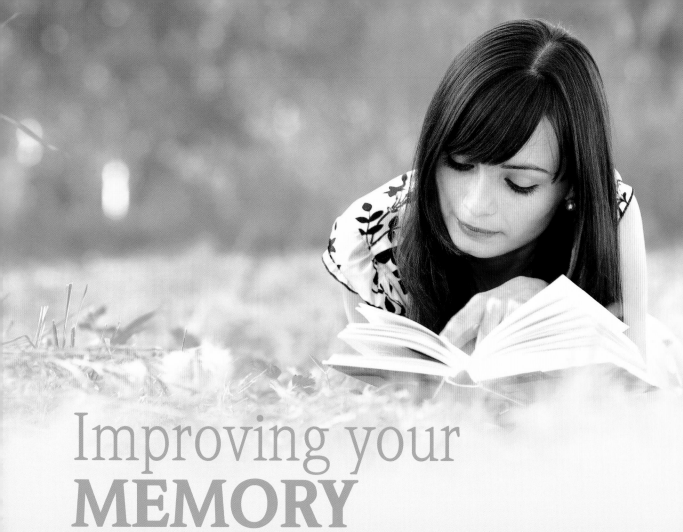

Improving your
MEMORY

Five things you need to buy at the supermarket – forgotten. The name of your neighbour's son – lost. The magazine you wanted to show a colleague – left at home. Relax. These little memory meltdowns are an inevitable part of life. In most cases, they have nothing to do with Alzheimer's, nothing to do with disease or injury, and everything to do with stress, too much work and daily chaos. The good news is that there has been massive research into the origins and maintenance of memory. If you think you have a serious memory decline, seek medical attention, of course. But if you're just trying to have fewer "senior moments," you'll find some help in the following 25 tips.

25 TRICKS TO KEEP YOUR BRAIN IN SHAPE

● **Use it or lose it: the golden rule of brainpower.** The brain functions like a muscle in that the more you use it, the stronger it gets. Watching lots of unstimulating TV, having a routine job, cooking, cleaning and shopping the same way over and over – all contribute to a loss of brainpower. Learning new things, varying your routines, having provocative discussions, going on exciting trips and playing a musical instrument all cause your brain to make new connections and function better.

☆ **Take a B-complex vitamin pill.** As you age, your body becomes less efficient at absorbing certain B vitamins from food. Yet the Bs are critical for maintaining a sharp memory. A study of 260 healthy men and women over the age of 60 found that those with low blood levels of vitamins C or B_{12} scored the worst on memory and cognitive functioning tests. Those with low levels of the B vitamins riboflavin or folic acid scored worst on a test of abstract thinking. Another study found that giving women a B-complex supplement improved their performance on memory tests. B vitamins also help to lower levels of artery-clogging homocysteine, linked to memory loss. Two other supplements to take along with your Bs are vitamins E and C. Studies find that taking the two together can protect against Alzheimer's. But taking the supplements separately (for example, one in the morning and one at night) had no effect.

● **Put whole-grain bread back into your diet.** If you've been following a high-protein, low-carb diet and simultaneously finding your memory going, it's probably not a coincidence. More than any other organ, the brain relies on glucose for fuel. And glucose comes from carbs.

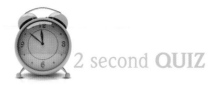

2 second QUIZ

Corn or canola oil?
ANSWER: **CANOLA OIL.**

Canola oil is high in omega-3 fatty acids, which help to reduce inflammation in the brain that can affect cognitive functioning (in other words, your ability to think clearly).

One study of 22 older people from the University of Toronto found that those whose diets contained the greatest percentage of calories as carbohydrates performed best on memory and task tests. Make sure you're getting your carbs from fruits, vegetables and whole grains, not ice cream, candy and cake.

● **Take up oil painting.** Or fishing, or needlework, or ballroom dancing, or piano. The idea here is to continue stretching your mind around new things and new experiences, which studies find can help to stave off dementia and improve memory.

● **Eat oil-rich fish at least once a week.** Fresh tuna, salmon, trout and mackerel are high in omega-3 fatty acids, important for maintaining memory. A delicious fresh tuna salad, for example, is a real brain treat. (Canned tuna contains some omega-3s).

● **Eat a vegetarian dinner at least once a week.** Low in saturated fat and high in fibre, a veggie meal will boost your efforts to maintain healthy cholesterol levels. That's important in terms of the memory, because high cholesterol levels eventually damage blood vessels, affecting long-term memory and speeding the progression of Parkinson's and Alzheimer's diseases.

Learn new skills like oil painting.

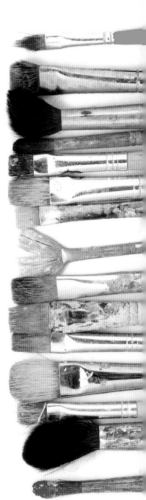

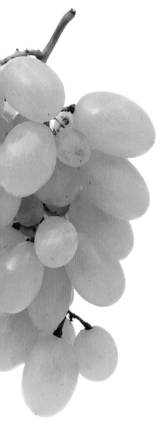

Munch on a delicious bunch of grapes, not cookies.

● Eat cereal mixed with blueberries for breakfast several days a week.
Not only do studies find that eating cereal in the morning can help your performance on certain cognitive tests, but a study in rats who had blueberries every day for two months found that the fruit boosted levels of enzymes which help brain cells communicate with each other. Although the study was done in rats, the lead researcher says the results were so compelling that he now eats a serving or two of blueberries every day – just in case.

● Skip dessert tonight. And tomorrow night as well. It might help you to lose some weight – a good thing when it comes to memory. Swedish researchers found that older women diagnosed with memory problems tended to be an average of 5 to 8 kg (11 to 17 lb) overweight compared to women who had fewer memory lapses. Other studies find that overweight women and men have a higher risk of developing Alzheimer's disease.

● Get a book on CD (or tape) and listen to it while you walk briskly, three times a week. A U.S. study found that older adults who walked that often had higher scores on memory tests than adults who just did stretching and toning exercises.

● Go to bed early the night after learning something important. So if you're learning a new computer program at work, make sure you get a good night's sleep after your training. A Harvard study found that a good night's sleep improves your ability to remember something you learned during the day.

☺ Stuff a chicken with sage and lemons and roast it in the oven at 350°F/180°C until it's done (about 2 hours). A couple of small studies suggest that the anti-inflammatory effects of sage may boost memory for several hours after eating the herb. Plus, lemons are chock-full of antioxidants important for maintaining healthy cell function. Other sage options: try a tea made with a teaspoon of the dried herb; or use it in salad dressing and rice dishes or add it to flavour pork or fish. Try growing some in your garden or in a small container in the kitchen.

☺ Snack on grapes instead of cookies.
Researchers find that people with a high intake of trans fats – found in baked goods like cookies – are more than twice as likely to develop Alzheimer's disease as those who eat the least. Grapes, on the other hand, have phytochemicals and antioxidants that help lead to improved blood flow and overall health.

● Have a glass of wine with dinner. A study of 746 men and women found that those who drank one to six alcoholic beverages (beer, wine or spirits) a week were 54 per cent less likely than abstainers to develop dementia (including Alzheimer's disease and vascular dementia) over six years. Stop at one, though; the same study found that 14 or more drinks a week increased the risk of dementia by 22 per cent.

● Whip up a batch of curried chicken tonight. An Italian study found that this common spice blend appears to enhance an enzyme that protects the brain against oxidative conditions which could lead to memory loss and Alzheimer's.

● Add some tofu cubes to your soup. Soy products such as tofu have isoflavones that also appear to help preserve memory and hinder protein changes which contribute to Alzheimer's.

☆**Read for an hour every day.** But forget Jackie Collins novels. Pick a topic about which you know very little and read five books on that topic. Then move on to the next topic. Your brain will soak up the knowledge like a parched rose bush, sending out blooms in the form of neurons to help to maintain a healthy memory.

● **Memorize a poem every day.** It may remind you of your schooldays, but it's also a great exercise for those memory muscles, aka the brain. Not into poetry? How about memorizing the phone numbers of all your friends, or the addresses of all your family members?

▐▐▌▶ **Do one thing every day that will force you out of your comfort zone.** It might be taking a different route to work, writing or using the mouse with your non-dominant hand, or approaching a total stranger and striking up a conversation (in a safe place, mind you). This kind of challenge is the perfect "weightlifting" exercise for brain cells.

● **Listen to music while you are exercising.** A study of 33 adults undergoing cardiac rehabilitation found that those who listened to music while they worked out improved their scores on a verbal fluency test – a test that measures overall brainpower.

● **Spend a day exploring in an unfamiliar town.** The challenge that comes from following a map, coupled with the novelty that new sights, sounds and smells bring, serves as a healthy wake-up call for your brain.

● **Get a course book from your local college and pick one class to take next term.** An American study found that people who had higher levels of education

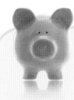

Healthy **INVESTMENT**

A book of crossword puzzles
Doing crossword puzzles is to the brain what a treadmill is to your heart and legs. Puzzles activate nearly every important area of the brain, including visual, language and memory systems.

exhibited fewer signs of Alzheimer's disease even when autopsies revealed that they had the disease.

● **Do one thing at a time.** If you're trying to have a phone conversation while checking e-mails, the chances are that you won't remember a word you spoke. A growing body of research finds our increasing tendency to multi-task hinders memory and concentration.

▐▐▌▶ **Pay better attention next time someone tells you his or her name,** or when you put down your keys or park your car. Often the reason we can't remember things is that we're on autopilot when we do them (or hear them). But if you stop for a second when someone introduces him or herself and repeat the name out loud, or stop when you get out of your car at the shopping centre and look – really look – at the spot in which you've parked, you'll remember it better.

● **Study, read and work in a quiet room.** Studies find that noise exposure can slow your ability to rehearse things in your mind, a way of building memory links.

● **Talk with your hands.** That doesn't mean use sign language. Rather, use your hands to emphasize what you're saying. It turns out it's easier for us to speak when we're gesturing, leaving more mental resources available for transferring information into the memory.

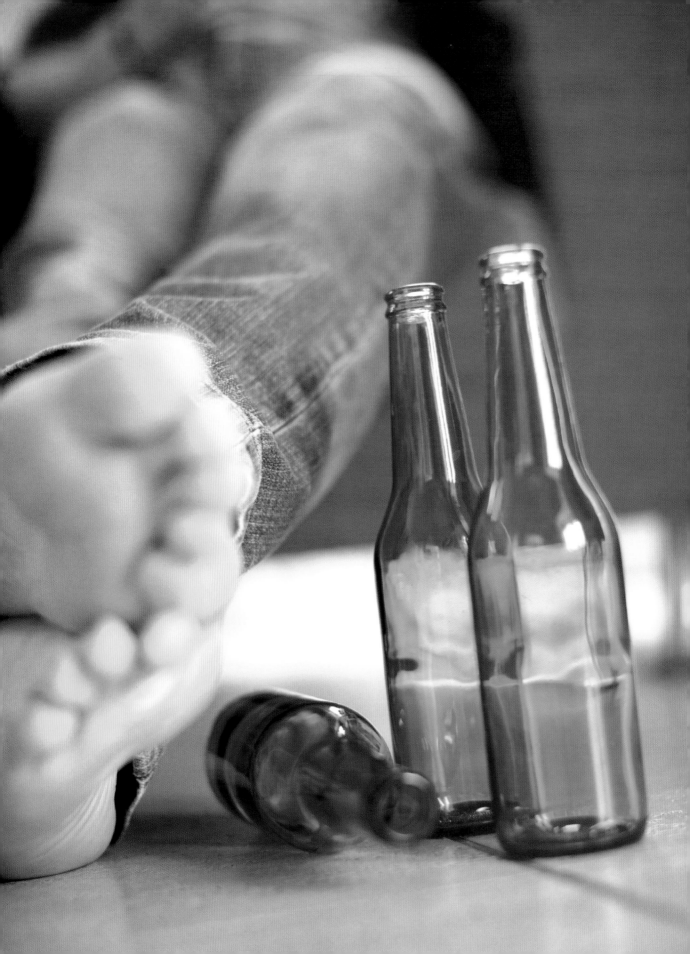

part *7*

STEALTH HABIT CONTROL

It's not the occasional binge or bender that causes lasting damage – it's the unhealthy habits we indulge in every day. Here's some practical advice for kicking bad habits that affect your long-term health.

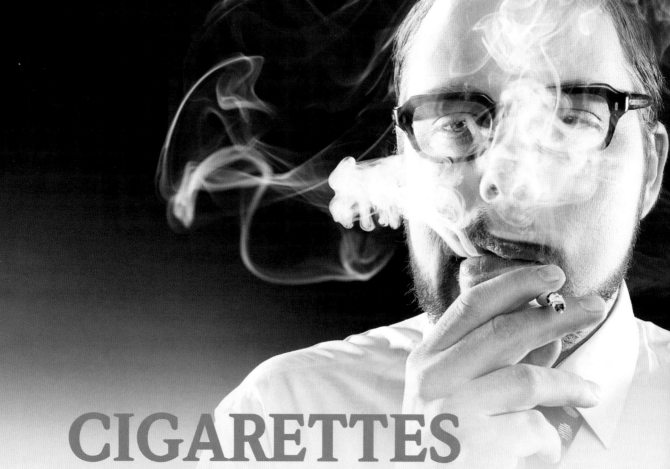

CIGARETTES

For all the intense efforts to reduce smoking over the past two decades, the progress has not been stellar. According to Health Canada, the smoking rate for Canadians 15 and older has gone from 23 per cent in 1999 to 18 per cent in 2008. Seventy-five per cent of Canada's smokers (or 3,670,767 people) light up every day, while the remaining 25 per cent are occasional smokers. The burden is high: Smoking kills over 47,000 Canadians every year, with 96 of those deaths being children under the age of one. And that's not even going into the other effects, like gastrointestinal problems, bone density loss, prematurely aging ... So why do millions still smoke? In part, because nicotine is highly addictive. But smoking also provides psychological comfort. The good news: never before have there been so many tools, systems and programs available to help you stop smoking. The following 23 tips will also help you to succeed.

23 WAYS TO PUT THE BUTTS BEHIND YOU

● **Make an honest list of all the things you like about smoking.** Draw a line down the centre of a piece of paper and write them on one side; on the other side list the things you dislike, such as how it can interfere with your health, work, family, etc. Think about the list over time, and make changes. If you're brave enough, get feedback from family and friends about the things they don't like. When the negative side outweighs the positive side, you're ready to quit.

● **Then make another list of why quitting won't be easy.** Be thorough, even if the list becomes long and discouraging. Next to each entry, list one or more options for overcoming that challenge. For instance, one item might be: "Nicotine is an addictive drug." Your option might be: "Try a nicotine replacement." Another reason might be: "Smoking helps me to deal with stress." Your option might be: "Take a walk instead." The more you anticipate the challenges to quitting, and the solutions, the better your chance of success.

● **Set a quit date** and write a "quit date contract" that includes your signature and that of a supportive witness.

● **Write all of your reasons for stopping** on an index card and keep it near you at all times. Here are some to get you started: "My son, my granddaughter, my partner …" You get the idea.

● **As you're getting ready to quit, stop buying cartons of cigarettes.** Instead, buy just a pack at a time, and carry only two or three cigarettes with you (put them in a small tin or a cigarette case). Eventually you'll find that when you want to smoke, you won't have any cigarettes instantly available. That will slowly wean you off.

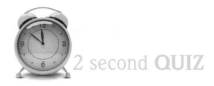
● **Keep a list of when you smoke,** what you're doing at the time and how bad the craving is for a week before quitting to see if specific times of the day or activities increase your cravings. Then arrange fun, absorbing or simply alternative things to do during those times. Suggestions include: take a walk, drink a glass of water, throw a ball for the dog, wash the car, clean out a closet, have sex, chew a piece of gum, brush your teeth, take a nap, get a cup of coffee or tea, practise deep breathing, light a candle.

● **When your date to quit arrives, throw out anything that reminds you of smoking.** That includes all smoking paraphernalia – leftover cigarettes, matches, lighters, ashtrays, even the lighter in your car. Check out Health Canada's On the Road to Quitting program at www.hc-sc.gc.ca for information and resources.

Choose sugarfree gum as your new habit.

Watch your savings increase when you stop smoking.
Use the money for something special you thought you could never afford.

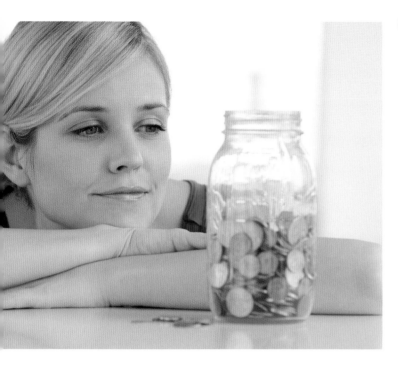

☺ **Put all the money you're saving on cigarettes in a large glass jar.** You want to see physically how much you've been spending. Earmark that money for something you've always dreamed of doing, but never thought you could afford, be it a Caribbean cruise or an exotic long-haul trip.

● **Make an appointment with an acupuncturist.** There's some evidence that auricular acupuncture (needles in the ears) curbs cigarette cravings quite successfully.

● **Think of difficult things you have done in the past.** Ask people who know you well to remind you of challenges you have successfully overcome. This will give you the necessary self-confidence to stick with your pledge not to smoke.

● **To minimize cravings, change your routine.** Sit in a different chair at breakfast or take a different route to work. If you usually have a drink and a cigarette after work, change that to a walk. If you're used to a smoke with your morning coffee, switch to tea, or stop at a coffee shop (where you know you can't smoke on the premises) for a cup of coffee.

● **Instead of a cigarette break at work, play a game of solitaire on your computer.** It takes about the same time and is much more fun (although, like cigarettes, it can get addictive). If your company prohibits playing games, find another 5 minute diversion: a phone call, a stroll or eating a piece of fruit outdoors (but not where smokers congregate).

● **Have a cup of herbal tea whenever you usually have a cigarette.** That might be at breakfast, midmorning or after meals. The act of brewing the tea and slowly sipping it as it cools will provide the same stress relief as a hit of nicotine.

☺ **Swap your cigarette habit for a nut habit** – eat four nuts in their shells for every cigarette you want to smoke. This way, you're using your hands and your mouth, getting the same physical and oral sensations you get from smoking.

● **Tell your friends, colleagues, boss, partner, children, etc. how you feel** about situations instead of bottling up your emotions. If something makes you angry, express it instead of smothering it with cigarette smoke. If you're bored, admit to yourself that you're bored and find something energetic to do instead of lighting up.

● **If you relapse, just start again.** You haven't failed. Some people have to try quitting as many as eight times before they're successful.

● **Switch to decaf** until you've been cigarette-free for two months. Too much caffeine while quitting can cause the jitters.

● **Create a smoke-free zone.** Don't allow anyone to use tobacco in your home or car. Make "No Smoking" signs for the house and car.

☺ **Find a healthy snack food** you can keep with you and use it in place of cigarettes to quench that urge for oral gratification. For instance, try pistachios, sunflower seeds, sugarfree lollipops or chewing gum, carrots or celery sticks. The last two are best if you're concerned about weight gain.

● **Picture yourself playing tennis.** Or go and play tennis. British researchers found that volunteers trying to quit smoking were better able to ignore the urge to smoke when they were told to visualize a tennis match.

● **Quit when you're in a good mood.** Studies find that you're less likely to be a successful quitter if you stop when you're depressed or under a great deal of stress.

● **Stick this list in a visible location in your house.** When you're tempted to light up, take a look at all the ways in which smoking can damage your health. It:
● Increases the risk of lung, bladder, pancreatic, mouth, esophageal and other cancers, including leukemia.
● Reduces fertility.
● Contributes to thin bones.
● Affects mental capacity and memory.
● Reduces levels of folate; low levels can increase your risk of heart disease, depression and Alzheimer's disease.
● Increases the likelihood of impotence.
● Results in premature babies of low birth weight.

● Increases the risk of depression in adolescents.
● Affects the ability to smell and taste.
● Raises the risk of heart disease, stroke, high blood pressure.
● Increases the risk of diabetes.
● Heightens your child's risk of obesity and diabetes later in life if you smoked while pregnant.

● **And put this list by your bedside to boost your morale.** Every day that you survive without a cigarette is a triumph. So just before you sleep, take a look at this list to encourage your efforts and help you to monitor the benefits. After:
● 24 hours, carbon monoxide is eliminated from your body.
● 48 hours, your ability to taste and smell improves.
● 72 hours, you'll notice your breathing gets easier.
● One month, your skin looks better.
● One year, your risk of a heart attack reduces by up to 50 per cent compared to that of a smoker.
● Five years, your risk of dying prematurely from heart disease or stroke is almost the same as that of someone who's never smoked.

Healthy INVESTMENT

A proven smoking-cessation aid
Get a recommendation from your doctor or pharmacist for a prescription or over-the-counter aid such as Zyban tablets, a nicotine inhaler or nicotine gum, lozenges or patches. Make sure you use as directed; too many smokers don't use large enough doses or stop using the aid too soon – and find themselves puffing away again.

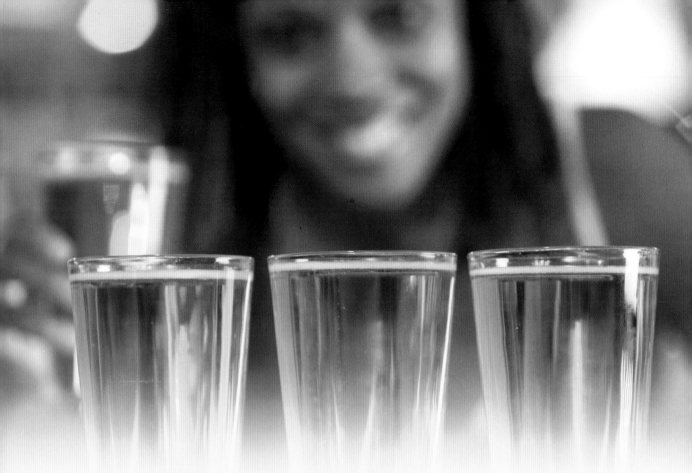

ALCOHOL

People often don't realize they have a drinking problem. Unlike other health-destroying habits, such as illegal drugs, drinking is something that most adults do, and it's quite healthy in moderation. Moreover, it's woven into our cultural fabric. So how do you know when your drinking has become a problem? Look for the small signs, such as waking in the middle of the night with a raging thirst or finding it harder to get out of bed in the morning. If this is you, it may be time to cut back. This chapter will help you to do it. One caveat, though: alcoholism is a serious disease. If you think you might be, or you know you are, an alcoholic, you need more help, so please see your doctor.

16 WAYS TO CUT BACK ON YOUR DRINKING

● **For optimal health, limit your drinking** to a level slightly lower than "Safe limits" (see below): up to two drinks a day for men, one for women with at least one day off alcohol each week. And no stockpiling: going without alcohol today doesn't increase the amount you can have tomorrow. In particular, you can't save up for a weekend binge.

● **Meet friends, dates or business associates at a coffee bar, not a pub.** If the point of the get-together is fun, casual conversation in a friendly environment, there are many ways to do that without the alcohol. Coffee shops and cafés are good places to meet. Other possibilities include bistro-style restaurants, bowling alleys and even sushi bars.

● **Never, ever drink alone.** Make it a rule. Not because it is so evil – indeed, there are plenty of times when a glass of wine by yourself is appropriate. Rather, do it for the discipline. If you get into the habit of drinking alone, it's too easy to start drinking excessive amounts.

✰ **Never, ever drink out of habit.** You know what that means: "7 o'clock, time for my martini," "Finished mowing the lawn, time for a beer," "Friday night, time to hit the pub with the gang and have my weekly drinks." Think through your week to see if you have a specific drinking routine or habit. If yes, commit to finding a substitute for it.

☺ **Never, ever drink for solace.** It's the old stereotype: sad-faced businessman, sitting at the bar, tie yanked down, clothes dishevelled, muttering, "Pour me another one, bartender." Sad, isn't it, numbing yourself from the challenges of the world through alcohol? Drink for joy, not pain. Drink to feel alive, not dead.

In PERSPECTIVE

Do I have a problem?

If you're wondering if your drinking – or a loved one's – has crossed the line, answer the following questions:

● Have you ever felt you should cut down on your drinking?
● Have people upset you by criticizing your drinking?
● Have you ever felt bad or guilty about your drinking?
● Have you ever had a drink first thing in the morning to steady your nerves or to get rid of a hangover?

One yes answer suggests a possible alcohol problem. More than one yes answer means it's highly likely that a problem exists.

✰ **Never, ever drink for courage.** People have long turned to drink to overcome social inhibitions. In fact, there's an old expression for alcohol: "Dutch courage." It's true – a few drinks can take the fright out of a party or business gathering but

SAFE limits

The Centre for Addiction and Mental Health in Toronto recommends a safe drinking limit of 2 standard drinks per day, up to 14 per week for men, or 9 per week for women. But not all drinks are created equal, so here's a small chart to clarify what's what with those after-dinner beverages. One standard drink is:

One 341 ml (12 oz) beer – 5% alcohol

One 142 ml (5 oz) glass of wine – 10–12% alcohol

One 89 ml (3 oz) glass of fortified wine – 16–18% alcohol

One 43 ml (1.5 oz) glass of spirits – 40% alcohol

Coolers and high-alcohol beers count as more than one standard drink.

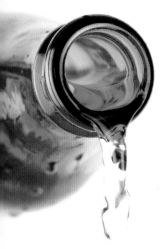

problems begin when you rely on alcohol for bravery. No one should need alcohol to function socially. So find other ways to bolster your confidence. It's harder, but healthier and more honest – and you're less prone to making alcohol-induced gaffes.

● **In particular, choose a pleasant alternative to your after-work drink.** It could be a non-alcoholic drink, such as an iced tea or fruit smoothie. Or it could be a walk, a hot bath, a sliced peach. Do it for two weeks so it becomes your new habit.

● **Switch to mixed drinks with a lower-proof alcohol.** There are lots of alternatives to the standard, high-power alcohols of gin, vodka or whisky. For example, a flavoured cognac with soda water has half the alcohol content of a gin drink, and probably twice the flavour.

▶ **Always drink two-fisted: your drink, and a large glass of water.** Don't use alcohol to quench your thirst. That's what water is for. Sip on alcohol for the flavour.

● **Dilute your drinks with soda water.** It doesn't contain the sugar in fruit juices or colas and still mixes well with wine

The bubbles in soda water will help you to cut your alcohol consumption.

and whisky. This can help you to cut down on alcohol consumption, not just because it dilutes your drink, but also because the bubbles make you feel full.

● **Keep the wine bottle off the dinner table.** It makes it too easy to keep pouring until it's empty. Instead, keep a jug of water on the table. Then pour one glass of wine, cork the bottle and put it away.

● **Create a list of rules for drinking.** For instance, no more than one drink a day. Drink only on the weekend. Drink only wine spritzers. Drink only when you're dressed up in your best clothes, etc. Post the list near the drinks cabinet/wine rack.

● **Keep a drinking diary.** Tracking how much you drink may provide you with some surprising information that will encourage you to cut down or quit.

● **Make a list of reasons why you want to cut back on drinking.** These could be: lose weight, sleep better, fewer headaches, get more done, improve blood sugar control, better sex, perform better at work. Stick the list in a prominent place and read through it every time you think about having a drink.

● **Work out how much money you're spending on alcohol every week.** Now commit to spending half that amount. Put the savings into a special account (or even a large glass jar) and use it for something special for you (not a bottle of 2006 shiraz).

● **Tell everyone you know that you're cutting back on your drinking.** The hope is that this will prevent people from urging you to have "just one" or "just one more."

2 second QUIZ

Wine or gin and tonic?
ANSWER: **WINE.**

Not only does a glass of wine provide more volume for the alcohol (meaning it lasts longer so you'll drink less), but the health benefits of wine are legendary. Choose red wine over white for maximum health benefits.

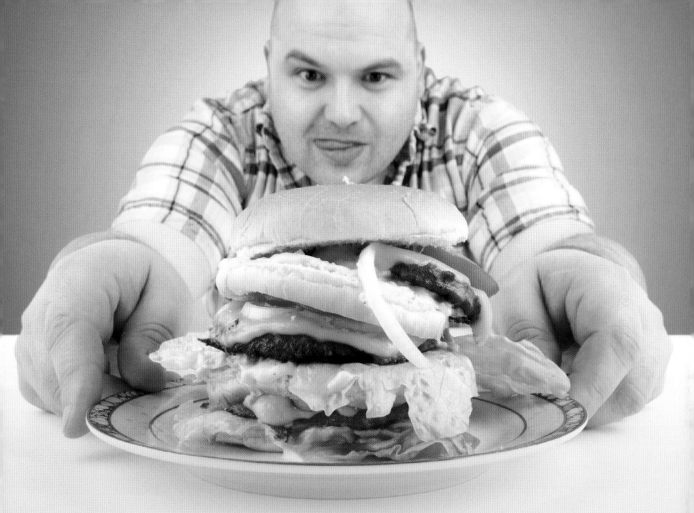

OVEREATING

What is it about food? Serve up a plate with a normal-sized portion and no other food on the table, and you'll eat it and probably be quite satisfied. But put yourself before an all-you-can-eat buffet and suddenly your hunger sensor goes on the blink and you eat until you have to loosen your belt. Whether you need to lose weight or you're just tired of leaving the table feeling as if you've swallowed a beach ball, the following tips will help you to curb your appetite and eat just enough – and no more.

24 WAYS TO STOP COMPULSIVE CONSUMPTION

⭐ **Purge your home of low-nutrition snack food.** That means ice cream, candy, chips, cookies, doughnuts, cake and any other salty or sugary snacks that you munch on between meals. Learn to live without this unhealthy stuff. Period. These are the foods that we eat compulsively and that make us overweight. From now on, eat these foods only when offered them at a social event, or when you and the family deserve a special treat.

● **In its place, stock your home with** mounds of fresh fruit, dried fruit, carrots, celery, tomatoes, granola bars and high-fibre breakfast cereal. These are your new snack foods.

In PERSPECTIVE

Binge-eating disorder

How do you know if you're simply eating too much or whether you have an actual eating disorder called binge-eating disorder? Well, how do you eat?

If your overeating generally occurs when you eat out, encounter a buffet or are served your all-time favourite food, you probably have nothing to worry about. But if you find you have episodes in which you eat faster than normal, eat until you're uncomfortably full, eat large amounts of food when you're not even hungry, eat alone because you're embarrassed by how much you're eating, feel disgusted with yourself, or depressed or very guilty after overeating, then you might have a problem.

Key symptoms are recurrent episodes of binge eating characterized by eating an excessive amount of food within a short period of time and by a sense of lack of control over eating during the episode.

If you think you might have binge-eating disorder – or if you make yourself vomit after bingeing, a condition called bulimia – see your doctor immediately. Therapy and medication can help you to bring it under control.

● **Never, ever stop at a store just to buy a snack.** Don't stop at the bakery for a quick Danish or doughnut. No candies or chocolate bars from the corner store on your way to or from work. No pizza slice from your local takeout. This kind of compulsive, unhealthy eating is contributing to many of our nation's widespread weight problems.

☺ **Make this simple salad to fill you up – the healthy way.** Feel desperate for a big bowl of crunchy food? Make a salad from half a head of shredded iceberg lettuce; a handful of bite-size carrots; half a tomato, sliced up; and half a cucumber, sliced. Drizzle on olive oil, shake on a little balsamic vinegar, sprinkle on some oregano, salt and pepper, and mix. This is a huge bowl of flavour-packed food for relatively few calories.

● **Yet another splurge food: vegetable soup.** Need comfort food? Heat up a large bowl of soup made with lots of vegetables and beans. It's flavourful, hearty and generally high in nutrition and low in fat.

☺ **One more great snack option: nuts in their shells.** The truth is, compulsive eating is often about boredom, stress and other non-food issues. The great thing about nuts is that the effort to crack the shells and extract the nut without breaking it is highly therapeutic and distracting. In addition, nuts are very healthy to eat (in moderation). Choose walnuts, almonds, pecans, Brazil nuts or hazelnuts. Peanuts and pistachios are too quick to open so you can easily overindulge.

● **Get picky.** Parents complain about children who are finicky eaters, but you're not a child, and you owe it to yourself to be a bit persnickety when it

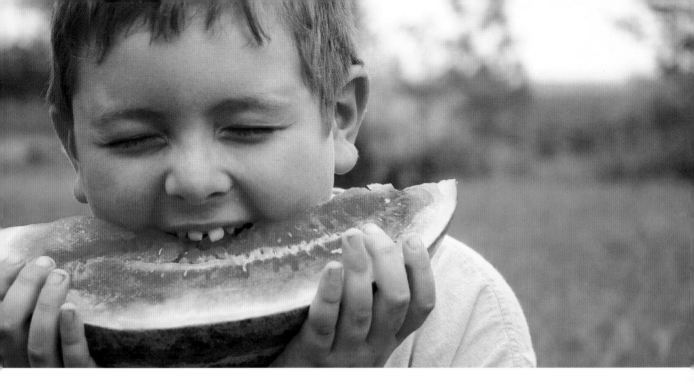

If you feel the need for a hearty helping of food, what could be healthier than a big slice of watermelon?

comes to what goes into your mouth. As a rule of thumb: if it doesn't look good, don't eat it. Watch naturally thin people: you won't see them scoffing down leftover cake or what's left in the bowl when the soup's gone cold. Follow their example.

● **Another splurge food: watermelon.** It's more than 90 per cent water, and the other 10 per cent has plenty of healthy nutrients and reasonable calorie levels. If you want to indulge in a hearty helping of food, dig deeply into a big slice of watermelon.

● **Get into the habit of ordering the small size.** There's no need to feel deprived. Today's small was the medium or large just a few decades back. Eat (or sip) slowly. Savour the flavours. Before long, small will feel just right. Besides, remember that ordering the small size leads to wearing the small size.

● **Always choose the best from what's available.** Sometimes you'll have lots of great choices – at a farmers' market, say, or a restaurant that specializes in healthy food. At other times you'll be on the road and have to choose from three fast-food places. Either way, pick the best in your current situation – a combination of what's most nutritious, most attractive, the right price and what you feel like eating.

▶ **When possible allow up to half an hour between your last bite of dinner and dessert.** A pause will give your brain time to get the fullness signal and make it easier for you to skip the sweet stuff.

● **Eat portions the size of the palm of your hand only.** Any more will be considered overeating.

☺ **Always put what you're eating on a plate or in a bowl.** Never eat out of the bag, package or box.

● **Have a healthy snack before going out to eat.** It will help you to avoid the tempting bread basket.

● **As soon as you feel the first stirrings of fullness,** remove your plate from the table or, if you're dining out, cover your plate with a napkin. This tells your brain that food time is over.

● **Dine to soothing music, not the television.** This signals that mealtime is to be enjoyed and savoured. You'll be more aware of what you're eating, will eat slower and will get the "full" signal sooner, thus eating less.

● **Put your snack foods into single-serving containers.** For instance, don't leave a huge tub of ice cream in your freezer; if you do, it's far too easy to add that second or third scoop when you're dishing it out. Instead, when you get home from the supermarket, scoop the appropriate serving size into individual containers and freeze. Make sure you're not hungry when you do it, so that you're not tempted to increase the size or sneak a bite. And buy only single-portion snacks for yourself.

Healthy INVESTMENT

A dinner belt
The idea is to have one belt that you wear while eating, to gauge your level of fullness. Wear it buckled firmly around your waist when you're about to eat dinner, using the same hole each evening. As soon as you feel the least amount of strain against the belt, put your fork down and cover your plate with your napkin. You've finished.

● **Don't talk while you're still chewing.** Instead, put your fork down, chew, then swallow your food before you begin talking. Again, this will force you to slow down while eating, and you'll be full (and feel full) before you know it.

● **Don't snack on leftovers.** Make it a habit immediately to cover and keep what you can re-use and toss what you can't.

● **Write down every morsel you eat in a food diary.** It's likely you've been overlooking some calories. Seeing all that you eat in black and white will help to keep you from overeating.

● **Ditch the restrictive or fad diets.** They will only make you crave certain foods, leading to binge eating.

● **Limit the amount of artificial sweeteners and artificially sweetened foods you eat.** One American study published in July 2004 found that consuming artificially sweetened foods and beverages may throw off your natural ability to monitor calories and increase your likelihood of overeating.

☺ **Practise the 20 minute distraction strategy.** When you find yourself looking for food, even though you're not hungry, do something else for 20 minutes, something that involves your brain as well as your hands, such as playing the piano. If you feel that you really are hungry, set your kitchen timer for 20 minutes – if you still want to eat when it rings, fine. If not, the urge will have passed.

● **Have a nutritious snack** such as a handful of peanuts, a piece of fruit and cheese or a yogourt about an hour before dinner. Keeping your appetite in check is one of the best ways to avoid binges.

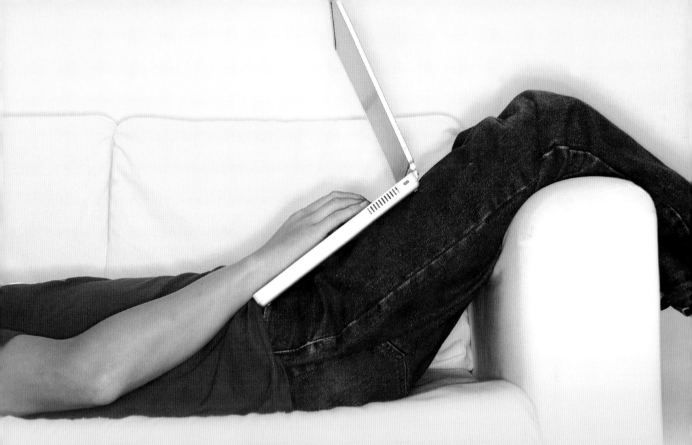

TV & PC addiction

Though the stats vary slightly from province to province or territory, Canadian adults average 23.25 hours of TV watching per week, and three-quarters of our households have computers. The Canadian Radio-television and Telecommunications Commission states that the average connected Canadian spends over 15 hours per week surfing the Net. Add on the time some people spend playing video games, and Canadians start to look like a pretty sedentary bunch. Just as TV watching has been linked to higher rates of obesity and diabetes, this extra sedentary computer time is bad news for the nation's health. Like kicking any habit, half the battle is acknowledging the problem and committing to change. Here are specific tips to help.

16 WAYS TO ESCAPE THE SCREEN

☆Give the extra TV to charity. Allow your home one TV in a room dedicated to nothing but reading or TV watching. Donate the rest to a school or charitable organization in your community. You'll feel good, and it will be that much harder to veg out in front of the TV.

🖵 Turn on the TV only to watch a particular show. In other words, don't just turn it on and go surfing for something worthwhile. Hours are quickly wasted, jumping from one show to the next, watching all and none at the same time. And, if your TV works without the remote, rather than surf, get up to change channels on the set.

🖵 Then, when you sit down to watch a particular program, set a timer or an alarm clock in another room for the length of the show. When it beeps, you'll have to get out of your chair to turn it off, a signal to turn off the TV as well.

⫸ Set a rule that you can't watch TV or surf the Internet if the sun is shining. Instead, you have to go for a walk, ride a bike or get some other kind of healthy physical activity for at least an hour before you can turn on the TV or PC. This rule also works well for your children or grandchildren.

Healthy INVESTMENT

Knitting needles and a ball of wool
Learn to knit while you watch television; it will keep you from eating your way through the evening, and you'll accomplish something productive.

🖵 Rearrange the furniture. Design your family room so that the television is no longer the focal point of the room, but an afterthought that requires twisting around or rearranging chairs to view it.

⫸ Hide the television. Put it behind a screen, hang a cover over it or stick it inside a cabinet. Do whatever you can to ensure it fades into the background and can't be seen when it's off.

⫸ Eat meals, especially dinner, with the television and computer firmly OFF. And ensure that every family member knows that eating at the computer is a no-no at any time. That goes for the game console as well.

🖵 Make a TV-watching plan each week. Sit down with the viewing guide and pick out the shows you want to watch that week. View only those shows and, when they're over, turn the TV off.

🖵 Set surfing, MSN and Facebook limits. Social networks have transformed computer use among the young and the old. Or you may just love to blog, check news websites or search for books or vacations. Time flies. But set yourself limits – no more than an hour an evening, say. And then try to do something more physical.

🖵 Make a rule that you must read 30 pages of a book or magazine before you can turn on the TV or PC. Pick the right reading matter and you'll soon find you've created a new addiction.

🖵 Create a list of 1 hour evening projects. List everything you can possibly dream of: cleaning a particularly messy closet, organizing recipes, touching up the paint on your bedroom walls, sharpening kitchen knives, sorting through your sewing materials. Then try to do one each evening.

 Choose games. With your partner and/or children, relearn the fun of Scrabble, backgammon or chess. Get out the playing cards and have a hearts or gin rummy battle. Play Ping-Pong, pool or darts. Go outside and work on your golf swing with practice balls. All of these are more fun, healthy and life-affirming than sitting in front of a TV or computer.

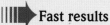 **Develop a fast-moving news routine.** Most news programs are scheduled down to the minute. So investigate the handful of programs you watch and figure out when they run the features you are most interested in, for example, the local weather, the recap of the day's headlines or the sports news. Watch when you get home, then turn off the television for the rest of the night.

 Say no to watching *Jaws* – yet again. Often we can be strangely drawn into watching things we've seen many times before. There's something comforting in the repetition. Well, resist it. Viewing the same thing again and again is unhealthy for your body and your brain.

Get outdoors every night. Make a point of leaving your home at least once after dinner, if only for a short walk. Too many of us consider the day pretty much done once we've eaten dinner when, in fact, evening can be a wonderful time for having fun, particularly on long summer evenings.

Change your TV-viewing chairs. Make them somewhat hard and upright – chairs you don't want to lounge in for hours. Move your most comfy chairs to the living room, for listening to music and reading.

Make the most of those long summer evenings.

Reminder

Fast results
These are tips that deliver benefits particularly quickly – in some cases, immediately.

Easy gains
These are health boosters that offer the best value for the least amount of effort.

Super-effective
This is advice that scientific research or widespread usage by experts has shown to be especially effective.

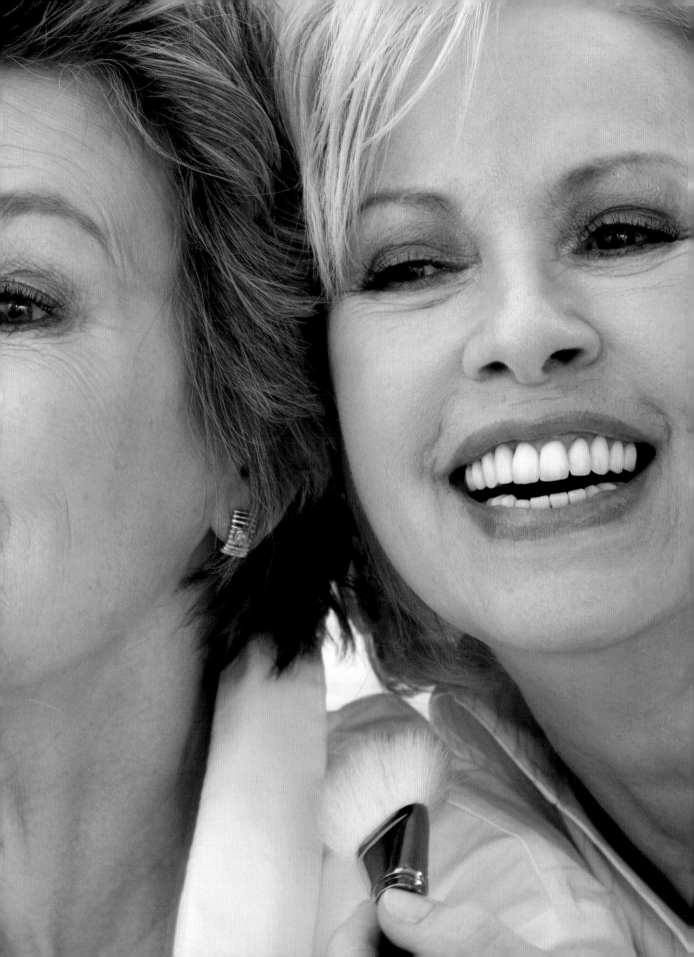

part 8

STEALTH HEALTHY LOOKS

Let's be honest. Looking good feels good. But appearance isn't just about vanity; healthy skin and teeth contribute to overall health. Here are easy, fast ways to look your best.

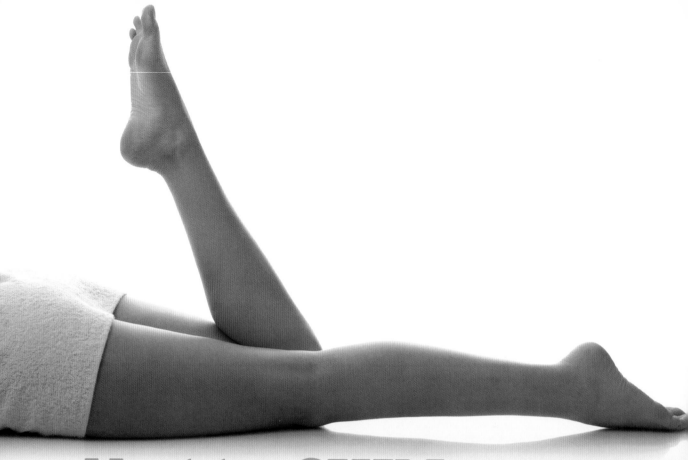

Healthy **SKIN**

Beauty, the saying goes, is only skin-deep. But the importance of skin goes a lot deeper. In particular, your skin is the first layer of your immune system, serving as a shield between you and legions of germs. And, of course, your sense of touch is crucial for everyday functions. Like any part of your internal body, though, your skin can be healthy or sick. In particular, aging causes the skin to become thinner and drier. While you can't control your age, you can control numerous other factors, such as a poor diet and cigarette smoking. Unlike your other organs, you can apply medicines, moisturizers and other potions directly to your skin. So, there's absolutely no reason why you can't have good skin throughout your life, especially if you follow these 37 tips.

37 QUICK TRICKS TO ENHANCE YOUR GLOW

● **Skip long, steamy showers** and opt for shorter, cooler sprays. Long, hot showers strip skin of its moisture and wash away the protective oils. So limit your showers to 10 minutes and keep the water cool.

▌▌▌➤ **Check the dryness of your skin** by scratching a small area on your arm or leg with your fingernail. If it leaves a white mark, your skin is indeed dry and needs both moisture and exfoliation (that is, removal of the outermost layer of dead skin cells).

● **Treat your neck and chest like an extension of your face.** Your neck and upper chest area is covered by very sensitive skin, making it a prime spot for telltale signs of aging — like dryness. To keep this area youthful, use facial cleansing creams that hydrate and cleanse gently rather than deodorant soaps, which can be drying. Top it all off with a good facial moisturizing cream. If this area is extra dry, use a facial moisturizing mask twice a month.

☺ **Run a humidifier every night in winter** to moisturize the air in your bedroom. Not only will it ease itchy, dry skin, but you'll be able to breathe the moist air more easily.

▌▌▌➤ **Switch from a deodorant soap to a special moisturizing product,** such as Dove or Neutrogena. Deodorant soaps can be drying, whereas these specially designed products leave an oily, yet beneficial, film on your skin.

● **Keep your beauty products simple,** particularly if you have sensitive skin. Stay away from anything with colour or fragrance, that produces bubbles or has "antibacterial" on the label.

Do **THREE** things...

If you do only three things to improve the look and feel of your skin, make them these three, agree several of our experts:

1 **Drink at least eight 250 ml glasses of** water a day to stay hydrated. This helps to flush toxins through your kidneys instead of your skin.

2 **Follow a healthy diet rich in fruits, vegetables and fish.** When researchers from Monash University in Australia studied the diets of 453 people aged 70 and older from Australia, Greece and Sweden to see if there was any correlation between what they ate and the number of wrinkles in their skin, they found that those who ate the most fruit, vegetables and fish had the fewest wrinkles. Conversely, the researchers found, foods high in saturated fat, including meat, butter and full-fat dairy products, as well as soft drinks, cakes, pastries and potatoes, increased the likelihood of skin wrinkling.

3 **Protect your skin from the sun all year round with a sunblock that has an SPF of 30 or greater.** Just because there's snow on the ground doesn't mean your skin can't be damaged by the sun. Time outdoors is time well spent, but be sure to keep your skin either well covered or well protected with sunblock. The sun is at its most damaging between 11 a.m. and 4 p.m.

● **Smooth a couple of drops of olive oil over your face, elbows, knees and the backs of your arms** every evening. The oil contains monounsaturated fat, which refreshes and hydrates the skin without leaving a greasy residue.

● **For soft, young-looking hands and feet,** put on plenty of moisturizing cream, then slip on thin fabric socks and gloves while you sleep.

● **Tone your skin with a sage,** peppermint and witch hazel combination. Sage helps to control oil, peppermint creates a cool tingle, and witch hazel helps to restore the skin's protective layer.

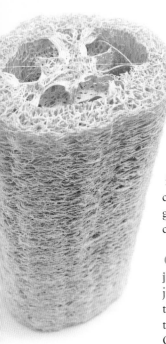

Your skin will thank you for a daily loofah scrub.

Combine 100 g of witch hazel with a teaspoon each of sage and peppermint leaves and steep for one to three days before applying to your skin.

● **Use a loofah every day** to keep ingrown hairs and scaly skin under control. While you're in the shower, gently scrub bumpy or scaly skin with a circular motion to remove dead cells.

● **Start the day with a glass of orange juice to help to build collagen.** Orange juice is rich in vitamin C, essential for the manufacture of collagen, which helps to keep the skin smooth and youthful. Other foods rich in vitamin C include guava, kiwis and red peppers.

● **Take a multivitamin every day.** Many nutrients are vital to healthy skin, including vitamins C, A and B. The most reliable way to get them all is to eat healthily, as well as taking a daily supplement.

● **Use unscented baby powder** to keep areas where skin meets skin – the inner thighs, underarms, beneath the breasts – clean and dry. This helps to prevent intertrigo, an irritating skin condition that occurs when such areas remain moist, allowing bacteria or fungi to grow.

● **If you're gearing up for a day in the sun,** steer clear of scented lotions and perfumes. Scented products can lead to blotchy skin when exposed to the sun.

☺ **To treat dry, rough, itchy skin, try these bath soaks:**
● 225 g of sea salt and 450 g of baking soda. Bathe until the water is cool to detoxify your skin and soothe the itch.
● 250 g of Epsom salts. In addition to soaking in it, while your skin is still wet, rub handfuls of Epsom salts on rough areas to exfoliate the skin.
● A few bags of your favourite tea. The tea provides antioxidants as well as a delicious scent.
● 100 g of uncooked oatmeal tied into an old stocking or muslin bag. Oats are not only wonderful for your inner health, they provide a healthy glow on the outside as well, leaving a film on your skin that seals in water.
● 115 g of powdered milk mixed with 1 tablespoon of grapeseed oil. The lactic acid in the milk will exfoliate your skin, and the grapeseed oil will provide a powerful dose of antioxidants.

● **Apply ice wrapped in a towel to dry, itchy skin.** A few minutes on, a few minutes off. Allow the moist cold to relieve your skin and draw warming blood to it, but don't let your skin get so cold that it stings or hurts.

▌▌▌▶ **Smooth aloe vera gel over extra-dry skin.** The acids in aloe eat away at dead skin cells and speed up the healing process. Buy a pre-prepared product or cut the end off of an aloe leaf, split it open and spread the gel on the dry area.

● **Cook with garlic every day.** A Danish study found that skin cells grown in a culture dish and treated with garlic had

Healthy **INVESTMENT**

A wide-brimmed hat
It provides an extra layer of protection from skin-damaging UVB and UVA rays. It also shields your eyes from direct sunlight. And it keeps the sun off your hair, which is another good thing.

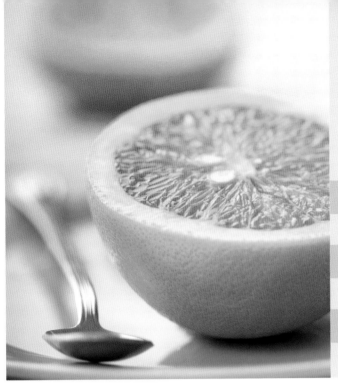

10 foods to eat
FOR GOOD SKIN

The following foods are all rich in antioxidants and other nutrients shown in laboratory studies to benefit skin health:

1 Salmon	6 Blueberries
2 Green tea	7 Flaxseeds
3 Olive oil and olives	8 Fat-free dairy products
4 Sardines	9 Citrus fruits
5 Brazil nuts	10 Avocados

Introduce dry elbows to the power of a grapefruit.

seven times the lifespan of cells grown in a standard culture. They also tended to look healthier and more youthful than untreated cells. Plus, garlic extract dramatically inhibited the growth of cancerous skin cells.

● **Hang room-darkening blinds in your bedroom.** They'll help you to avoid sleep disturbances or insomnia caused by ambient light. Sleep is critical to your skin's health because most cell repair and regeneration occurs while you're out for the count; if you're not getting enough rest, your skin cannot renew itself.

● **Place rough, dry elbows on grapefruit halves.** First exfoliate your elbows in the bath or shower, then cut a grapefruit in half and rest one elbow on one half, one on the other, letting them soak for 15 minutes. The acid in the grapefruit provides extra smoothing power.

● **Go for a run, ride your bike or work in the garden on a hot day** – anything to get you sweating. Sweating is nature's way of eliminating toxic chemicals that can build up under the skin. Plus, regular exercise maintains healthy circulation and blood flow throughout your body, including your skin. If you're exercising outdoors, though, remember to wear a sunscreen on your face that protects against UVA and UVB rays, or a moisturizer with sunscreen protection.

☆ **Grill salmon brushed with olive oil and sprinkled with toasted, crushed walnuts.** You've just had a skin-healthy dose of poly and monounsaturated fats, particularly omega-3 fatty acids, which studies suggest may affect the amount of sun damage and aging your skin experiences. By extension, make sure olive oil is the primary source of fat in your cooking each and every day, and try to have salmon twice a week.

A skincare GLOSSARY

Confused about skincare terminology? Here's what several common terms mean:

● **Collagen.** A protein that contributes to the elasticity of skin tissue.

● **Emollient.** A lotion or cream that helps to make skin smoother and softer.

● **Exfoliant.** Any product that helps to remove dead cells from the skin's surface.

● **Humectant.** A product that promotes the retention of moisture in the skin.

● **Hydration.** The process of bringing more water into the skin tissues.

● **SPF.** Stands for "sun protection factor," a numeric scale used to establish how effective a product is at blocking the harmful rays of sunlight, stopping them from reaching the skin. The higher the number, the greater the protection.

● **AHA.** Stands for alpha-hydroxy acid. A natural acid, often derived from fruit, that helps to slough off dead skin and speed up cell renewal. AHAs have emerged as one of the most important ingredients in skincare.

● **Brew a pot of tea, chill it, then store it in the fridge and drink it throughout the day.** Tea, as you probably know, is a great source of antioxidants, molecules that fight the free-radical damage caused by sun exposure and cigarette smoking. One U.S. study, for instance, found that the more tea people drank (particularly tea with lemon), the less likely they were to develop squamous cell skin cancer.

● **Here's one for men:** recognize that skin-preserving products, such as cleansers and moisturizers, aren't just for women. Men need skincare just as much as their partners and sisters. To prevent wrinkles and skin cancer, use a daily moisturizer containing a sunscreen with an SPF (see left) of at least 30. Also use a gentle exfoliant every week and a nighttime moisturizer.

● **Change your moisturizer every time the season changes.** Your skin needs more moisture in winter than in summer. So when it's time to wear a heavy sweater, it's time to buy a heavier moisturizer. When you swap your sweater for a T-shirt, switch to a lighter one.

● **Prepare a homemade oat scrub** and use it on your face every other day. Oats moisturize and exfoliate your skin at the same time. Grind enough rolled oats in a food processor or coffee grinder to fill $^1/_2$ cup. Mix with $^1/_3$ cup ground sunflower seeds, $^1/_2$ teaspoon of peppermint leaves and 4 tablespoons of ground almonds. Mix 2 teaspoons with a little double cream. Scrub your face and neck with the mixture, then rinse well with cool water.

● **Add a teaspoon of grapeseed oil to your toner.** The oil acts as an anti-aging serum by helping your skin cells to repair and rejuvenate themselves.

☺ **For double protection, apply a cream containing vitamin C to your face over your sunblock.** The cream helps to prevent facial skin damage, dehydration and wrinkles. Also try creams containing vitamin E or beta carotene.

● **Use a spray of rose, sandalwood or bergamot essential oils mixed with water.** These oils are great for hydrating the skin. To create a herbal spray, mix a few drops of essential oil with water in a small spray bottle and spritz on your face whenever your skin needs a little boost. Your skin is more pliable when it's hydrated, so a spray helps to stave off frown lines and general movement wrinkles. The hydrator also keeps pollutants out and retains your skin's natural lubricants. An added bonus: your make-up will stay on for longer and look more natural.

● **Avoid these three skin destroyers:** smoking, tanning salons and sunbathing. All three will age your skin prematurely, many doctors agree.

● **Make your own cleansing, moisturizing masks.**
• Mix 1 tablespoon of plain yogourt with a few dashes of sesame oil. Leave on for 15 minutes, then rinse.
• Mash a banana well and mix with a little honey for an instant dry-skin fix. Leave on for 15 minutes, then rinse.
• Mix together $1/4$ cup (50 ml) of whipping cream, $1/2$ teaspoon of olive oil, 2 tablespoons of ripe, mashed avocado and 1 teaspoon of calendula petals. Leave on for 5 minutes, then rinse. A study completed at the Technion-Israel Institute of Technology found that avocado oil significantly increased the collagen content in skin, maintaining its youthful look. Not only does the oil in avocado act like an emollient, but the fruit also contains moisturizing vitamin E. Another good avocado mix is 1 tablespoon of mashed avocado, 2 egg whites and 2 tablespoons of honey blended until smooth. Leave on for 15 minutes, then rinse.
• Mash peeled mango flesh until it turns soft and pulpy. Then massage it into the skin and leave on for a few minutes before rinsing. This helps to clean and tighten the pores.
• Add 1 tablespoon of peppermint, yarrow, sage or hyssop to 1 cup of boiling water. Steep for 30 minutes, then strain and cool before dabbing it on your face. This is a great skin toner for oily skin.

● **Clean your face and neck with a natural cold cream** and follow with a rose water and glycerine rinse twice a day to remove skin-damaging pollutants.

☺ **Keep your hands off your face.** Because your hands touch so many surfaces, they are a magnet for dirt and germs. Rub your eyes, stroke your chin, cup your cheek and you've transferred everything on your hands to your face. As an extension of this, use headphones or a headset when talking on the phone.

● **Stop with one glass of wine or one alcoholic drink.** Overdoing it enlarges the blood vessels near the surface of your facial skin.

● **De-shine your face throughout the day** by periodically dabbing on loose powder to blot excess oil. Don't use pressed powder, which actually contains oil as an ingredient.

● **Never, ever rub your eyes – apply compresses instead.** The skin on your face is extremely delicate, especially under your eyes. So use a very light touch on your face at all times. If your eyes itch, apply a cold compress or cloth to the area, or try a cotton-wool pad moistened with toner or witch hazel.

● **Use one brand of skincare products.** If you buy and use lots of different skincare products, some will probably contain the same ingredients, thus making them redundant. And some brands aren't very compatible with others, though you have no way of knowing that until you've already paid for and opened them. You'll get better results if you use products that are formulated to work together. You may have to shell out a little more cash, but experts agree you'll get better results.

Dab on loose powder to blot excess oil.

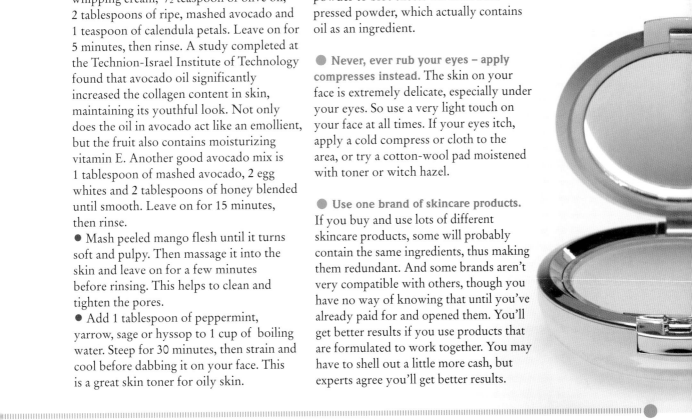

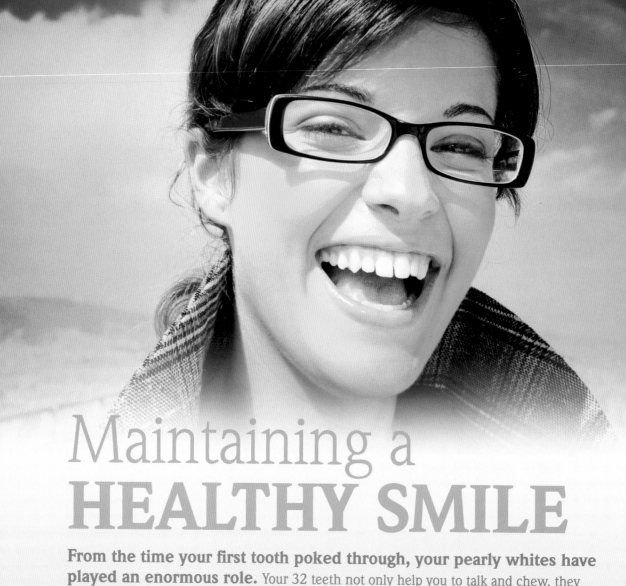

Maintaining a
HEALTHY SMILE

From the time your first tooth poked through, your pearly whites have played an enormous role. Your 32 teeth not only help you to talk and chew, they can make or break your appearance. Although aesthetics are important, of more concern is tooth and gum health. In the past few years, researchers have found a link between periodontal (gum) disease and an increased risk of heart disease. One study found that men with periodontitis had a whopping 72 per cent greater risk of developing coronary artery disease than men with healthy gums. Read on for 16 tips to keep you smiling.

16 WAYS TO KEEP YOUR GUMS AND TEETH CLEAN

Go on a white-teeth diet. What goes in shows up on your teeth. So if you're drinking a lot of red wine and black tea, or smoking cigarettes, expect the results to show up as not-so-pearly whites. Other culprits include colas, gravies and dark juices. The bottom line: if it's dark before you put it in your mouth, it will probably stain your teeth. Step one: brush your teeth immediately after having foods that stain. Step two: regularly use a good bleaching agent, either from the pharmacy or your dentist. Step three: be conscious of tooth-staining foods and drinks, and have them only when a toothbrush is around. If not, have an apple for dessert.

Hum while you brush. The ideal amount of time to brush to get all the bacteria-packed plaque out is at least 2 minutes, researchers found. Use your watch or keep a timer in the bathroom and set it for 2 minutes. Or find a tune that lasts about 2 minutes and hum it to the end.

☺ **Grip your toothbrush like a pencil.** Does your toothbrush look as if it's been used to clean the car? If so, you're probably brushing too hard. Contrary to what some scrub-happy people think, brushing with force is not the best way to remove plaque. The best way is to place your toothbrush at a 45 degree angle against your gums and gently move it in a circular motion, rather than a back-and-forth motion. Grip the toothbrush like a pencil so you won't scrub too hard.

Drink a cup of tea every day. Flavonoids and other ingredients in tea seem to prevent harmful bacteria from sticking to teeth, and also block production of a type of sugar that contributes to cavities. Tea also contains high amounts of fluoride.

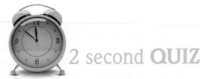

2 second QUIZ

Manual or electric toothbrush?
ANSWER: **ELECTRIC.**

A major review of studies on the subject conducted over the past four decades found that rotational oscillation devices (that is, electric toothbrushes) were more effective than manual toothbrushes in reducing plaque and gingivitis.

Throw away your toothbrush or change the head of your electric toothbrush at least every two to three months. Otherwise, you're just transferring bacteria to your mouth.

Use alcohol-free mouthwash to rinse away bacteria. Most over-the-counter mouthwashes have too much alcohol, which can dry out the tissues in your mouth, making them more susceptible to bacteria. Some studies even suggest a link between mouthwashes containing alcohol and an increased risk of oral cancer. To be safe, be a teetotaller when it comes to choosing a mouthwash.

Do **THREE** things...

If you do only three things to keep your teeth healthy, make them these three, most dentists agree:

1 Brush at least twice a day.

2 Floss at least once a day.

3 See your dentist for a thorough cleaning every six months.

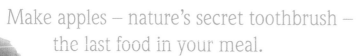

Make apples – nature's secret toothbrush – the last food in your meal.

● **Clean your tongue** with a tongue scraper every morning to remove tongue plaque and freshen your breath. A major cause of bad breath is the build-up of bacteria on the tongue, which a daily tongue scraping will help to banish. Using a tongue scraper is more effective than brushing your tongue with a toothbrush.

● **Even if you're an adult, avoid sugary foods.** Sugar plus bacteria equals oral plaque. Plaque then leads to bleeding gums, tooth decay and cavities. Plus, the acid in refined sugars and carbonated beverages dissolves tooth enamel.

▐▐▐➡ **Instead, eat "detergent" foods.** Foods that are firm or crisp help to clean the teeth as they're eaten. Apples have already been mentioned; other choices include raw carrots, celery and (unsweetened) popcorn. For best results, make "detergent" foods the final food you eat in your meal if you know you can't brush your teeth straight after eating.

☆ **Drink one 250 ml glass of water for every hour that you're at work.** That way, when you get home, you'll have had your recommended daily eight glasses. If you work at home or part-time, be sure to drink at least one glass every hour for 8 hours. Not only does the water help to keep your digestive system healthy and hydrate your skin, but it also helps to keep your teeth white. The more water you drink, the more bacteria you flush off your teeth and out of your mouth, meaning less risk of gum disease, fewer cavities and fresher breath.

☺ **Brush with baking soda once a week** to remove stains and whiten your teeth. Use it as you would toothpaste. You can also use salt as an alternative toothpaste. Also, if your gums start to feel raw, brush with salt every other day.

● **Keep a bottle opener and a small pair of scissors in your bag or desk drawer.** If you have the right gadgets to hand, you won't be tempted to use your teeth as tools, which can damage them. In fact, never, ever use your teeth as tools for anything except eating.

● **To check the freshness of your breath,** lick your palm and smell it while it's still wet. If you smell something, it's time for a sugar-free breath mint.

● **Suck – don't chew – very hard foodstuffs** such as hard candy or ice. Chewing hard foods creates tiny fractures in the enamel of your teeth that, over the years, combine to result in major cracks.

● **Women: choose a medium-coral or light-red lipstick.** These colours make your teeth look whiter, whereas lighter-coloured lipsticks tend to bring out the yellow in your teeth.

● **Eat a container of fat-free yogourt every day.** Think of your teeth as external bones; just like your bones, they need adequate calcium to remain strong.

Healthy INVESTMENT

A dental water jet
Dental water jets clean your teeth three times deeper than brushing and flossing alone. Fill the machine with mouthwash, water or an antibacterial rinse and let the jet's pulsation go to work on your teeth once a day.

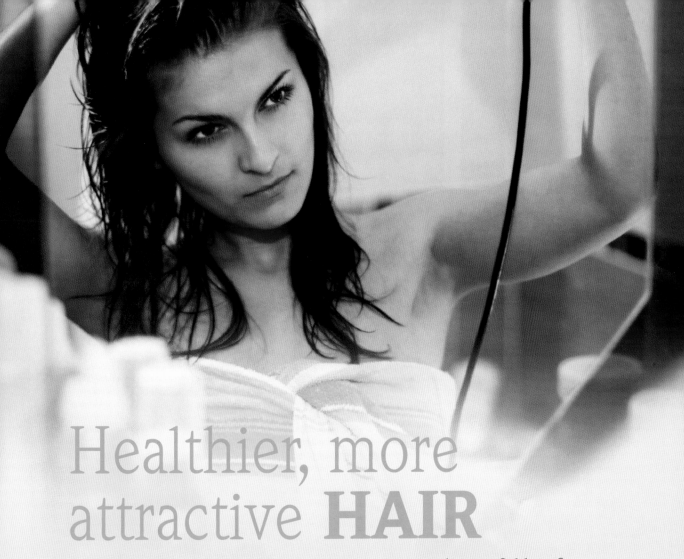

Healthier, more attractive **HAIR**

Considering it's technically dead tissue, we spend an awful lot of time, money and energy on our hair. And well we should. In addition to being fun to style and colour, hair serves a valuable biological purpose: it keeps your head warm and helps to regulate your body temperature. The typical hair cell stays with you for three to five years until it falls or grows out. Most of the time, it gets replaced.

Because you spend so much time on your hair, particularly if you're a woman, it makes sense to give it the best care. These tips will help you to keep your tresses shiny and healthy.

20 WAYS TO ADD BODY, PERSONALITY AND LONGEVITY

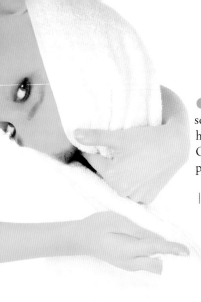

● **For soft, natural highlights,** squeeze some lemon juice on your hair before heading into the sun. Or use shampoos and styling products that contain citrus fruits.

▶ **Wrap wet hair gently in a towel** and let the cotton absorb the moisture for a few minutes instead of rubbing. This helps to prevent split ends.

● **Check the drain after each shower for the amount of hair.** The typical person loses between 50 and 200 hairs a day (out of 80,000 to 120,000 hairs on the head). So it's normal to have a very small clump of hair left in the drain after washing. But if that amount starts to increase, see your doctor about it. It could mean your scalp has an infection, that baldness is beginning to set in or, more rarely, that you have a nutritional deficiency.

Wrap,
don't rub,
wet hair.

2 second QUIZ

Brunette or blonde?
ANSWER: **BRUNETTE.**

The "blondes have more fun" message comes directly from those who market hair-colouring products. Most people on this planet have black or dark hair. From a health point of view, people with naturally blonde hair are more susceptible to sunburn and skin cancer. And, let's face it, there are plenty of negative stereotypes about blondes. If becoming a blonde will really change your self-esteem for the better, pursue it. Otherwise, brunette is just fine.

● **Mix a few drops of your favourite fragrance** into your hair gel before applying. You'll end up with hair that not only looks good, but smells great, too.

● **Transform ordinary shampoo into a herbal experience** by mixing in a few drops of essential oils. Dilute a 250 ml bottle of shampoo by half with water and add 20 drops of essential oil of lavender.

● **Men: if you're going bald, go short.** One of the worst mistakes balding men make is the comb-over. A sexier, more modern style is to keep it closely trimmed. An added bonus: your hair will be easy to maintain.

● **Bathe your hair in botanical oils.** Available at health-food stores, olive, jojoba and sweet almond oils are all wonderful hair elixirs. If your hair is thick and heavy, coconut oil works wonders. Dampen your hair and apply small amounts of the botanical oil until your hair is thoroughly covered. Cover with a shower cap and warm towel for half an hour, then rinse and shampoo as usual.

● **Shampoo grey hair every day with a blue-coloured shampoo.** By the very nature of its light colour, grey hair gets duller, dirtier and drier than darker shades, which is why it's so important to shampoo and condition it daily. The bluish shampoo helps to hide any yellowish tinge, which can be aging.

● **If you want to hide your roots** and try a new hairdo at the same time, zigzag your part.

● **Allow at least four weeks** between single-process colour treatments and at least eight weeks between high- or low-light treatments.

● **Create effective, instant highlights** by applying champagne or gold-hued eyeshadow to your hair using an ordinary make-up sponge.

● **Use a humidifier at night in your bedroom, especially in cold weather.** Your central heating probably keeps the air very dry, which can dry out your hair.

▷ **To reduce damage to your tresses and add bounce to your hairdo,** dry your hair until 90 per cent of the moisture is removed, then stop. Most people falsely believe they must use a hairdryer until their hair is bone dry. Not true. The style should fall into place if your hair is healthy and well cut.

● **If you usually wear your hair in a ponytail,** take it out for a few hours a day to give your hair a break. Also, try not to pull hair back too tightly. And never sleep with any sort of accessories in your hair.

▷ **Comb conditioner through your hair before going swimming** to protect it from the harsh chemicals. Do the same before going to the beach.

● **Use moisturizing conditioner two to three times a week to combat fine, thin hair.** Many people think conditioners will flatten thin hair, but, actually, using a moisturizing conditioner a few times a week will help your hair to block out humidity, which can make the hair flat.

● **Use styling gel correctly.** Here's how to get the hold you want while avoiding a greasy look. Place a dime-sized dollop of gel in the palm of one hand, then dab a tiny amount onto the fingertips of your other hand, leaving most of the gel in your palm. Starting at the back of your head near your scalp line, work the gel

CORRECT
shampooing technique

Few people realize that there's a correct way to shampoo your hair. Yet proper shampooing not only improves the look of your hair but also helps to slow down hair loss and promote healthier hair growth. Try these tips:

● Before you step into the shower, brush your hair from front to back with a stiff boar-bristle brush. This will stimulate the circulation and prevent the build-up of styling products.

● Wet the hair with warm water. (Hot water can strip your hair of protective oils.) Apply shampoo at the nape of the neck and shampoo the hairline first, then do the top of your head.

● Massage your entire scalp at least three times to push nutrients into the hair bulb and free your hair follicles of clogging deposits.

● After rinsing your hair thoroughly, apply your conditioner. If you're doing all of this outside the shower, wrap a "steam towel" (a wet towel that's been microwaved for 2 minutes) around your head and leave it on for 30 to 60 seconds. The steam allows the conditioner to be more evenly absorbed.

● Finish with a cool-water rinse, which helps to tighten scalp pores, firm hair fibres, reduce limpness and increase sheen.

from your fingertips into the root area of your hair. Continue until you've used up the dollop of gel.

● **Flip your head over,** spray the underneath layers with hairspray, and shake it out to style your hair instantly without having to rewash and blow-dry.

● **Pick a hair colour that's just a few shades lighter than your complexion,** which tends to lighten as you age. Highlight or bleach grey hair to give your hair a more uniform look and brighten your skin tone at the same time.

● **Use a gentle shampoo for oily hair.** Ironically, harsh shampoos can actually lead to more oil because your scalp tries to compensate. Use a shampoo that's gentle enough for everyday use.

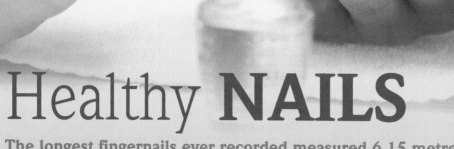

Healthy **NAILS**

The longest fingernails ever recorded measured 6.15 metres on a single hand and took more than 40 years to grow. Imagine the difficulties their owner had with everyday tasks! No one really knows why we have nails, but whatever the reason, they make it easier to do many things, such as pick up small items. They also provide an external sign of health: weak, brittle nails often signal a nutritional deficiency. Ignore them and you could end up with painful ingrown nails or a fungal infection. Follow these tips to ensure you have 20 healthy nails on your fingers and toes.

11 WAYS TO KEEP THEM STRONG

- To keep your nails hydrated, rub a small amount of petroleum jelly into your cuticle and the skin surrounding your nails every evening before you go to bed or whenever your nails feel dry. Not a fan of petroleum jelly? Substitute castor oil. It's thick and contains vitamin E, which is great for your cuticles. Or use olive oil – it also works to moisturize your nails.

- ☺ Wear rubber gloves whenever you do housework or wash the dishes. Most household chores, from scrubbing the bathroom to washing the dishes, as well as gardening, are tough on your nails. To protect your fingers from dirt and harsh cleaners, cover them with rubber gloves at chore time. For extra hand softness, apply hand cream before you put on the gloves.

- Trim your toenails straight across to avoid ingrown toenails. This is extra important if you have diabetes.

- Dry your hands for at least 2 minutes after doing the dishes. Also dry your toes thoroughly after swimming or showering. Leaving them damp increases your risk of fungal infection.

- Air out your work boots and running shoes. Better still, keep two pairs of each and switch between them so you're never putting your feet into damp, sweaty shoes, which may lead to fungal infections.

- Wear 100 per cent cotton socks. They're best for absorbing dampness, thus preventing fungal infections.

- To make your nails as strong and resilient as a horse's hoofs, take 300 mcg of the B vitamin biotin four to six times a day. Long ago, vets discovered that biotin strengthened horses' hoofs, which are made from keratin, the same substance as

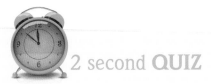

2 second QUIZ

Quick-drying or standard nail polish?
ANSWER: **STANDARD.**

Quick-drying nail polishes may save time, but at the expense of your nails. Most of these formulas contain more formaldehyde and alcohol than standard polishes, both of which are drying and make nails prone to splitting. To fast-dry nails naturally, chill them. Empty a tray of ice cubes into your bathroom sink and fill it with cold water. After each coat of nail polish, dip your wet nails into the cold water for a minute or two. Miraculously, they'll be dry when you take them out.

human nails. Swiss researchers found that people who took biotin every day for just over five months had firmer, harder nails. In a U.S. study, 63 per cent of people who took biotin developed stronger nails.

- File your nails correctly. To keep your nails strong, avoid filing in a back-and-forth motion – go in one direction only. Never file just after a shower or bath – wet nails break more easily.

- Massage your nails to keep them extra-strong and shiny. Nail buffing increases blood supply to the nail, which stimulates the matrix of the nail to grow.

- Polish your nails, even if it's just with a clear varnish. It protects them. If you prefer colour, use a base coat, two thin coats of colour and a top coat. The colour should last at least seven days but should be removed after ten days.

- Avoid polish removers containing acetone or formaldehyde. They're very drying to the nails. Use acetate-based removers instead.

Let your rubber gloves take the punishment, not your nails.

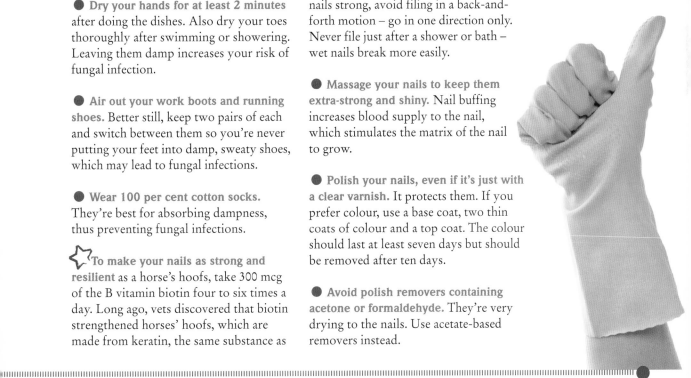

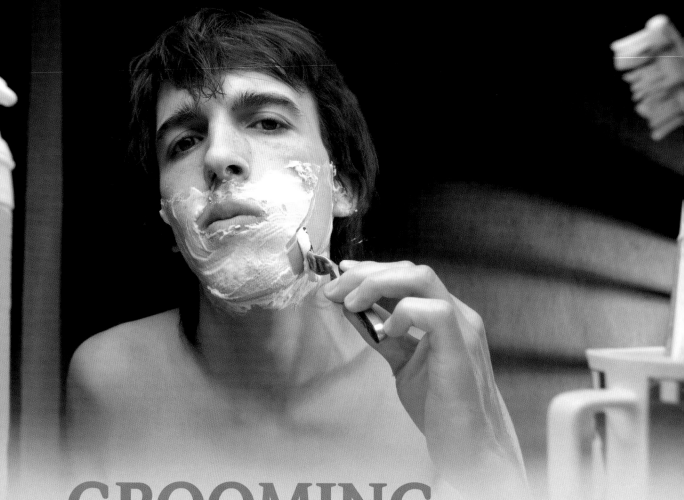

GROOMING

When it comes to grooming, little things can make a big difference.
A cleanly plucked brow, clipped nose hairs, neatly filed fingernails and toenails, or a close shave can mean the difference between looking good and looking great.

Few of us want to spend hours in front of the mirror primping or spend hundreds of dollars at a salon. So here are some easy grooming tips that will help you to look polished, refined and youthful – without investing a lot of money or time. Some are for men only, some for women only, and some are for both.

30 WAYS TO LOOK (AND SMELL) YOUR BEST

Unisex grooming

● **Keep track of the amount of time you spend "grooming,"** and stop at 45 minutes. That's the most it should ever take to shower, take care of your skin, apply make-up and style your hair. Any longer, and you need to get an easier haircut, use less make-up and cut down to one skincare product.

● **If you're prone to ingrown hairs,** lather with shaving cream or gel for 5 minutes to soften the hairs. Then shave in the direction of the hair growth with a new blade. Follow with a gentle moisturizer.

● **Shave slowly, with short strokes, and rinse the blade often in hot water.** Your skin is not flat, so long strokes increase your chances of cuts or scrapes. Try not to press down with the blade, especially around sensitive areas.

● **Apply your shaving cream with a shaving brush** for an extra-lustrous shaving session (whether on your legs or your face). It will create tons of lather, which will make the hairs softer and easier to remove.

☆ **If you have no time for a shower but need to be at your freshest,** fill your sink with water and add 4 tablespoons of baking soda. Then dip a sponge or washcloth in the sink and rub yourself down.

● **Ward off smelly feet with odour-absorbing insoles.** Foot odour is a very common problem. Keep your feet smelling fresh by scrubbing them daily and drying them completely when you get out of the shower. Then insert odour-absorbing insoles into your shoes.

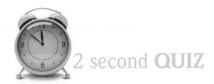

2 second QUIZ

Antiperspirant or deodorant?
ANSWER: **ANTIPERSPIRANT.**

If you want maximum protection, choose an antiperspirant. Bacteria that feed on the chemical components in underarm sweat cause odour. A deodorant works by controlling the bacteria, but does nothing to control wetness. An antiperspirant, on the other hand, controls both.

● **Schedule a weekly manicure and a monthly pedicure.** This works for men and women. You can do it yourself, but a professional will always do a better job. The simple detail of well-filed nails, clean cuticles and smooth toenails (if you're wearing open-toed shoes) tells bosses, colleagues and clients that you care about the little as well as the big things.

● **Wear loose-fitting clothes to allow air to circulate** around your body and perspiration to evaporate. Tight-fitting clothing causes sweat to be trapped in a film on your skin, which can result in body odour or embarrassing perspiration stains.

● **Buy clothes made from natural fibres such as cotton.** They allow skin to breathe, reducing body odour. Avoid synthetic, man-made fibres, such as nylon or Lycra, which may limit ventilation.

● **Apply antiperspirant when your underarms are a little moist and wet,** for example, just after a warm shower or bath. It enables the active ingredients to enter the sweat glands more readily.

Banish smelly feet with odour-absorbing insoles.

● **Avoid sitting in direct sunlight.** It heats your body and causes perspiration, especially in warmer weather.

● **Apply baby powder** in the morning to help your skin stay drier throughout the day and to reduce odour.

● **Take up yoga.** The stress management training will help you control perspiration and body odour better. After heat, stress is probably the top cause of sweating.

● **Wipe a cotton ball soaked in rubbing alcohol** onto your underarms during the day to cut down on odour-causing bacteria. Or try witch hazel or tea tree oil, both of which help to keep you dry, kill bacteria and deodorize.

☺ **Prepare some greens for dinner each night.** Dark-green leafy vegetables such as spinach, chard, parsley and kale are rich in chlorophyll, which has a powerful deodorizing effect on the body.

For women only

● **Pluck your eyebrows as soon as you step out of the shower.** Your pores are open then, enabling the hairs to slide out when you pluck. Avoid brow-shaping

Healthy INVESTMENT

A magnifying make-up mirror
Even if you're not planning on using make-up, it gives you an up-close-and-personal look at any nose, ear or chin hairs that need to be plucked, wax build-up in ears, large pores, blackheads or other stuff that only you want to know about.

when your skin is most sensitive: first thing in the morning, after you've been outside in extremely hot or cold weather, or during your period, when your nerve endings are at their most sensitive.

● **Carry a make-up touch-up kit with you wherever you go.** Look for multi-purpose products, such as a lip/cheek/eye cream or a two-ended wand with mascara on one end and eyeliner on the other. Other good kit items include cotton balls soaked in make-up remover, then stored in a film canister, pressed powder, a nail file and lip gloss.

● **Check out your face in a hand mirror in front of a window once a day.** You'll catch a glimpse of any sun spots or wrinkles you need to cover up or facial hairs you need to pluck, uneven make-up, even long nose hairs. Natural sunlight makes the inspection more revealing.

☺ **Apply make-up in natural light.** Even if this means bringing your make-up and a mirror into the living room. The light from a bulb is often a different shade from that of natural light, and rarely does a bulb-lit room have evenly distributed light. If you must work in a bulb-lit room, be sure to use the correct wattage – at least 60 watts for overhead lights and 25 watts for make-up mirrors.

● **Rub some olive oil on your bikini line** to keep it soft and free of unsightly red bumps. For best results, apply the olive oil to the area immediately after shaving.

● **For instantly fresh feet,** spray your soles with chilled cologne, chilled peppermint or rose geranium herbal water. Make your own by adding a couple of drops of the essential oils to a spray bottle of water and storing it in the fridge.

● To make your eyes appear closer together, tweeze your brows on the outer edges and let them grow in closer towards the nose. To make your eyes appear farther apart, tweeze your brows to expand the open space above the nose. In other words, make the brows shorter.

For men only

● If you have a unibrow, consider laser hair removal to tidy up the area. This procedure can also be used to remove stray nose and ear hairs. Excessive facial hair is generally considered unattractive.

● Shave after your shower. Steam and hot water soften the bristles of your beard and open up the pores of your skin, making shaving easier and less painful.

● Or, shave in the shower. Most men can get a terrific shave without any lather or cream by shaving as the last part of a shower. Just 5 minutes of hot, steamy water provides all the moisture and hair softening your beard needs, and the rinse-off and clean-up take just seconds.

● Change the blade in your razor every three or four days. You could be shaving with the most expensive razor on the market, but if the blade is dull, it will leave you with a red, blotchy face.

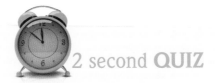

2 second QUIZ

Electric or conventional razor?
ANSWER: **CONVENTIONAL.**

It may be faster and simpler to shave with an electric razor, but it's harsher on your skin and can strip away natural oils. It also doesn't shave quite as effectively as a conventional razor.

● Shave off some or all of your facial hair for a more youthful look. If you have a full beard, try a goatee. If you have a goatee, go for the clean-faced look.

● Trim the other hair on your body. Many men losing the hair on their heads start to gain it in other places, such as the ears, nose or back. To look clean and contemporary, trim, wax or pluck unwanted hair.

● When the weather gets warmer, trim your armpit hair. There will be less hair to trap bacteria and, hence, less odour.

● Extend the life of your razors by soaking them in mineral oil. Fill a shallow dish with mineral oil and soak them for a few minutes – the oil stops the oxidation process that can dull the edges. Then use a little rubbing alcohol to clean it off.

Reminder

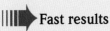 **Fast results**
These are bits of advice that deliver benefits particularly quickly – in some cases, immediately.

 Easy gains
These are health boosters that give the biggest value for the least amount of effort.

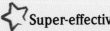 **Super-effective**
This is advice that scientific research or widespread usage by experts has shown to be especially effective.

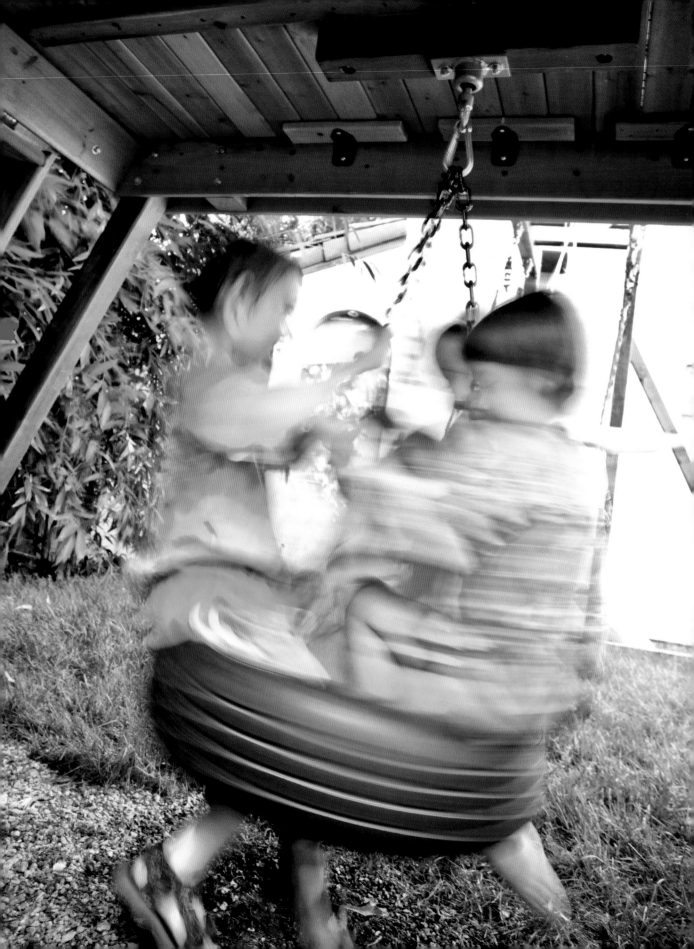

part 9

PEOPLE & PLACES

Your relationships have a very real effect on your physical health. Here's how to make sure the people around you are helping – not hurting – your well-being.

A better, healthier
RELATIONSHIP

Most couples come together expecting their relationship to remain as warm, loving and intimate as it was at the start. And, for many couples, that's the case. There's no secret and no luck involved: they've simply learned to devote time and attention to their relationship. Not just sometimes, but every day. You see, it's not diamonds and flowers that make a relationship, but the little things. Like taking a Saturday afternoon to explore the countryside and stop at an out-of-the-way pub for lunch. Above all, it's learning through the years to accept your partner's shortcomings and to forgive one another for transgressions both large and small. The good news is that taking small, simple steps can bring big results. So check out the tips that follow.

28 WAYS TO GROW CLOSER

● **Praise your partner for the little things.** If there's something you appreciate about your partner, from the way he or she makes scrambled eggs to how hard he or she's working on decorating the bedroom, speak up. Praise provides a reminder of your love.

● **Do things that show you care.** The good we do tends to come back to us. When you're thoughtful to your partner, he or she's more inclined to be thoughtful in return. So remember to buy each other's favourite dessert, cut out or e-mail articles you think your partner might like, take on the other's jobs, arrange for your partner to have a day off, with no housework or expectations.

● **Keep your promises.** Failing to keep your word can destroy the unity and trust in a relationship. It's better to say "Let me think about it" than to say you'll do something but fail to deliver.

● **Share your passions.** Take turns choosing an arts or cultural event to attend together each month. The point is to show your partner what you love, so that he or she can experience it as you do (or close enough). To make this work, both of you have to be flexible: you may have to attend a hockey game, and your partner may have to go to the theatre with you. The reward lies in experiencing each other's passion. And who knows – you may have a lot more fun than you ever imagined.

● **Kiss under a full moon.** On a fine evening, spread a blanket under the night sky and drink in the beauty and quiet of your surroundings together. You can talk if you wish, or simply savour the silence and the experience of being together, side by side, under the stars.

Do **THREE** things...

If you do only three things to strengthen your relationship with your partner, make it these three, say relationship experts:

1 Be kind to him or her. Every day there are opportunities for simple gestures that demonstrate your love. A compliment, a hug, a note or a favour takes only a moment, and yet these can brighten your partner's day and your special bond.

2 Give a full pardon. When your partner has hurt you, extending forgiveness frees you from the bitterness and hurt that can eat away at your relationship. But don't think you have to forgive him or her instantly. Forgiveness is a process, rather than an event, so be as kind as you can be to your partner while you heal.

3 Say, "I'm sorry." If you hurt your partner, swallow your pride and offer a simple but sincere apology. Make it clear that you didn't mean to cause pain. At the same time, show that you take your mistake seriously by asking, "What can I do to make it up to you?"

● **Play the newlywed game.** Do something for your partner that you did when you were newlyweds or first got together. Make a special meal. Send some flowers after a night of lovemaking. Tuck notes in unexpected places or leave sexy messages on your partner's cellphone.

▌▌▶ **Have a conversation about the big things in life.** When you were courting, did you talk for hours about current events or the meaning of life? If all you seem to talk about now is the grocery shopping or how much to spend on a new sofa, reintroduce meaningful conversation into your relationship. Try this: one night, while you're in front of the TV or in the car, make a provocative (but not hurtful) remark about something your partner cares deeply about – the government, an athlete – something that will get his or her dander up. He or she will disagree, of course, which will get the ball rolling. Keep it rolling!

☺ **Say thank you at least once a day.** You thank others for the little courtesies they do for you. But do you thank your partner for his or hers? If he or she makes you breakfast every morning, say thank you – and mean it. If your partner took out the garbage without being asked, say thank you – even if it's his or her allotted chore. Thank yous keep you from taking each other for granted.

● **Get active together.** Are you both a few pounds heavier than when you first met? Engaging in a physical activity that you both enjoy can be as good for your relationship as it is for your body, and can reinforce the fact that you're a team of two. You needn't run a marathon together (although training for one could provide a lot of couple time). How about tennis? Golf? Swimming? Even gardening can be a good workout, if you're landscaping the garden or tending a large flower bed or vegetable plot.

● **Develop a common interest.** The couple that plays together, stays together. To keep your relationship fresh and vibrant, think of an activity that both you and your partner enjoy, and do it together. The possibilities are endless: gardening, sports, attending classes or cultural events together, walking, hiking, home-improvement projects.

● **Do charitable work together.** Helping others takes you out of yourself and your own problems and gives you a broader, more spiritual view of life. Again, try to pick a cause or an organization that appeals to you both, whether it's a mentoring program for disadvantaged children or working on weekends in the local soup kitchen.

● **Walk through your disagreements.** When you and your partner are at loggerheads, ask him or her to go for a walk to work things through. Being outdoors and walking at a steady pace can melt away the tension, so it's easier to talk honestly, form compromises or apologize.

● **Organize film nights once a month.** All right, so you both prefer different types of films – one likes sci-fi, the other prefers historical dramas. It doesn't matter. To find common ground, select films for the characters, not the genre. So, for example, if you choose to watch Ralph Fiennes in *The English Patient*, there's espionage and adventure as well as a love story.

● **Each morning, ask, "What are you doing today?"** Does your partner have a big meeting or lunch with an old friend? Is he or she dreading a phone call to an important client? Talking about the daily details of life is just as important as sharing hopes, dreams and fears, so

Remember to say thank you – and mean it.

showing a genuine interest is a great way to build understanding and rapport. And don't forget to ask how that meeting, phone call or lunch turned out. Your thoughtfulness will make your partner feel loved and cared for.

☺ **Treat your partner with respect and admiration in public.** Whether you're at a party, a business meeting or just strolling down the street, give him or her subtle signals of your connection. Hold hands or put an arm around one another. Smile at him or her. And never, ever, make fun of your partner in public.

● **Give your demands a makeover.** If you want a job done, such as a shelf put up, make sure you ask, rather than demand. We all tend to respond better to requests than orders. For example, instead of saying, "You should …" say, "Could you …?" And instead of saying, "Why didn't you …?" say, "Next time it would help me if you could try to …"

● **Try to air grievances at the same time each week.** This may at first seem odd. But consider this: if you and your partner discuss what's bothering you in a structured, formal way, these issues won't come up so often at other times. Make the meeting formal. Sit down, turn off the television or computer and let the voicemail handle any calls.

||||► **Cuddle in the morning.** You may associate snuggling up with bedtime, and it is a lovely way to end the day. But cuddling in the morning will keep you feeling close to each other all day. So set the alarm clock 5 minutes early and snuggle up. You can talk, or not. What's important is that you both start the day connecting physically and feeling secure and loved.

● **Schedule time for lovemaking.** Yes, you're both busy. But don't let it stand in the way of an activity that's so crucial to a loving relationship. It may not be as spontaneous as you'd like, but there's something nice about looking forward to a night (or morning, or afternoon) of sex.

● **Always turn in together.** This may take some compromise on both parts. If your partner is tired, give up your nightly ritual (television, surfing the Internet, whatever) and follow him or her to bed at least a few nights a week. Talk about the day, or simply snuggle up while each of you reads. And if you're the morning person, maybe you can stay up for something after the 10 o'clock news. The point is to be together when the house is quiet and the demands of the day are done.

☆ **Make sure your bedroom is a sanctuary.** Your bed is not the place to argue, bring up complicated subjects or discuss difficult parenting issues. Your bed is a place for good things only – sleep, companionship, romance. If it becomes a place for hard talks and criticism, one of you will eventually feel your bedroom is emotionally unsafe, and you'll start to avoid each other. If this is already going on, you need to stop it – declare the bedroom a safe zone, and make sure all serious discussions take place earlier and elsewhere.

● **Pursue your own interests.** Go ahead, take that writing class – or pursue any other interest you might have outside those you share with your partner. It makes you more interesting to your partner and everyone else. Moreover, a little "me time" allows both of you to grow as individuals and reduces the pressure on each of you to fill the other's every need.

● **Take a weekend getaway.** If you present the idea to your partner as an adventure, he or she'll be more inclined to get in on the act. Then the fun begins: deciding where you'll go, what you'll do, and how you'll get there. Plan it together. Pore over maps and the travel section of the newspaper together. Discuss whether you should splurge on a room with a hot tub or a four-poster.

Healthy INVESTMENT

A CD you both love
One study found that when couples listened to music they both liked, they felt more caring towards their partner. It's just something else they can share.

● **Renew your vows.** Renewing your vows renews your commitment not only to your partner but also to keeping passion and intimacy in your relationship. You can do it once a year by taking a romantic getaway on your anniversary or make it a once-in-a-lifetime event.

● **Read the comics out loud to each other** and share funny stories. A 2004 study found that sharing humorous experiences significantly reduced the amount of conflict couples felt.

● **Go shopping (or watch a soccer game) with a close friend.** One study found that couples who have individual friendships outside their relationship were more satisfied with their marital relationships than those who didn't.

● **Demonstrate your love by trying to improve something about yourself** that upsets your partner. For instance, if your partner likes order and tidiness, stop throwing your dirty socks on the floor and leaving your dishes in the sink. Saying "I love you" is always nice, but showing it is really fundamental.

☆ **Always put your marriage first,** even if you have a houseful of children. This is a golden rule: of all your relationships, your partner must come first. After all, the children are going to leave some day; hopefully, your partner isn't. Plus, giving up your life as a couple to indulge your children simply sets an uninspiring example: grow up, become an adult, then you, too, can subjugate your existence to that of your children. Putting your marriage first means things like deliberately setting aside time for the two of you, whether it's a weekly date, a nightly bath together or dinner alone a few nights a week (feed the children early).

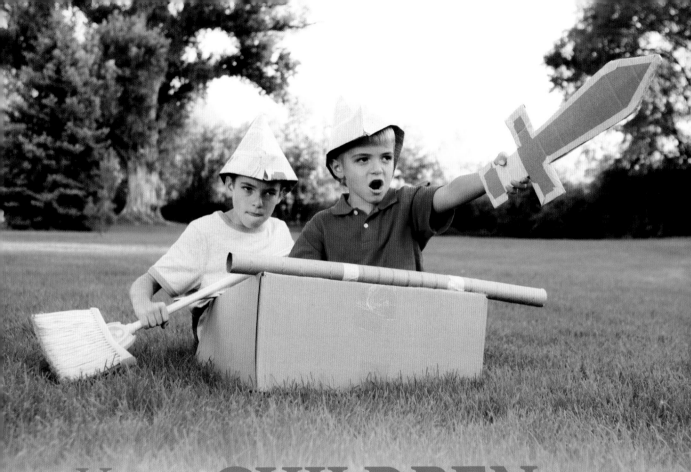

Your **CHILDREN**

You remember them in diapers. You recall their first words. You cherish the days when they were innocent, loving and eager for your hugs. And yet, as your children grow and evolve, so must your relationship with them. You need to be supportive but not intrusive; offer emotional back-up without being overly involved in their lives; and hope they make wise choices, while understanding that those choices are theirs to make. The tips that follow can help you to bond with your children even if they're no longer children. This, too, is a matter of health: nothing can break your heart as much as a strained relationship with your child. And nothing can make your heart soar as much as watching their lives prosper – and them wanting you to be part of it.

13 WAYS TO SUSTAIN THE LOVE AND RESPECT

☆ **Set a standing dinner date.** There's something comforting about the family gathered around the dinner table, perhaps because that tradition is disappearing. Yet the evening meal is often the one time of day when the family can get together in one place. So make dinner a family affair, even if you're just having a takeout at the dinner table. Use the time to share news of your day, make weekend plans and enjoy one another's company. Research shows that adolescents who dine with their family at least several times a week are less likely to smoke and use drugs and they tend to get better exam results.

In PERSPECTIVE

For a better relationship, lay down the law(s)

If you're the parent of a teen, be a parent rather than a pal. Chances are, your teen will welcome your rules and expectations – even if he or she grumbles about them.

Teens whose parents establish house rules have better relationships with their parents – and a lower risk of smoking, drinking and using drugs – than the typical teen, according to one U.S. study.

The study, which analyzed a hands-on versus a hands-off approach to parenting, found that teens living in hands-on environments have parents who monitor their children's TV and Internet use, know and restrict the CDs they buy, know where their teens are after school and on weekends, impose a curfew, eat dinner with their teens six or seven nights a week and assign them chores, among other actions.

What's more, the survey found that 57 per cent of the teens with hands-on parents reported having an excellent relationship with their mothers and 47 per cent reported an excellent relationship with their fathers. Only 24 per cent of the teens with hands-off parents reported an excellent relationship with their mothers and just 13 per cent said they had an excellent relationship with their fathers.

● **Back off, but stay close.** It's normal for teens to want to spend more time with friends than parents. But don't take this to mean your job as a parent is diminished. Find ways to remain involved in your child's life. For example, while tea parties may be a thing of the past, you can still get to know your children's friends by making them welcome after school. Staying involved may be more challenging, but it's an important way of enhancing your relationship with your child.

● **Share your own feelings with your teen.** Of course, spare the intimate details of very personal subjects, but confiding that you, too, occasionally feel angry, insecure or awkward shows your teenager that you're not just a parent – you're human. Not only will your child feel closer to you, but he or she may feel safe enough to disclose uncomfortable issues or feelings when they arise.

☺ **Seek their opinions.** Teenagers have opinions about, well, everything, and they aren't shy about sharing them. So allow them to make more independent decisions. For instance, let them decide when and where to study, what to wear, what after-school activity to pursue. However, keep in mind that some decisions are non-negotiable. Parents need to set limits that protect their child's health, safety and well-being – at every age. These might include curfews, decisions about drinking and sexual activity, issues around grades and university.

● **Trust your children to make smart choices.** Of course, they'll make the wrong ones occasionally. But, especially if they're over 18, give them the chance to work out solutions to problems on their own. Didn't you want the same from your parents at that age?

● **Phone before you drop in.** If you have an adult child, always call before you go to his or her home, unless it's absolutely necessary. If you're the parent of a teen, knock before you enter his or her room.

● **Accept their holiday absences with grace.** Yes, you may be disappointed that your children – and their children – spend Christmas without you. But don't nag or complain about it. You may win a battle over which in-law's house they visit for Christmas, but end up losing your child's respect – and an enduring relationship.

☺ **State your views, then invite reaction.** "Does that seem fair to you?" "Can you think of a better way to deal with this?" "What would you do in my position?" You're more likely to find a middle ground that you can both accept.

● **Be there when they want you or need you, rather than when you want to be.** A lifetime of love, trust and respect will ensue if you are reliably around whenever a reasonable or acceptable request is made of you.

● **Respect your teen's privacy.** Don't read his or her diary, eavesdrop on phone conversations or badger him or her with questions. If any behaviour is troubling you, address it directly, using five little words: "Can we talk about it?" Here's an example: "You seem very quiet lately, and I'm worried about you. Can we talk about it?"

● **Be honest.** Many parents offer praise when they shouldn't, as well as when they should. That just undermines trust. If both your praise and criticism are heartfelt and valid, your child will learn to trust you.

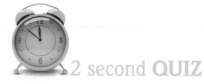

2 second **QUIZ**

Argue back, or walk away?
ANSWER: **ARGUE BACK.**

Choose battles with your children selectively – don't ever start an argument that's not worth having. But if you get into one that is worth it, stay in it to win it. And try to be right. That helps a lot, too!

● **Cultivate love, but demand respect.** Don't try so hard to be your child's friend that you fail to set limits, protect your own integrity and earn respect. You can be friends long after your child is grown up as long as you are the parent first.

☆ **Acknowledge that things have changed since you were their age.** And they have. Music, clothes, technology, language, style, educational methods, the job market, even sexual mores and attitudes have evolved significantly in recent years. And the speed of change is only accelerating. You cannot keep up with it all, and nor should you. But you do need to strike a balance: don't live in the past, but equally don't try to bluff that you know exactly what's going on among teens today. Your children will respect you if you are contemporary in a mature way.

Allow your teen some private time.

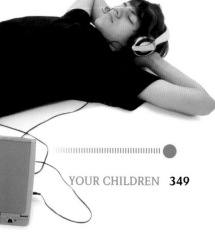

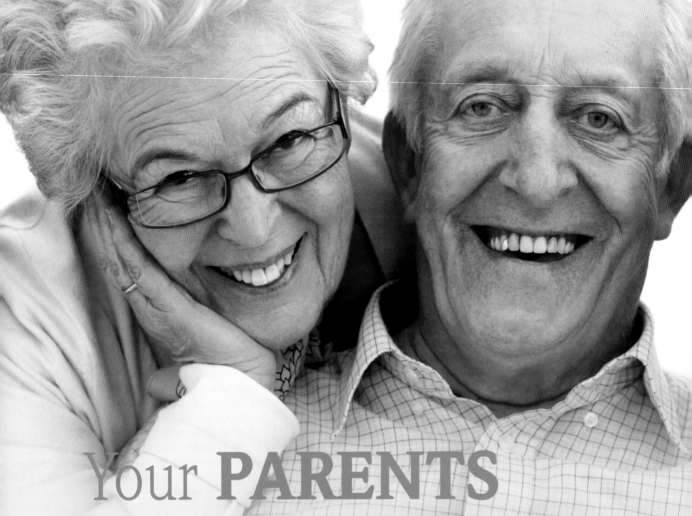

Your **PARENTS**

Of course you love your parents, but, at times, maintaining the bond between parent and adult child can be as challenging as that between parent and teenager. These days, both of you are confronting new challenges – retirement or career changes, health issues, concerns about the future. It's to be expected that these matters will affect you and change your relationship. Part of that evolution requires forging a new bond, one between mature adults rather than "parent" and "child." You already have love and shared memories. Add mutual respect and common interests and you may find a more fulfilling relationship than any you've had since childhood. Here are 13 ways to stay close to your parents.

13 WAYS TO MAINTAIN A HEALTHY PEACE

Think of them as fellow adults, rather than your parents. If your parents still treat you like a child, despite the fact that you have children of your own, you may have to help them let you "grow up." Feeling and acting like an adult around your parents is the cornerstone of having an adult relationship with them. If you treat them as fellow adults, they're more likely to treat you like one. A simple way to do this is to ask yourself a question before each interaction with them: "How would I act in this situation if Mom or Dad was a friend or an acquaintance?" Then behave accordingly.

● **Talk to your parents as friends.** If your parents still treat you as though you're 6 or 16, it may feel funny to give up your role as the child. A good start is to model your conversations with them on those you have with friends. Don't limit your chats strictly to family memories, or gossip about family members or your personal life. There's a whole wide world out there – why not explore it with your mom and dad as you would with a friend? Current events, sports, work, local neighbourhood issues or politics (if you happen to share the same views) are all fair game.

● **Keep your sense of humour.** When you're dealing with your parents, laughter can be a lifesaver – both to help you to handle the stress of dealing with sometimes crotchety individuals and to help you to bond together. Tell a few jokes you know they'll enjoy, share some comics from the paper, watch a comedy together. If you can laugh together, you're doing OK.

● **Tell your parents what bothers you.** If you love your parents, but they drive you crazy, your resentment can eat away at

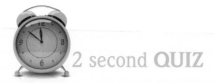
your relationship. So don't seethe silently. Communicate, with gentleness and respect. For instance, if your mom keeps calling you at work, tell her that your boss is starting to notice and, while you love talking to her during the day, it's beginning to affect your job performance. Arrange a call at a mutually convenient time.

☺ **Don't ask your parents' advice or opinion unless you really want it.** Sometimes, asking for a parent's advice is really a way of asking for approval. If so, remember that you're an adult now, perfectly capable of choosing a living room carpet or a car on your own. If your parents are bent on offering you advice whether asked for or not, smile, nod and take it in. Then, make your own choice – without guilt.

● **Don't ask your parents to help bail you out of your latest personal or financial crisis.** While you may depend on their emotional support, relying too much upon their resources, rather than your own, can lead to mutual resentment. So get used to solving your problems, big or small, on your own. You'll be amazed how good doing it all by yourself can make you – and them – feel.

8 great ways
TO GET CLOSER

1 Teach older parents to use e-mail or surf the Internet.

2 Introduce your parents to your friends, and include them in social gatherings when appropriate.

3 Eat out together. Try a cuisine you've never tried before.

4 Join a book or investment club together.

5 Read the same books and talk about them in your own book club.

6 Start a new family tradition with the grandchildren, such as once-a-month picnics.

7 Challenge your parents to a round of golf or a hand of gin rummy.

8 Go bike riding or for a walk together.

● **Create opportunities for exploring and uncovering memories.** If your parents are older, look through their photo albums with them, asking them for stories about the people in the photos. You can help your parents to discover the meaning in their lives by encouraging them to talk about their accomplishments, the high points, and their joys and sorrows.

● **Help your parents to preserve their memories on film, CD or in a scrapbook.** The finished product will not only be a testament to a renewed closeness between you, but also provides a wonderful legacy.

● **Express your appreciation for all your parents have done for you.** Yes, they may do things that annoy you, but they also come to your rescue when you need help.

The point is, your parents still do things for you that deserve your notice – and your gratitude.

● **Rediscover and share mutual interests.** When you were a child, did you and your dad share a passion for a particular hockey team? Did you and your mom spend time each summer making jam? Make these happy memories the foundation for new, shared activities.

● **Be honest about who you are and what you want.** Maybe there are things about the way you grew up that your parents regret. But as long as *you* don't regret anything, they have to adjust. Be clear about who you want to be and help your parents to accept you as you are.

● **Do not allow them to channel guilt at you.** If your parents are the type to complain about you never calling, never visiting, forgetting an uncle's birthday, not sending enough pictures or whatever irks them that day, don't take the bait and feel guilty – unless you honestly regret the oversight. In which case, apologize immediately and seek a way to make amends. Otherwise, let it wash over you. You are mature and independent, and you act on your own volition. For more on this, see "Dealing with guilt," page 290.

● **Grant them their independence, too.** Sometimes it's the grown-up child who doesn't want to cut off the nurturing relationship. If you are past 25 and still find it necessary to talk to your mom every night, or immediately turn to your dad for a house repair rather than your partner, or automatically assume your parents will babysit the children whenever you need to go out, then you may be the problem, not your parents. They deserve freedom, too.

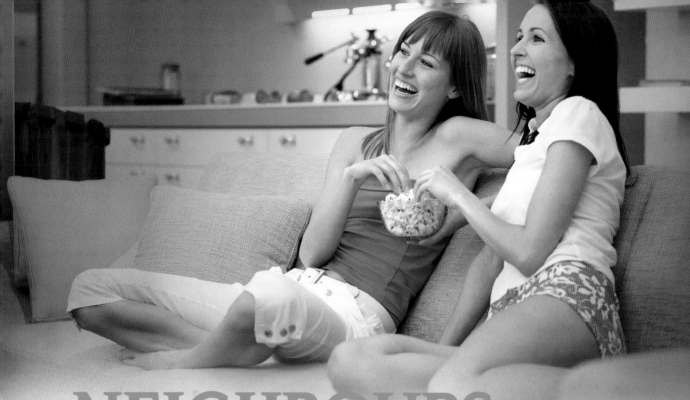

NEIGHBOURS and FRIENDS

Modern life is a lot less conducive to friendships and neighbourliness than it used to be. In the course of lifetime many of us will move house several times. And, these days, we often drive everywhere instead of walking, and spend time in front of the TV or computer instead of socializing. Often, we don't even know our neighbours' names. We don't usually realize how much we depend on good neighbours and friends until we lose them. They make our lives more pleasant and give us a sense of who we are. And all it takes to enhance your relationship with them is respect for their feelings, concern for their property and a willingness to offer a helping hand when it's needed. Here's how to nurture your relationships with two types of vitally important people in your life.

10 WAYS TO MAINTAIN A HEALTHY CIRCLE AROUND YOU

To be a popular neighbour

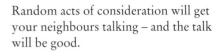 **Strike up a conversation over the fence or in the street.** It's OK to be the one to break the ice, even if you've lived next door for years. Most neighbours enjoy making small talk with other people. So as you see them in the backyard, smile and say hello. Ask how their children are or whether they could use some extra carrots from your garden.

● **Introduce yourself to the new family down the road.** Your new neighbours may be feeling lonely and unsure, especially if they're far from home, and might appreciate a friendly face bearing a homemade cake or a plant. If they have children, tell them where the other local children live. Give advice on the best places to eat and shop.

☺ **Be considerate, especially of elderly people.** Return anything that you borrow from a neighbour, such as tools, in good repair and as soon as you're finished with them. Replace anything that belongs to your neighbour that you, your children or your pets break or soil. If your neighbour hasn't brought in his or her recycling bin yet, do it as a favour.

Random acts of consideration will get your neighbours talking – and the talk will be good.

● **Invite your neighbours to your next bash – or throw one in their honour.** What better way to meet your neighbours than to invite them to an informal barbecue or party? If you deliver the invitations in person, you'll get a chance to have a chat before moving on to the next house.

To be a better friend

☺ **On your computer at home or work, make a note to "call friends" regularly.** Or, keep a Post-it note on the phone, the bathroom mirror, the car dashboard, anywhere you're likely to see it. Also make sure your friends' phone numbers are programmed into your phone. Then call a friend when you have a spare 10 minutes. Alternatively, schedule a regular once-a-month lunch – same time, same place.

● **Make time for friendships.** Nothing makes closeness fade away more than never talking to or seeing each other. While some bonds of friendship may be strong enough to span long silences, most aren't. If you cherish a person's friendship, make time for him or her, whether it's just the occasional phone call, e-mail or a weekly get-together.

● **Remember: a true friend doesn't flee when changes occur.** Nothing is sadder for new parents than to find that their single friends have abandoned them because of the baby. A good friend is one who stays true through it all – marriage, parenthood, new jobs, new homes, any losses. Just because a situation's changed doesn't mean the person has.

Healthy **INVESTMENT**

A pressure washer
You might use a pressure washer only two or three times a year, but being able to lend your tools to neighbours and friends comes back a hundred times in terms of the benefits. Everyone needs a pressure washer: for cars, the outside of the house, decking, patios, paths and sidewalk.

● **Make sure you aren't being a burden to a friend.** Friendships fade away if there isn't an equilibrium between the give and the take. Be sensitive to how much your friend can and can't offer you – be it time, energy or help – and don't overstep the mark. And vice versa: friendships that drain you will not last. If a friendship is out of balance, talk the situation through.

✩ **Be a good listener.** It can be the hardest thing in the world to do – simply to listen as he or she pours it all out or is seeking your advice or opinion. To be a better listener, follow this advice:
● Maintain eye contact. Offer nods and murmurs to indicate that you understand his or her point of view.
● Don't finish your friend's sentences. If you catch yourself planning your response while your friend is still talking, gently remind yourself to focus.
● Minimize distractions – don't write or read e-mails, open the mail or watch television while you're on the phone to your friend. He or she will hear the lack of interest in your responses.
● Be careful with advice. Assume your friend wants to let off steam, not necessarily ask for a plan of action.

● **Be in your friend's corner if he or she's not there to defend him or herself.** If you're at a gathering at which someone

mentions your friend disparagingly, defend him or her against gossip or criticism. Say, "Mary is my friend, and it makes me feel bad to hear you talk this way." Sooner or later, news of your loyalty will travel back to your pal, and it will deepen your friendship.

Do **THREE** things…

If you do only three things to be a good neighbour, make it these three, experts tell us:

1 **Be house-proud.** Part of what makes a "good neighbourhood" is that the people have a common interest – and a personal and financial investment – in keeping their neighbourhood looking neat and clean. So do your part to maintain your lawn and the outside of your home. Or hire someone to do it. Ask a neighbour for a recommendation for painting or landscaping.

2 **Don't park in your neighbour's parking space.** On-street parking can be a sensitive issue for neighbours who don't have a garage, so don't thoughtlessly take "their" space. And don't let any visiting friends do it.

3 **Understand that not all your neighbours love children or animals.** Don't assume it's acceptable for your children to run wild with their skateboards, or allow your dog to roam free. Teach your children the neighbourhood boundaries they must live by, be it noise, geography or time of day. Likewise, promptly clean up any mess your pet makes, either on your property, theirs or on the sidewalk. Talk to your neighbours occasionally to make sure your family aren't infringing on them.

Reminder

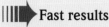 **Fast results**
These are tips that deliver benefits particularly quickly – in some cases, immediately.

 Easy gains
These are health boosters that offer the best value for the least amount of effort.

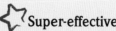 **Super-effective**
This is advice that scientific research or widespread usage by experts has shown to be especially effective.

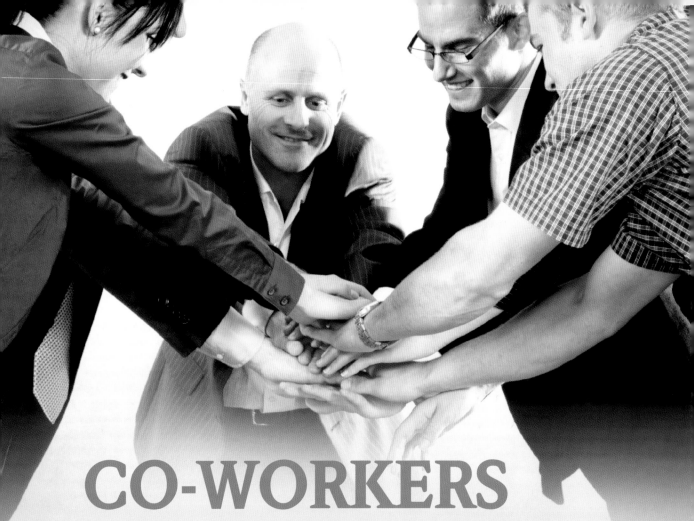

CO-WORKERS

You can pick your friends, but you can't pick your co-workers. Yet you
need them in more ways than one. First, you need their goodwill and cooperation in order
to perform your own job well. Second, studies find that disagreements with co-workers
and bad working relationships deflate morale and impair performance even more than
rumours of layoffs. And third, if you're like most people, you spend more waking hours
at work than anywhere else. Reaching out to your co-workers – or extending an olive
branch, if need be – can make your work environment a much nicer place in which to
spend so many hours a day. You don't have to be friends with your co-workers, but you do
need to be friendly. Read on for fresh ways to make work a happier place to be.

16 WAYS TO KEEP THE PEACE AND HAVE FUN AT WORK

☺ **Say a cheery "Hello!" in the morning.** Do you plod into the office, eyes down, shoulders slumped, and immediately start work? If so, you're likely to find that co-workers ignore you (at best) or avoid you (at worst). Get into the habit of smiling and greeting everyone as you arrive in the morning or begin your shift. It's amazing how fast this little courtesy can thaw chilly workplace relations.

● **Learn the art of small talk.** Ask your co-workers about their interests – their favourite music, films, books, hobbies. Showing a genuine interest in them will make them feel comfortable around you.

● **Join the office sports team.** Many offices have a sports team, be it hockey, soccer, tennis or softball, and joining in is a great way to enjoy some exercise while you get to know your co-workers.

● **Accept good-natured teasing.** Other workers sometimes play jokes and tease to test what kind of person you are. So if they poke fun at your new shoes or mischievously put a funny screensaver on your computer, don't get angry. Let them know that you enjoy a good joke – even if it's sometimes on you. Of course, if the teasing is personal (about your weight or ethnicity, for example), and makes it difficult for you to do your job or makes you feel uncomfortable because of its sexual implications, you may need to take up the matter with your supervisor.

● **Ask what they think.** People love to be asked their opinion, so go out of your way to ask, "What do you think is missing from this report?" or "How do you think I should handle this situation with X?" Then give the advice-giver a sincere thank you, even if the ideas are less than helpful.

In PERSPECTIVE

Office friendships benefit your work

Do you have a best pal at work? Chances are, if you do, you're a better, more productive worker than the office loner or grouch, research shows.

If you have a strong office friendship, you're more likely to be engaged with your work. And a 2009 Gallup poll found that a sense of engagement really matters. According to Gallup, 60 per cent of employees without a good pal are not engaged, and 36 per cent are actively disengaged. Only 4 per cent of those without a good work friend are content and productive at work. Engaged employees are those who know what's expected of them and who have what they need in order to do their job. They also feel that they are involved in making a difference, along with co-workers whom they can trust. Not only that, they have chances to improve and develop at work.

At the opposite end of the spectrum are people described as CAVE dwellers – Consistently Against Virtually Everything – the people who are actively disengaged at work. Unfortunately, these negative people are often the most vocal.

The advice to employers to ensure their employees feel engaged is to work at raising and maintaining morale, hope and trust among workers, to concentrate on employees' strengths and to improve workplace communication.

☆ **Avoid gossip.** You don't want anyone talking about you behind your back, so return the favour. When a co-worker sidles up to you bearing some gossip about an office romance or someone's impending firing, respond with, "Really?" Then change the subject or get back to work. If you don't respond, the gossiper will move on – and you'll retain the trust and respect of your co-workers.

▐▶ **When dealing with a difficult co-worker,** pretend your children are watching. This simple visualization technique will help you to keep a cool head. After all, you've taught your children to have good manners. With them "watching," it will be difficult to stoop to the level of your infuriating co-worker.

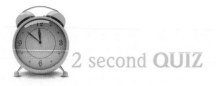

2 second QUIZ

Show your emotions or keep your cool?
ANSWER: **KEEP YOUR COOL.**

A U.S. study in 2002 found that many employees don't want their co-workers to express any type of strong emotion – positive or negative – on the job.

● **Ladle out the compliments.** Did Tom fix the office photocopier – again? Has Ann stopped smoking? By all means, compliment your co-workers on their achievements – personal or professional. Too often, we focus on what people are doing wrong.

● **Spread your good cheer.** You don't have to be a Pollyanna, but try to perform one kindly act a week, choosing a different co-worker each time. For example, one week you might bring in muffins for no reason. Another week, it might be a card for a co-worker – maybe a thank-you note for helping you out the week before, or a light, humorous card for a co-worker who seems to be a bit down.

● **Return calls and e-mails promptly.** To win friends at work, a good place to start is good office etiquette. There's nothing more frustrating to busy people than to have their e-mails and phone messages ignored. Your silence doesn't just make their job harder to do; it also conveys an unpleasant message to them: you're unimportant to me.

▮▮▮▶ **Give credit where credit is due.** Don't withhold credit from deserving co-workers. You'll alienate them, and they won't be there for you when you need them (or when they all go out for lunch). Embrace the attitude that we all win together, and let others know when someone has done something above and beyond the call of duty on a project. Also, if someone incorrectly gives you credit and praise, acknowledge your co-worker who does deserve the accolades. It will be remembered.

● **Here's one for the boss:** always work at least as hard as anyone working with or for you. Make it clear that you would never ask anyone to do a level of work you wouldn't be willing to take on yourself.

● **Always be on time** to show you respect other people's time.

● **Express your good ideas** in a way that makes it clear that they are not the only good ideas, and that others may have equally good insights to add.

● **Talk about your life outside the office when it's appropriate.** This will remind the people you work with that you're a person first, not just an employee or employer.

☆ **Assume the positive about what you don't know.** Isn't it funny how a team of workers often think they're working harder than another team elsewhere in the building? Or that the bosses are clueless? Don't subscribe to that kind of toxic thinking, even if it's rampant. It's a negative attitude that makes work become miserable. Instead, assume that everyone else is working hard and doing their best, even if you don't know what their work is. You should believe both in the work you're doing and the organization you're doing it for. If you can't, perhaps it's time to move on.

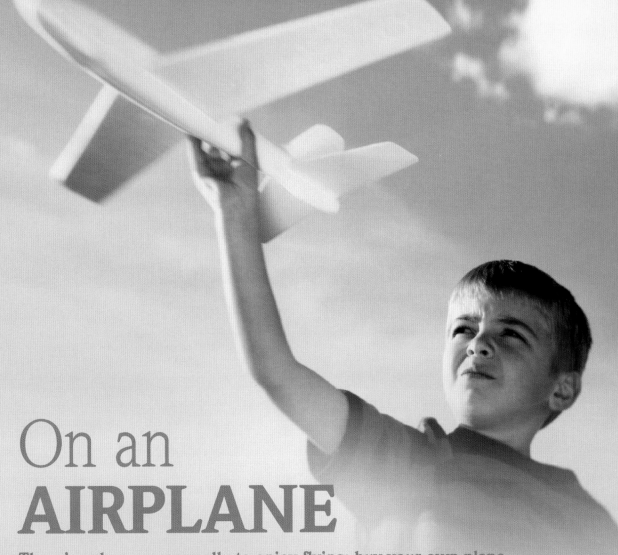

On an
AIRPLANE

There's only one way really to enjoy flying: buy your own plane.
The rest of us are stuck with missed and cancelled flights, tightly packed cabins and
humiliating security procedures, all of which are enough to send stress levels soaring.
Add to that the physical tolls extracted by cabin air that's literally drier than the air in the
Sahara, the changing cabin pressure and the hours of sitting in a chair barely wider than
your hips, with someone's seat back in your lap, and you'll understand why the following
tips are so critical when you take to the skies.

16 STRATEGIES FOR A HEALTHY FLIGHT

☺ **Pack three camomile tea bags in your carry-on bag.** When the flight attendant comes around with drinks, ask for a cup of hot water and dunk in your tea bag. The herbal tea will soothe any travel jitters and relax you enough to get some sleep on the plane, ensuring you arrive refreshed.

Use a carry-on backpack so that you can take the stairs in the airport instead of the elevator or escalator. You'll probably have the stairs all to yourself, and it's a great way to stretch your legs and burn a few calories before you get on-board. As you wait for your flight, power walk through the terminal. You can have a good workout just by striding to and from the gates and circling the baggage carousel.

Buy a pair of flight socks. You can purchase special flight socks (called compression stockings), which improve blood flow during the journey, helping to relieve aching legs and prevent deep vein thrombosis (DVT). Make sure you choose the correct size, not just for your foot, but for your ankle and calf. The socks should not be too loose or restrictive or cause you any discomfort or pain.

Get up and walk between meals, and use that time to stretch. Do the following stretching exercises at least once every hour during the flight:
- Standing in the aisle, stretch your calves by taking a large step back with one leg and reaching into the floor with your back heel.
- Also while standing, stretch your torso and back by twisting gently from side to side.
- Then, when seated, stretch your arms, shoulders and upper back by extending one arm overhead, bending it and placing your palm against your shoulder blade. You can use the other arm to increase the stretch.

In your seat, perform these six exercises every half-hour. They will keep the blood flowing and help to prevent stiffness.
- Raise your shoulders and rotate them front to back, then back to front.
- Drop your chin to your chest. Nod yes, then shake no, pointing your chin to one shoulder, then the other.
- Clasp your fingers together, palms facing each other, then stretch your arms out straight in front of you, palms facing out.
- With your heels on the floor, pull your toes up as far as possible. Hold for a few seconds, then release.

In PERSPECTIVE

Jet lag

Nothing's worse than arriving at your vacation destination only to spend the first three days feeling like you've been hit by a truck as you try to recover from jet lag. To reset your internal clock more quickly, follow this advice:

- Allow a day for every time zone you've passed through to recover fully from your jet lag.
- If you're flying east, book an early flight. If you're flying west, however, book a later flight.
- Begin preparing for time changes a few days before your departure by getting up half an hour to an hour earlier or by going to bed later (depending on where you're heading).
- When you get on the plane, immediately adjust your watch to the time of your destination. If it's nighttime, try to sleep.
- Use sunlight to reset your clock. After flying west, spend a few hours outdoors in the afternoon; after heading east, take a half-hour walk outside in the morning.

- Lift one foot slightly off the floor and make small circular motions in each direction with your foot. Repeat with the other foot.
- Lift one heel as high as possible while keeping your toes on the floor. Hold for a few seconds, then release. Repeat with the other foot.

Avoid sitting with your legs crossed. Instead, prop up your feet on a carry-on bag to make yourself more comfortable.

If you can, travel business class. The usual fabric seats in economy class are havens for dust mites and other allergens and germs. The seats in business class are often leather, which is more hygienic.

Bring a fully charged cellphone pre-programmed with airline reservation telephone numbers. If your flight is delayed or cancelled, you can immediately call reservations to rebook. This is much quicker (and less stressful) than standing in the customer-service line.

Carry a large, empty plastic coffee cup (the kind with a top you can sip through). On the plane, ask the attendant to fill it with water. Much better than the tiny cup they usually provide.

When booking flights, book the first flight of the day. Particularly if you're flying east (see advice on jet lag, opposite) It's most likely to be on time, so you're less likely to get stressed. An early flight is also more likely to be freshly cleaned.

Keep your nasal passages and ears clear by taking a decongestant as directed for 24 hours before your flight. This will shrink the membranes in your sinuses and ears, reducing the painful pressured sensation flying can often produce.

Healthy INVESTMENT

An inflatable neck pillow
It will enable you to sleep on the plane without waking up with the proverbial pain in the neck.

Chew some chewing gum, swallow vigorously or yawn widely when the plane is taking off or landing. This will equalize the pressure in your middle ear.

Skip the alcohol during the flight. The air in the plane is dry enough; alcohol just dehydrates you even more. It's the same for caffeinated drinks. Water is best.

Bring a bag of healthy snacks in your hand luggage even for what should in theory be a short flight. And buy a bottle of water once you're through security. Not only do fewer airlines serve complimentary food these days, but unexpected delays (such as sitting on the tarmac for 90 minutes while the wings of the plane are being de-iced) can send your blood sugar plummeting.

Resist the temptation to remove your shoes during the flight. You'll end up with swollen feet due to the low air pressure in the cabin, and your shoes will be uncomfortable when you have to put them back on.

Dress in layers. Planes are often too hot or too cold. Stay in control of your own temperature by wearing layers that you can put on or take off.

The bigger the cup, the more water you'll drink.

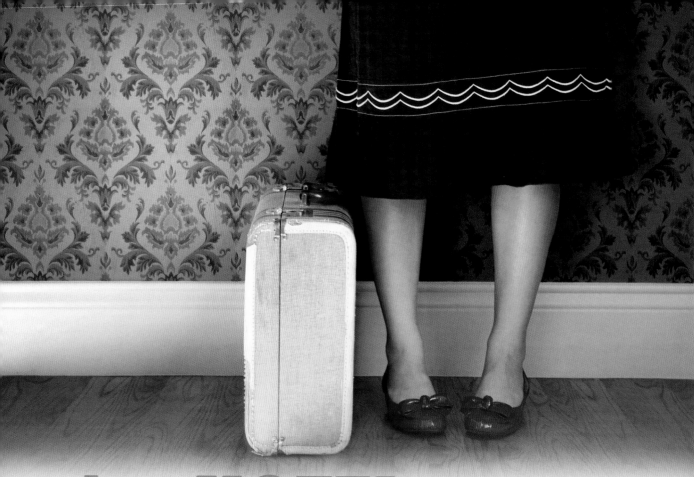

In a HOTEL

Let's say you're lucky enough to take two weeks' vacation away from home each year. Or perhaps your job sends you on a training course for a few days. Then there's your niece's wedding, a weekend getaway or two to the country – or New York or farther afield. All in all, we may spend 10 to 20 nights a year in a hotel room. That's not to be sneezed at. Or, more accurately, that's a lot to sneeze at. We'd all love to stay at five-star hotels with immaculate cleanliness, but the reality is most of us can afford only smaller, cheaper hotels – and hygiene and cleanliness may not be quite up to par. Here are 16 ideas on how to make your vacation home more pleasant, healthier and safer.

16 WAYS TO STAY HEALTHIER AND SAFER

Choose modern over old. Yes, older bed and breakfasts are far superior in terms of charm and personal touches, but their rooms and public sitting areas also tend to accumulate more allergens and dust. So if health is a real concern while travelling, go for good modern hotels.

● **Pack a long-sleeved pyjama top and long PJ pants.** If you are concerned about the hygiene of bedding in a budget hotel, reduce contact by wearing body-covering PJs and light socks to bed.

Use your bed for sleeping only. Don't work or eat on it and don't watch TV on it. Not only is this more hygienic, but you'll probably find it easier to fall asleep.

● **Ask for an allergy-free room.** Some hotels offer rooms that are designed to minimize the amounts of dust mites and other allergens. Even if you don't have allergies, this might be a good choice if you're prone to colds and flus. Other hotels provide allergy packs, including face masks, special pillows and mattress covers. But you have to ask for them.

● **Ask for a room on the third floor or higher.** Most thefts occur on the first two floors.

● **Divide your breakfast and lunch breaks in two.** Whether away on vacation or business, use half the time for eating and the other half for walking outside. Just as you should always do.

● **If you're staying for several days, book a hotel with a pool or gym room.** Exercising will ease any stiffness from travelling and burn off some of the calories from the breakfast buffet, business lunch or wedding cake.

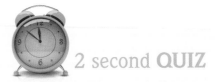

2 second QUIZ

A hotel or a busy relative's home?
ANSWER: **HOTEL.**

But it's about relationships rather than cleanliness. If you plan to stay for a single night or two, a busy relative will no doubt be delighted to see you but for longer stays it is often better to find a nearby hotel and drop in on your relative for meals or go out together for pure enjoyment.

● **Pack insect and pest repellent.** In tropical and sub-tropical countries your hotel room could be invaded by mosquitoes, particularly if it is close to open water. Always take an effective insect repellent (and make sure you've taken any necessary precautions in advance, such as anti-malaria pills). Some people also find that taking 100 mg vitamin B_1 or 300 mg of brewer's yeast keeps mosquitoes at bay – take it in advance as the benefits are only apparent after about a week. In some cheaper hotels you may also need protection against bedbugs which leave itchy welts on the skin. The evidence is tiny bloodstains on pillows or mattress liners and seams. If you see any, you should immediately contact the management, ask for a change of room and make sure it's bedbug clear.

Cover up with a long-sleeved pyjama top and long PJ pants.

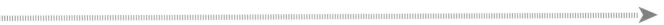

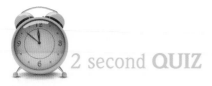

2 second QUIZ

Sagging mattress or sleeping on the floor?
ANSWER: **THE FLOOR.**

If you have back problems of any kind and the hotel bed has seen better days, pull the mattress onto the floor. You'll get better support and be less likely to wake up with a crick in your back that could cramp your style for days.

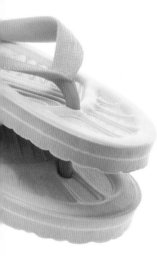

Keep bugs at bay with a pair of flip-flops.

● **Check your luggage for alien bugs and insects when you get home.** If you find any, put your clothes straight into the washing machine, then dry them on high heat for at least 15 minutes. Anything that isn't washable should be put into the freezer for a couple of days.

☺ **Moisten the dry air with the help of a kettle.** If your room has a kettle, fill it with plenty of water, heat it until it steams, then let the steam escape into the room until the water's almost gone. Your sinuses will thank you.

● **Pack a photograph of someone you love (even your dog).** If, when you come back to your room after a stressful day, you begin to feel lonely or get that "What city am I in?" confusion that often comes with long trips, you can cheer yourself up by looking at the picture and reminding yourself of home.

● **Use a battery-operated travel alarm clock.** You'll fall asleep quicker and sleep better if you don't have to worry about missing an important appointment because you set the hotel alarm clock wrongly or someone at reception has forgotten your wake-up call.

● **Pack a pair of flip-flops.** Use them in the bathroom, on the carpet (who knows the last time the carpet was properly cleaned) and in the pool area to prevent any fungal (or worse) infections.

● **Be wary of a hotel's hot tub.** There's no doubt that hot tubs are luxuriously soothing and, if you're fit and healthy, go ahead and plunge in. Just be aware that hot tubs can foster bacteria such as the one that causes folliculitis (itchy red bumps). And occasionally people have developed bronchitis and even serious forms of pneumonia from breathing in air contaminated by bacteria in the water.

● **Play it safe.** One of the easiest ways to stay healthy is to make sure that you're not physically attacked in a strange place. Here are some important tips on how to protect yourself when staying in a hotel:
● When registering, make sure the receptionist doesn't say your room number aloud, but instead writes it down and hands it to you. If he or she does say it out loud, ask for another room and ask for the number to be written down.
● If someone knocks on your door, ask who it is and verify before opening. If you didn't order room service, or don't know why the "employee" is there, call the front desk to verify they sent someone.
● Use the main entrance of the hotel when returning in the evening.
● Use all of the locking devices for your door, and lock all of the windows and sliding glass doors.

● **Don't leave the "Please Clean the Room" sign** outside your door unless you want to tell the whole world you're not there. Instead, put the "Do Not Disturb" sign on the door. If you want your room cleaned while you're out, call reception and let them know.

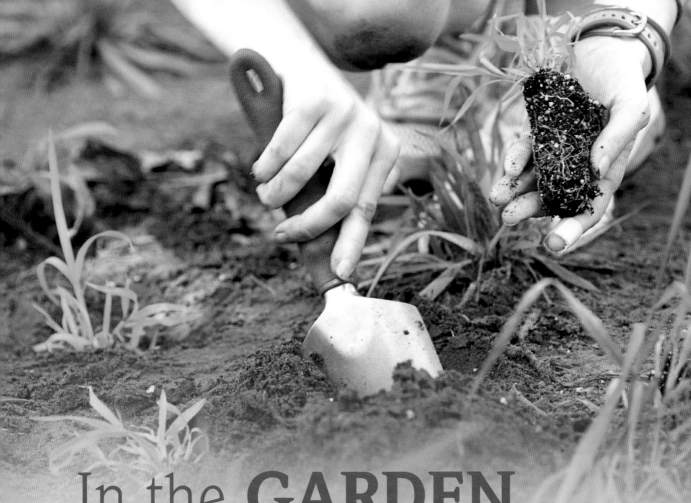

In the GARDEN

Quick: what is one of the best ways to reduce your risk of hypertension, osteoporosis and depression? How about digging in the dirt? Studies find that gardening is one of the best physical activities of all when it comes to preventing or improving chronic health conditions. Plus, the stress-relieving benefits of watching something grow, of breathing in the scent of flowers, of picking a sun-kissed tomato from your own garden, are legion.

The key is not to overdo it or do it incorrectly. These 13 tips will enable you to remain healthy while gardening.

13 SECRETS FOR HEALTHIER DIGGING

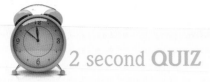

Electric mower or manual?
ANSWER: **FOR MOST YARDS, MANUAL.**

You'll get a much better workout every time you cut the grass, and the intensity isn't that great if your yard is small to medium-sized. If you have a larger yard, you can go with an electric- or gas-powered mower, but make it a push, not ride-on, mower.

❀ **Stretch for 5 minutes before heading out to the garden.** Focus on your hamstrings, back and arms. For specific moves, see "Stretching," page 134.

❀ **Dress for gardening.** That means wearing sunscreen with an SPF of 30 or higher and reapplying it every couple of hours. Also put on insect spray, a hat, sunglasses and a light, long-sleeved shirt that covers most of your neck.

❀ **Bend from your knees and take frequent breaks from bending over.** Back strain is a common gardening injury. Other ways to avoid it are to carry a small stool with you to sit or lean on while weeding, and to use knee pads to protect your kneecaps from hard ground.

❀ **Check the pollen count before heading out,** particularly if you suffer from allergies or asthma. Also, forgo gardening on days of high heat and humidity. The heavy air could cause problems if you have respiratory issues.

❀ **Choose gardening tools with padded handles** to protect the joints in your hands and fingers from excess pressure. Tools such as shears or clippers with a spring-action, self-opening feature are particularly helpful if you have a weak grasp.

❀ **Divide large bags** of mulch, dirt or fertilizer into smaller, more manageable loads and use a cart or wheelbarrow to move materials. When lifting, use the muscles in your legs, not your back.

❀ **Vary your tasks to avoid overstressing any one part of your body.** For instance, don't spend the entire day stooping and weeding. Instead, pick one section of the garden and complete it: weeding, laying the mulch, then raking. Tackle another section the following day.

❀ **Carry a cellphone** Garden accidents do occasionally occur. It can be a painful strain or worse. Make sure you can quickly summon help if need be, especially if you're at the community garden away from home.

❀ **Plant at least one vegetable in your garden.** You'll be more likely to eat it. Also plant some herbs to use for flavouring food in place of salt.

❀ **Keep all your gardening tools, gloves,** etc. in a backpack that you can carry with you as you move from bed to bed.

❀ **Keep your garden manageable.** If you take on too much too soon, you'll find you ache the next morning (and risk a more serious injury), and you'll quickly become overwhelmed and stop altogether.

❀ **Carry a water bottle with you** if you're spending the day in the garden. And be sure to sip on it every 30 minutes or so. It's easy to become dehydrated when you're working outdoors.

❀ **Take time after gardening** to sit in a shady spot and admire your accomplishments. Sip a cool drink and enjoy the beauty around you.

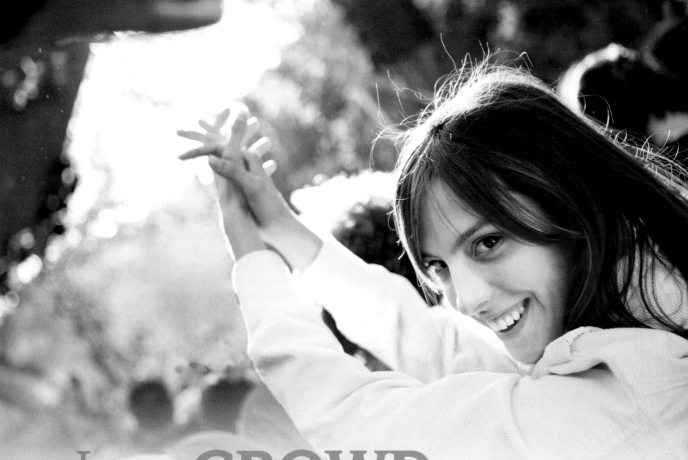

In a CROWD

You're seated in a venue with a thousand other people. Which do you feel more threatened by: a fire or a stranger sneezing on you?

The chances are, most of us aren't very concerned about either. Which is an acceptable attitude to have – the first is unlikely, the second poses a relatively minor health risk. But they pose risks nonetheless. And with a little more forethought, you can better protect your health and safety in the rare event that something goes wrong at the concert hall or football game. The advice here is not to avoid crowds. Rather, be sure to follow these tips to keep yourself and your loved ones safe and healthy while you're out living life to the fullest.

11 WAYS TO STAY SAFE AND HEALTHY

☆ **Keep your hands in your pockets.** The formula for getting ill: germs get on hands, hands touch face, germs enter body, you are infected. Where there are crowds, there are germs – millions of them – on every surface. Don't touch them and they won't make you ill.

● **Carry a bottle of hand sanitizer.** Use it after portable toilet visits, before eating and any time you feel contaminated by the microbes of the masses.

● **Put a pair of earplugs in your handbag or pocket.** If the event gets too loud, or you get stuck standing next to the speakers, use the earplugs.

● **Look for the emergency-exit signs as you enter a large venue.** It takes only seconds – and those seconds could turn out to be the most worthwhile ever. One study found that more than half of fatalities at concerts occurred when people were trying to get out of the building or concert setting.

● **Arrange a place to meet** your family or friends in case you get separated. Actually, you should choose two places: one inside and one outside.

● **In the rare event of a stampede,** try to move sideways to the crowd until you get to a wall. Then press yourself against it until the crowd dissipates, or you find a better exit. It doesn't happen often, but people do get trampled to death. If you've memorized the emergency exits, you'll have a better chance of getting to one that the rest of the crowd may not have noticed.

Be prepared – save money and avoid germs by packing your own lunch.

● **Pack your own lunch.** Peanut butter and jam sandwiches and apples will keep for the whole day and will help to forestall your children's pleas for junk food from the vendors at the event site. If you can't avoid buying from food stalls, check out the vendor. Does the stall look clean? Are the cook's hands clean? Is the vendor handling the food with gloves? Does he or she handle money, then touch the food? It's hard to tell just by looking at it if food will make you ill, but you should definitely avoid undercooked (pink) meats and meat that is not hot when served. The last thing you need when you're in a place that has only portaloos is food poisoning.

● **Remember to put a wad of tissues in your handbag or pocket.** Now you have emergency toilet paper if you have to use the portable toilets.

● **Put water bottles in the freezer the night before.** You'll save money on overpriced bottled water at the event and, as the ice melts, you'll have nice cold water on hand to stay hydrated.

● **Dress in layers.** The crowd is pressing in around you, you feel overly warm … and suddenly the ground comes up to meet you. Don't let it happen. If you've dressed in layers, you can shed one of them if you get too hot. If you're wearing only one layer to start with, you might just get arrested! Of course, layering your clothing works the other way, too. If the temperature drops as the game goes into overtime, you'll be prepared.

● **Sit and wait when the curtain comes down.** Let the crowd go first. You'll get out of the parking lot more easily and avoid ruining your great time out with a bout of blood pressure-raising stress.

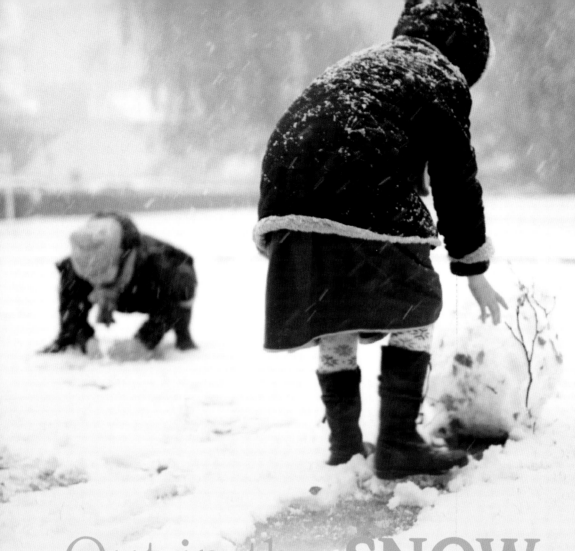

Out in the SNOW

What is it about a snowstorm that brings out the child in all of us?
Suddenly we're ready to bundle up and head outside to play. Plus, snow is great for a winter workout, what with all the sledding, skiing, snowboarding and snowshoeing you can do. Whether you're outside shovelling the walk, digging out the car or just making a snowman, follow the tips here to keep safe and warm.

12 WAYS TO KEEP SAFE AND WARM

● **Apply a Vaseline shield.** If it's cold and windy, your face may suffer a case of windburn. A thin coating of Vaseline on exposed skin – particularly your cheeks, nose, chin, ears and neck – will help to prevent it.

● **Don't walk with your hands in your pockets.** It's pretty basic advice, but that way, you can use your arms to regain your balance if you slip.

In PERSPECTIVE

Frostbite

Cold winters make it a concern for Canadians. Quite often, the worst might be permanent numbness, but you can end up with gangrene – and lose a toe, finger, ear or even your nose as a result – if you're not careful. So it's important to recognize symptoms:

● A pins-and-needles sensation, then numbness.
● Hard, pale, cold, numb skin. When frostbitten skin has thawed, it becomes red and painful (early frostbite). More severe frostbite results in white and numb skin.

If you or someone you're with has frostbite:
● Get the person to a warmer place. Remove any constricting jewellery and wet clothing and, if possible, wrap the affected areas in sterile dressings (remember to separate affected fingers and toes) then get the person to the nearest emergency department.
● If immediate care is not available, immerse affected areas in warm – never hot – water or repeatedly apply warm cloths to affected ears, nose or cheeks for 20 to 30 minutes. The warming is complete when the skin is soft and sensation returns.
● Move thawed areas as little as possible.
● If the frostbite is extensive, give warm drinks, but never alcohol, to the person in order to replace lost fluids.
● Don't thaw a frostbitten area if it cannot be kept thawed. Refreezing may make tissue damage even worse. Also, don't use direct dry heat (such as a radiator, campfire, heating pad or hairdryer). Direct heat can burn already-damaged tissues.
● Don't rub the area, or disturb blisters on frostbitten skin.

● **Beware: ice.** If it's icy, wear rubber-soled boots with good traction, go slowly, don't carry too many bags and give yourself extra time to get wherever you're going, whether on foot or in a car.

● **Or buy traction devices for your shoes.** It's possible to buy antislip spikes or stretchable traction devices that fit over your shoes to prevent you from slipping on ice or snow. Yaktrax, for example, are rubber and wire devices that fit over the bottom of your boots. Go to www.yaktrax.ca or www.mec.ca for more information.

● **Look out for patches of white or pale-grey, waxy-textured skin.** These are signs of frostbite. Go indoors and get immediate medical attention. (See the panel about frostbite, left.)

● **It might look silly, but pull large rubber dishwashing gloves over woollen gloves.** This will keep your woollen gloves dry.

● **Make sure your boots aren't too tight,** either because they're too small or because you've stuffed them with too many pairs of bulky socks. You won't have enough blood circulating to your feet and they'll get even colder. Wool or thermal socks are a good choice.

● **Dress in layers.** Depending on how active you are, and the outside temperature, you will be able to add or remove layers as needed. Avoid cotton, which gets wet and stays wet. Top your first layer with a fleece garment, then a windproof jacket.

● **Equip your car for driving in snowy conditions.** Clean the snow off the car before you start driving, make sure your windshield wipers work well, clean your headlights and, in extreme conditions, use chains. Stock your car trunk with a shovel, tow rope, ground sheet (for fitting chains), rubber gloves, plastic ice scraper, blanket and flashlight.

● **If you're not in good-enough shape to shovel,** pay someone else to do it for you. Shovelling snow can be very strenuous. Think twice before doing it if you have a history of heart disease, heart attack or high blood pressure.

● **Stretch for 5 minutes and walk outside for 5 to 10 minutes before you start shovelling.** Here are some more tips:
● Drink plenty of water so that you're well hydrated. Don't drink caffeine or alcohol, or use nicotine products immediately before shovelling.
● Shovel early and often. Newly fallen snow is lighter than heavily packed or partially melted snow. Starting out early allows you extra time to take breaks.
● Take your time. Never remove deep snow all at once. Shovel a layer 5 to 10 cm thick, then take off another 5 to 10 cm.
● Pick the right shovel. A smaller shovel will require you to lift less snow, putting less strain on your body.
● Protect your back with good technique. Stand with your feet about hip-width apart for balance, and keep the shovel close to your body. Bend from the knees, not the back, and tighten your stomach muscles as you lift. Avoid twisting movements. If you need to move the snow to one side, reposition your body so your feet face the direction in which the snow will be going. Always throw the snow in front of you, not over your shoulder.
● If you experience any shortness of breath, dizziness or chest discomfort, stop immediately and seek medical attention.

WHEN COLD sets in

One of the best ways to guard against hypothermia (lowered body temperature) is to recognize the early warning signs. If someone you're with exhibits any of these, get him or her to a warm place right away. Severe cases require medical attention.
● **Shivering.** An early sign of hypothermia, shivering starts mildly, but can become more severe and finally convulsive before ceasing.
● **Slurred speech.**
● **Loss of coordination.** This might begin as difficulty tying your shoelaces or zipping your jacket, and eventually include stumbling or falling.
● **Confusion.**
● **Apathy** (for example, not caring about your own needs).
● **Irrational behaviour.**

☺**Smear on some sunscreen and lip balm if you're out in the snow on sunny days.** And slip on a pair of sunglasses or goggles to protect your eyes from the snow's glare. A sunny day in winter is often brighter and more dangerous to your eyes than the summer sun, thanks to the reflection from the ice and snow.

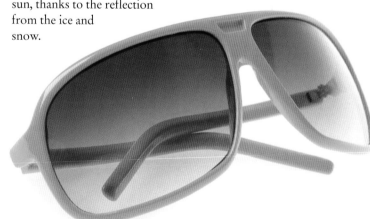

Sunglasses form a vital part of your winter wardrobe.

Index

A

B

Back Cover: Fotolia.com/© Yuri Arcurs

Throughout, Green Alarm Clock: Fotolia.co.uk/ Dmitry Koksharov;
Pink Piggy Bank: Fotolia.co.uk/ Robyn Mac

2-3 iStockphoto.com/Jordan Philips; 4 iStockphoto.com;13 iStockphoto.com/Neustockimages; 14 iStockphoto.com/Thomas Vogel; 16 Fotolia.com/Alexey Stiop; 18 Fotolia.com/Renata Osinska; 20 Corbis/Manceaux/SoFood; 21B ShutterStock, Inc/tkemot; 23 ShutterStock, Inc/Max Krasnov; 24 ShutterStock, Inc/Diego Cervo; 25 Fotolia.com/Natalia Klenova; 27 ShutterStock, Inc/Chas; 28 iStockphoto.com/René Mansi; 30 ShutterStock, Inc/Andresr; 32 Fotolia.com/Yuri Arcurs; 35T Fotolia.com/Express 3300; 36 ShutterStock, Inc/Konrad Bak; 40T ShutterStock, Inc/Michaela Stejskalova; 42 iStockphoto.com; 43 ShutterStock, Inc/Robyn Mackenzie; 46 iStockphoto.com/Carey Hope; 47 ShutterStock, Inc/Beata Becla; 48 ShutterStock, Inc/Norman Pogson; 50 Fotolia.com/Glenda Powers; 52B ShutterStock, Inc/Tomasz Trojanowski; 54 Fotolia.com/LV Design; 55 Fotolia.com/Victures; 56 ShutterStock, Inc/Perov Stanislav; 58 iStockphoto.com/Nagy-Bagoly Ilona; 61 ShutterStock, Inc/Timothy Geiss; 63 ShutterStock, Inc/Poleze; 64 Fotolia.com/Anatoly Tiplyashin; 66 ShutterStock, Inc/Eric Isselée; 68 Fotolia.com/Mood Board; 70 ShutterStock, Inc/Carlos Caetano; 72 Fotolia.com/Yuri Arcurs; 73 ShutterStock, Inc/Petoo; 76 iStockphoto.com/KEMAL BAS; 78 ShutterStock, Inc/Stanislav Crnjak; 82 ShutterStock, Inc/iofoto; 83 ShutterStock, Inc/Franz Pfluegl; 84T ShutterStock, Inc/Andrey Armyagov; 88 ShutterStock, Inc/Olga Solovei; 89R ShutterStock, Inc/Mikael Damkier; 91 ShutterStock, Inc/Whaldener Endo; 92 Fotolia.com/Fotolia1; 93B ShutterStock, Inc/Alex Staroseltsev; 94 ShutterStock, Inc/Sarah Johnson; 95B ShutterStock, Inc/Vikiri; 98 Fotolia.com/3w.LMSTRANS.pl; 100 iStockphoto.com/Dori Oconnell; 101 Fotolia.com/Ruth Black; 102T ShutterStock, Inc/Thomas M Perkin; 104T ShutterStock, Inc/ampFotoStudio; 105 ShutterStock, Inc/Robyn Mackenzie; 106T ShutterStock, Inc/Marc Dietrich; 109B ShutterStock, Inc/Dino O; 110 iStockphoto.com; 111 Getty Images/Punchstock/Westend61; 114 iStockphoto.com/Kevin Russ; 116 ShutterStock, Inc/Yuri Arcurs; 118 iStockphoto.com/Jill Chen; 120 iStockphoto.com/Norman Chan; 121 ShutterStock, Inc/Egypix; 122 iStockphoto.com/Joe Gough; 124 iStockphoto.com/Jill Chen; 125T iStockphoto.com/Jack Jelly; 126 iStockphoto.com/Scott Karcich; 127 iStockphoto.com/Jim Jurica; 128T iStockphoto.com/Brian McEntire; 130 iStockphoto.com/Kristian Gehradte; 131B iStockphoto.com; 132 iStockphoto.com/Pascal Genest; 134 iStockphoto.com/Neustockimages; 135-139 © Reader's Digest/Russell Sadur; 140 ShutterStock, Inc/Yuri Arcurs; 141B iStockphoto.com/Arpad Benedek; 142 iStockphoto.com; 145 iStockphoto.com/Don Bayley; 146 Getty Images/Punchstock; 147 iStockphoto.com; 148 iStockphoto.com/Eric Hood; 149R iStockphoto.com/Claudia Dewald; 150 iStockphoto.com; 151 iStockphoto.com/Jacob Wackerhausen; 152 iStockphoto.com/Zhang Bo; 154 iStockphoto.com/Catherine Yeulet; 157 iStockphoto.com/Chris Price; 159T iStockphoto.com/Gremlin; 164-165 © Reader's Digest/Russell Sadur; 167 iStockphoto.com/Dori Oconnell; 168 iStockphoto.com/Pali Rao; 170-176 © Reader's Digest/Russell Sadur; 177 ShutterStock, Inc/Diego Cervo; 179-183 © Reader's Digest/Russell Sadur; 184 iStockphoto.com/DNY59; 185 iStockphoto.com/Lise Gagne; 187-189 © Reader's Digest/Russell Sadur; 190 ShutterStock, Inc/Tiplyashin Anatoly; 192 ShutterStock, Inc/Feng Yu; 194 iStockphoto.com/Sawayasu Tsuji; 196 iStockphoto.com/Lise Gagne; 197 ShutterStock, Inc/Katusha; 198 ShutterStock, Inc/Val Thoermer; 199 iStockphoto.com/Angelika Schwarz; 201 iStockphoto.com/Doug Berry; 202 iStockphoto.com/Timothy Boomer; 205 iStockphoto.com/Steven von Niederhausern; 206 ShutterStock, Inc/Eduard Stelmakh; 208 ShutterStock, Inc/Monkey Business Images; 210 iStockphoto.com/Liv Friis-Larsen; 211B iStockphoto.com/Teresa Pigeon; 212 iStockphoto.com/Eric Simard; 214 iStockphoto.com; 215 ShutterStock, Inc/Igor Leonov; 216 ShutterStock, Inc/Shebeko; 217 ShutterStock, Inc/GoodMood Photo; 218 iStockphoto.com/Jeannette Meier; 219 iStockphoto.com/Eva Serrabassa; 222 iStockphoto.com/Justin Horrocks; 223 iStockphoto.com/Robyn Mackenzie; 224B iStockphoto.com; 226 iStockphoto.com/Davide Fiorenzo De; 227 ShutterStock, Inc/Nazira G; 229 iStockphoto.com/Julie Kendall; 231 iStockphoto.com; 232T iStockphoto.com/Liv Friis-Larsen; 234B Fotolia.com/Elzbieta Sekowska; 235 iStockphoto.com/Andrew Rich; 236 iStockphoto.com/Benjamin Brandt; 237T iStockphoto.com/Joe Biafore; 240 iStockphoto.com/John Boylan; 241B iStockphoto.com/Dean Birinyi; 242 iStockphoto.com; 243 iStockphoto.com/Pali Rao; 244T iStockphoto.com/James McQuillan; 245 ShutterStock, Inc; 246 ShutterStock, Inc/Paul Paladin; 247 iStockphoto.com/Lise Gagne; 249T Getty Images/Punchstock/Digital Vision; 250T iStockphoto.com/Gustaf Brundin; 251 ShutterStock, Inc/Yuri Arcurs; 252 iStockphoto.com/Simon Askham; 253B iStockphoto.com/Suprijono Suharjoto; 254B iStockphoto.com/Dimitrije Paunovic; 255 ShutterStock, Inc/Hanzl; 257B Fotolia.com/Gabi Moisa; 258 iStockphoto.com/Kim Everuss; 259B iStockphoto.com/Andy Medina; 260 iStockphoto.com/Matt Porteous; 261T iStockphoto.com; 262 iStockphoto.com/Nicolas Loran; 263B iStockphoto.com/Ed O'Neil; 264 iStockphoto.com/Valentin Casarsa; 265 iStockphoto.com/Nikada; 266 Getty Images/George Doyle/Stockbyte; 268 iStockphoto.com/Elian Dric; 270 ShutterStock, Inc/Yuri Arcurs; 272 ShutterStock, Inc/Cilla; 274T iStockphoto.com/Dmitry Bomshtein; 276 ShutterStock, Inc/Raluca Teodorescu; 278T ShutterStock, Inc/Stanislav Popov; 280B ShutterStock, Inc/Bidouze Stéphane; 281 iStockphoto.com; 282 iStockphoto.com/Catherine Yeulet; 284B ShutterStock, Inc/Luciano Mortula; 285 iStockphoto.com/Aldo Murillo; 287 ShutterStock, Inc/Denis Babenko; 288T ShutterStock, Inc/Siberia; 289B ShutterStock, Inc/Indigo Fish; 290 ShutterStock, Inc/Arenacreative; 292B iStockphoto.com/Helder Almeida; 294 ShutterStock, Inc/Liudmila P. Sundikova; 296 iStockphoto.com/Tatiana Melnikova; 297 ShutterStock, Inc/Peter Zurek; 298T iStockphoto.com/Kutay Tanir; 300 ShutterStock, Inc/Eduard Titov; 301B ShutterStock, Inc; 302 ShutterStock, Inc/Serg64; 304 iStockphoto.com/Enrico Fianchini; 306,307B iStockphoto.com; 308 ShutterStock, Inc/JGP-NYC; 310 Fotolia.com/Monkey Business; 312 T iStockphoto.com/Rüstem GÜRLER; 313 iStockphoto.com/Kati Neudert; 315 iStockphoto.com/Tracy Tucker; 317 iStockphoto.com/Jay Mast; 319 iStockphoto.com/Carmen Martínez; 320 iStockphoto.com/H-Gall; 322 ShutterStock, Inc/Millann; 324T iStockphoto.com/Ryan Jones; 325 ShutterStock, Inc/Liv Friis-larsen; 327 iStockphoto.com/Louis Aguinaldo; 328 iStockphoto.com/Izabela Habur; 329R ShutterStock, Inc/Helen Imberechts; 330 ShutterStock, Inc/Emilia Stasiak; 331 iStockphoto.com/Igor Balasanov; 332 ShutterStock, Inc/Aetherial Images; 334T iStockphoto.com/Andrey Armyagov; 335B iStockphoto.com/Shantell; 336 iStockphoto.com/Cevdet Gökhan Palas; 337B iStockphoto.com/Yuriy Borysenko; 340 iStockphoto.com; 342 iStockphoto.com/Rich Legg; 344 ShutterStock, Inc/Yuri Arcurs; 347 iStockphoto.com/Andrew Rich; 349B ShutterStock, Inc/Jaimie Duplass; 350 ShutterStock, Inc/Yuri Arcurs; 353 iStockphoto.com; 356 iStockphoto.com/Anja Hild; 359 iStockphoto.com/Andrew Rich; 361B iStockphoto.com/Pavlen; 362 iStockphoto.com/David Cox; 363B iStockphoto.com/Daniel Kourey; 364B ShutterStock, Inc/HomeStudio; 365 iStockphoto.com/Jill Chen; 367 iStockphoto.com/©webphotographeer; 368 ShutterStock, Inc/Andi Berger; 369 iStockphoto.com/Franky De Meyer; 371 iStockphoto.com/Michal Rozanski

NOTE TO OUR READERS
The information in this book should not be substituted for, or used to alter, medical therapy without your doctor's advice. For a specific health problem, consult your physician for guidance.

Stealth Health is published by Reader's Digest Association (Canada) ULC, 1100 René-Lévesque Blvd. West, Montreal, QC H3B 5H5

ISBN: 978-1-55475-048-1

Copyright © 2010 Reader's Digest Association (Canada) ULC
Copyright © 2010 The Reader's Digest Association, Inc.
Copyright © 2010 The Reader's Digest Association Limited
Copyright © 2010 Reader's Digest Association Far East Limited.
Philippines Copyright © 2010 Reader's Digest Association Far East Limited
Copyright © 2010 Reader's Digest (Australia) Pty Limited
Copyright © 2010 Reader's Digest India Pvt Limited
Copyright © 2010 Reader's Digest Asia Pvt Limited

We are committed both to the quality of our products and the service we provide to our customers. To order additional copies of this book, please contact us at **1-800-465-0780.** For more information about our products, please visit us at our website at **www.readersdigest.ca**

If you have any comments or suggestions about the content of our books, please write to the Book Editor at the address above.

Library and Archives Canada Cataloguing in Publication
    Stealth health : how to sneak age-defying, disease-fighting habits into your life without really trying / the editors of Reader's Digest. -- 1st Canadian ed.
Includes index.
ISBN 978-1-55475-048-1
    1. Health. 2. Physical fitness. 3. Mind and body. I. Reader's Digest Association (Canada)
RA776.S795 2010   613.7   C2010-901106-6

CANADIAN PROJECT TEAM
Editor Robert Ronald
Assistant editor Jesse Corbeil
Art Designer Andrée Payette
Proofreader Judy Yelon
Production Coordinator Gillian Sylvain
Production Manager Gordon Howlett

For Reader's Digest Association (Canada) ULC
Vice-President, Book Editorial Robert Goyette
Manager, English Book Editorial Pamela Johnson

For The Reader's Digest Association, Inc.
President and Chief Executive Officer Mary Berner
President, Canada and Latin America Patricia Hespanha

Printed in China